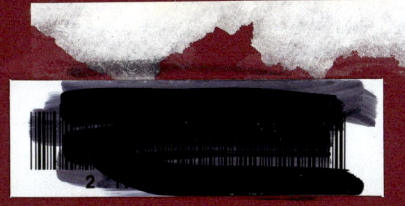

**WITHDRAWN**

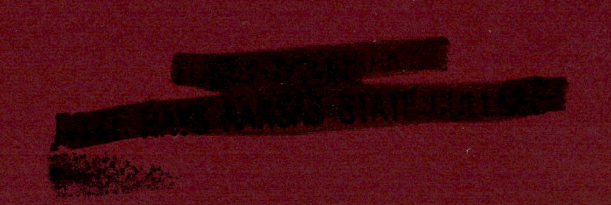

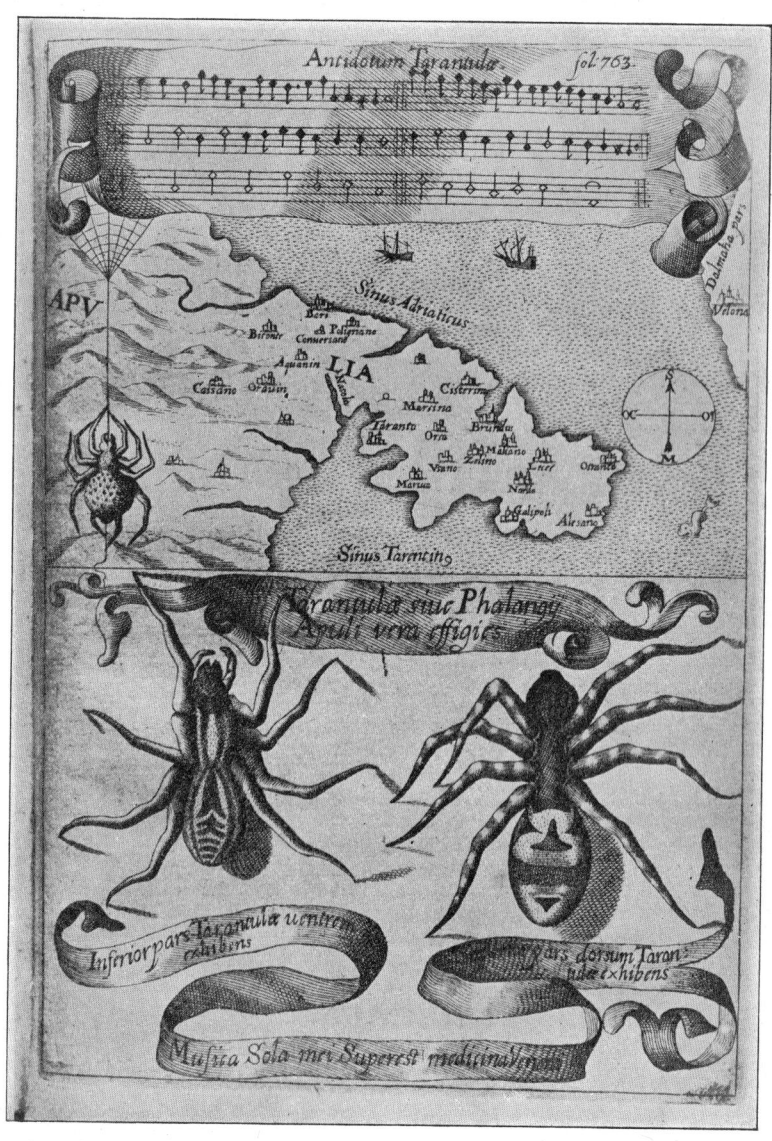

Some early medical entomology. Athanasius Kircher's illustration of the Italian tarantula and the music prescribed as an antidote for the poison of its bite. (1643).

# HANDBOOK OF MEDICAL ENTOMOLOGY

WM. A. RILEY, Ph.D.
Professor of Insect Morphology and Parasitology, Cornell University

and

O. A. JOHANNSEN, Ph.D.
Professor of Biology, Cornell University

ITHACA, NEW YORK
THE COMSTOCK PUBLISHING COMPANY
1915

COPYRIGHT, 1915
BY THE COMSTOCK PUBLISHING COMPANY,
ITHACA, N. Y.

Press of W. F. Humphrey
Geneva, N. Y.

# PREFACE

THE Handbook of Medical Entomology is the outgrowth of a course of lectures along the lines of insect transmission and dissemination of diseases of man given by the senior author in the Department of Entomology of Cornell University during the past six years. More specifically it is an illustrated revision and elaboration of his "Notes on the Relation of Insects to Disease" published January, 1912.

Its object is to afford a general survey of the field, and primarily to put the student of medicine and entomology in touch with the discoveries and theories which underlie some of the most important modern work in preventive medicine. At the same time the older phases of the subject—the consideration of poisonous and parasitic forms—have not been ignored.

Considering the rapid shifts in viewpoint, and the development of the subject within recent years, the authors do not indulge in any hopes that the present text will exactly meet the needs of every one specializing in the field,—still less do they regard it as complete or final. The fact that the enormous literature of isolated articles is to be found principally in foreign periodicals and is therefore difficult of access to many American workers, has led the authors to hope that a summary of the important advances, in the form of a reference book may not prove unwelcome to physicians, sanitarians and working entomologists, and to teachers as a text supplementing lecture work in the subject.

Lengthy as is the bibliography, it covers but a very small fraction of the important contributions to the subject. It will serve only to put those interested in touch with original sources and to open up the field. Of the more general works, special acknowledgment should be made to those of Banks, Brumpt, Castellani and Chalmers, Comstock, Hewitt, Howard, Manson, Mense, Neveau-Lemaire, Nuttall, and Stiles.

To the many who have aided the authors in the years past, by suggestions and by sending specimens and other materials, sincerest thanks is tendered. This is especially due to their colleagues in the Department of Entomology of Cornell University, and to Professor Charles W. Howard, Dr. John Uri Lloyd, Mr. A. H. Ritchie, Dr. I. M. Unger, and Dr. Luzerne Coville.

They wish to express indebtedness to the authors and publishers who have so willingly given permission to use certain illustrations. Especially is this acknowledgment due to Professor John Henry Comstock, Dr. L. O. Howard, Dr. Graham-Smith, and Professor G. H. T. Nuttall. Professor Comstock not only authorized the use of departmental negatives by the late Professor M. V. Slingerland (credited as M. V. S.), but generously put at their disposal the illustrations from the MANUAL FOR THE STUDY OF INSECTS and from the SPIDER BOOK. Figures 5 and 111 are from Peter's "Der Arzt und die Heilkunft in der deutschen Vergangenheit." It should be noted that on examining the original, it is found that Gottfried's figure relates to an event antedating the typical epidemic of dancing mania.

WM. A. RILEY.
O. A. JOHANNSEN.

CORNELL UNIVERSITY,
January, 1915.

# CONTENTS

## CHAPTER I

**INTRODUCTION** .................................................. 1–5
    Early suggestions regarding the transmission of disease by insects.
    The ways in which arthropods may affect the health of man.

## CHAPTER II

**ARTHROPODS WHICH ARE DIRECTLY POISONOUS** ............ 6–56
    The Araneida, or Spiders.
        The tarantulas. Bird spiders. Spiders of the genus Latrodectus. Other venomous spiders. Summary.
    The Pedipalpida, or whip-scorpions.
    The Scorpionida, or true scorpions.
    The Solpugida, or solpugids.
    The Acarina, or mites and ticks.
    The Myriapoda, or centipedes and millipedes.
    The Hexapoda, or true insects.
        Piercing or biting insects poisonous to man.
            Hemiptera, or true bugs.
                The Notonectidæ or back-swimmers. Belostomidæ or giant water-bugs. Reduviidae, or assassin bugs. Other Hemiptera reported as poisonous to man.
            Diptera; the midges, mosquitoes and flies.
        Stinging insects.
            Apis mellifica, the honey bee. Other stinging forms.
        Nettling insects.
            Lepidoptera, or butterflies and moths. Relief from poisoning by nettling larvæ.
        Vesicating insects and those possessing other poisons in their blood plasma.
            The blister beetles. Other cryptotoxic insects.

## CHAPTER III

**PARASITIC ARTHROPODS AFFECTING MAN** ................... 57–130
    Acarina, or mites.
        The Trombidiidæ, or harvest mites.
        The Ixodoidea, or ticks.
            Argasidæ. Ixodidæ. Treatment of tick bites.
        The mites.
            Dermanyssidæ. Tarsonemidæ. Sarcoptidæ, the itch mites. Demodecidæ, the follicle mites.
    Hexapoda, or true insects.
        Siphunculata, or sucking lice.
        Hemiptera.

The bed-bug. Other bed-bugs.
Parasitic Diptera, or flies.
Psychodidæ, or moth flies. Phlebotominæ. Culicidæ, or mosquitoes. Simuliidæ, or black-flies. Chironomidæ, or midges. Tabanidæ, or horse-flies. Leptidæ or snipe-flies. Oestridæ, or bot-flies. Muscidæ, the stable-fly and others.
Siphonaptera, or fleas.
The fleas affecting man, the dog, cat, and rat.
The true chiggers, or chigoes.

## CHAPTER IV
**ACCIDENTAL OR FACULTATIVE PARASITES**.................. 131-143
Acarina, or mites.
Myriapoda, or centipedes and millipedes.
Lepidopterous larvæ.
Coleoptera, or beetles.
Dipterous larvæ causing myiasis.
Piophila casei, the cheese skipper. Chrysomyia macellaria, the screw-worm fly. Calliphorinæ, the blue-bottles. Muscinæ, the house or typhoid fly, and others. Anthomyiidæ, the lesser house-fly and others. Sarcophagidæ, the flesh-flies.

## CHAPTER V
**ARTHROPODS AS SIMPLE CARRIERS OF DISEASE**........... 144-163
The house or typhoid fly as a carrier of disease.
Stomoxys calcitrans, the stable-fly.
Other arthropods which may serve as simple carriers of pathogenic organisms.

## CHAPTER VI
**ARTHROPODS AS DIRECT INOCULATORS OF DISEASE GERMS** 164-174
Some illustrations of direct inoculations of disease germs by arthropods.
The rôle of fleas in the transmission of the plague.

## CHAPTER VII
**ARTHROPODS AS ESSENTIAL HOSTS OF PATHOGENIC ORGANISMS** ..................................................... 175-185
Insects as intermediate hosts of tape-worms.
Arthropods as intermediate hosts of nematode worms. Filariasis and mosquitoes.
Other nematode parasites of man and animals.

## CHAPTER VIII
**ARTHROPODS AS ESSENTIAL HOSTS OF PATHOGENIC PROTOZOA** ...................................................... 186-211
Mosquitoes and malaria.
Mosquitoes and yellow fever.

## CHAPTER IX
**ARTHROPODS AS ESSENTIAL HOSTS OF PATHOGENIC PROTOZOA** .................................................. 212–229
Insects and trypanosomiases.
  Fleas and lice as carriers of Trypanosoma lewisi.
  Tsetse-flies and nagana.
  Tsetse-flies and sleeping sickness in man.
  South American trypanosomiasis.
  Leishmanioses and insects.
Ticks and diseases of man and animals.
  Cattle tick and Texas fever.
  Ticks and Rocky Mountain Spotted fever of man.

## CHAPTER X
**ARTHROPODS AS ESSENTIAL HOSTS OF PATHOGENIC PROTOZOA (Continued)**.......................................... 230–240
Arthropods and Spirochætoses of man and animals.
  African relapsing fever of man.
  European relapsing fever.
  North African relapsing fever of man.
  Other types of relapsing fever of man.
  Spirochætosis of fowls.
  Other spirochæte diseases of animals.
Typhus fever and lice.

## CHAPTER XI
**SOME POSSIBLE, BUT IMPERFECTLY KNOWN CASES OF ARTHROPOD TRANSMISSION OF DISEASE**............. 241–256
Infantile paralysis, or acute anterior poliomyelitis.
Pellagra. Leprosy. Verruga peruviana. Cancer.

## CHAPTER XII
**KEYS TO THE ARTHROPODS NOXIOUS TO MAN**.............. 257–317
  Crustacea.
  Myriapoda, or centipedes and millipedes.
  Arachnida (Orders of).
    Acarina or ticks.
  Hexapoda (Insecta).
    Siphunculata and Hemiptera (lice and true bugs).
    Diptera (mosquitoes, midges, and flies).
    Siphonaptera (fleas).

## APPENDIX
Hydrocyanic acid gas against household insects..................... 318–320
  Proportion of ingredients. A single room as an example. Fumigating a large house. Precautions.
Lesions produced by the bite of the black-fly...................... 321–326
BIBLIOGRAPHY ............................................... 327–340
INDEX ...................................................... 341–348

# CHAPTER I.

# INTRODUCTION

## EARLY SUGGESTIONS REGARDING THE TRANSMISSION OF DISEASE BY INSECTS

Until very recent years insects and their allies have been considered as of economic importance merely in so far as they are an annoyance or direct menace to man, or his flocks and herds, or are injurious to his crops. It is only within the past fifteen years that there has sprung into prominence the knowledge that in another and much more insiduous manner, they may be the enemy of mankind, that they may be among the most important of the disseminators of disease. In this brief period, such knowledge has completely revolutionized our methods of control of certain diseases, and has become an important weapon in the fight for the conservation of health.

It is nowhere truer than in the case under consideration that however abrupt may be their coming into prominence, great movements and great discoveries do not arise suddenly. Centuries ago there was suggested the possibility that insects were concerned with the spread of disease, and from time to time there have appeared keen suggestions and logical hypotheses along this line, that lead us to marvel that the establishment of the truths should have been so long delayed.

One of the earliest of these references is by the Italian physician, Mercurialis, who lived from 1530 to 1607, during a period when Europe was being ravaged by the dread "black death", or plague. Concerning its transmission he wrote: "There can be no doubt that flies feed on the internal secretions of the diseased and dying, then, flying away, they deposit their excretions on the food in neighboring dwellings, and persons who eat of it are thus infected."

It would be difficult to formulate more clearly this aspect of the facts as we know them to-day, though it must always be borne in mind that we are prone to interpret such statements in the light of present-day knowledge. Mercurialis had no conception of the animate nature of contagion, and his statement was little more than a lucky guess.

Much more worthy of consideration is the approval which was given to his view by the German Jesuit, Athanasius Kircher in 1658.

One cannot read carefully his works without believing that long before Leeuwenhook's discovery, Kircher had seen the larger species of bacteria. Moreover, he attributed the production of disease to these organisms and formulated, vaguely, to be sure, a theory of the animate nature of contagion. It has taken two and a half centuries to accumulate the facts to prove his hypothesis.

The theory of Mercurialis was not wholly lost sight of, for in the medical literature of the eighteenth century there are scattered references to flies as carriers of disease. Such a view seems even to have been more or less popularly accepted, in some cases. Gudger (1910), has pointed out that, as far back as 1769, Edward Bancroft, in "An Essay on the Natural History of Guiana in South America," wrote concerning the contagious skin-disease known as "Yaws": "It is usually believed that this disorder is communicated by the flies who have been feasting on a diseased object, to those persons who have sores, or scratches, which are uncovered; and from many observations, I think this is not improbable, as none ever receive this disorder whose skins are whole."

Approaching more closely the present epoch, we find that in 1848, Dr. Josiah Nott, of Mobile, Alabama, published a remarkable article on the cause of yellow fever, in which he presented "reasons for supposing its specific cause to exist in some form of insect life." As a matter of fact, the bearing of Nott's work on present day ideas of the insect transmission of disease has been very curiously overrated. The common interpretation of his theory has been deduced from a few isolated sentences, but his argument appears quite differently when the entire article is studied. It must be remembered that he wrote at a period before the epoch-making discoveries of Pasteur and before the recognition of micro-organisms as factors in the cause of disease. His article is a masterly refutation of the theory of "malarial" origin of "all the fevers of hot climates," but he uses the term "insect" as applicable to the lower forms of life, and specific references to "mosquitoes," "aphids," "cotton-worms," and others, are merely in the way of similes.

But, while Nott's ideas regarding the relation of insects to yellow fever were vague and indefinite, it was almost contemporaneously that the French physician, Louis Daniel Beauperthuy argued in the most explicit possible manner, that yellow fever and various others are transmitted by mosquitoes. In the light of the data which were available when he wrote, in 1853, it is not surprising that he erred by thinking that the source of the virus was decomposing matter which the mosquito took up and accidentally inoculated into man. Beauperthuy not only discussed the rôle of mosquitoes in the transmission of disease, but he taught, less clearly, that house-flies scatter pathogenic organisms. It seems that Boyce (1909) who quotes extensively from this pioneer work, does not go too far when he says "It is Dr. Beauperthuy whom we must regard as the father of the doctrine of insect-borne disease."

In this connection, mention must be made of the scholarly article by the American physician, A. F. A. King who, in 1883, brought together an all but conclusive mass of argument in support of his belief that malaria was caused by mosquitoes. At about the same time, Finley, of Havana, was forcefully presenting his view that the mosquito played the chief rôle in the spread of yellow fever.

To enter more fully into the general historical discussion is beyond the scope of this book. We shall have occasion to make more explicit references in considering various insect-borne diseases. Enough has been said here to emphasize that the recognition of insects as factors in the spread of disease was long presaged, and that there were not wanting keen thinkers who, with a background of present-day conceptions of the nature of disease, might have been in the front rank of investigators along these lines.

## THE WAYS IN WHICH ARTHROPODS MAY AFFECT THE HEALTH OF MAN

When we consider the ways in which insects and their allies may affect the health of man, we find that we may treat them under three main groups:

A. They may be directly poisonous. Such, for example, are the scorpions, certain spiders and mites, some of the predaceous bugs, and stinging insects. Even such forms as the mosquito deserve some consideration from this viewpoint.

B. They may be parasitic, living more or less permanently on or in the body and deriving their sustenance from it.

Of the parasitic arthropods we may distinguish, first, the *true parasites*, those which have adopted and become confirmed in the parasitic habit. Such are the itch mites, the lice, fleas, and the majority of the forms to be considered as parasitic.

In addition to these, we may distinguish a group of *accidental, or facultative parasites*, species which are normally free-living, feeding on decaying substances, but which when accidentally introduced into the alimentary canal or other cavities of man, may exist there for a greater or less period. For example, certain fly larvæ, or maggots, normally feeding in putrifying meat, have been known to occur as accidental or facultative parasites in the stomach of man.

C. Finally, and most important, arthropods may be transmitters and disseminators of disease. In this capacity they may function in one of three ways; as *simple carriers*, as *direct inoculators*, or as *essential hosts* of disease germs.

As simple carriers, they may, in a wholly incidental manner, transport from the diseased to the healthy, or from filth to food, pathogenic germs which cling to their bodies or appendages. Such, for instance, is the relation of the house-fly to the dissemination of typhoid.

As direct inoculators, biting or piercing species may take up from a diseased man or animal, germs which, clinging to the mouth parts, are inoculated directly into the blood of the insect's next victim. It it thus that horse-flies may occasionally transmit anthrax. Similarly, species of spiders and other forms which are ordinarily perfectly harmless, may accidentally convey and inoculate pyogenic bacteria.

It is as essential hosts of disease germs that arthropods play their most important rôle. In such cases an essential part of the life cycle of the pathogenic organism is undergone in the insect. In other words, without the arthropod host the disease-producing organism cannot complete its development. As illustrations may be cited the relation of the Anopheles mosquito to the malarial parasite, and the relation of the cattle tick to Texas fever.

A little consideration will show that this is the most important of the group. Typhoid fever is carried by water or by contaminated milk, and in various other ways, as well as by the house-fly. Kill all the house-flies and typhoid would still exist. On the other hand, malaria is carried only by the mosquito, because an essential part of the development of the malarial parasite is undergone in this insect. Exterminate all of the mosquitoes of certain species and the dissemination of human malaria is absolutely prevented.

Once an arthropod becomes an essential host for a given parasite it may disseminate infection in three different ways:

1. By infecting man or animals who ingest it. It is thus, for example, that man, dog, or cat, becomes infected with the double-pored dog tapeworm, *Dipylidium caninum*. The cysticercoid stage

occurs in the dog louse, or in the dog or cat fleas, and by accidentally ingesting the infested insect the vertebrate becomes infested. Similarly, *Hymenolepis diminuta*, a common tapeworm of rats and mice, and occasional in man, undergoes part of its life cycle in various meal-infesting insects, and is accidentally taken up by its definitive host. It is very probable that man becomes infested with *Dracunculus (Filaria) medinensis* through swallowing in drinking water, the crustacean, *Cyclops*, containing the larvæ of this worm.

2. By infecting man or animals on whose skin or mucous membranes the insect host may be crushed or may deposit its excrement. The pathogenic organism may then actively penetrate, or may be inoculated by scratching. The causative organism of typhus fever is thus transmitted by the body louse.

3. By direct inoculation by its bite, the insect host may transfer the parasite which has undergone development within it. The malarial parasite is thus transferred by mosquitoes; the Texas fever parasite by cattle ticks.

# CHAPTER II.

## ARTHROPODS WHICH ARE DIRECTLY POISONOUS

Of all the myriads of insects and related forms, a very few are of direct use to man, some few others have forced his approbation on account of their wonderful beauty, but the great hordes of them are loathed or regarded as directly dangerous. As a matter of fact, only a very small number are in the slightest degree poisonous to man or to the higher animals. The result is that entomologists and lovers of nature, intent upon dissipating the foolish dread of insects, are sometimes inclined to go to the extreme of discrediting all statements of serious injury from the bites or stings of any species.

Nevertheless, it must not be overlooked that poisonous forms do exist, and they must receive attention in a consideration of the ways in which arthropods may affect the health of man. Moreover, it must be recognized that "what is one man's meat, is another man's poison," and that in considering the possibilities of injury we must not ignore individual idiosyncrasies. Just as certain individuals may be poisoned by what, for others are common articles of food, so some persons may be abnormally susceptible to insect poison. Thus, the poison of a bee sting may be of varying severity, but there are individuals who are made seriously sick by a single sting, regardless of the point of entry. Some individuals scarcely notice a mosquito bite, others find it very painful, and so illustrations of this difference in individuals might be multiplied.

In considering the poisonous arthropods, we shall take them up by groups. The reader who is unacquainted with the systematic relationship of insects and their allies is referred to Chapter XII. No attempt will be made to make the lists under the various headings exhaustive, but typical forms will be discussed.

## ARANEIDA OR SPIDERS

Of all the arthropods there are none which are more universally feared than are the spiders. It is commonly supposed that the majority, if not all the species are poisonous and that they are aggressive enemies of man and the higher animals, as well as of lower forms.

That they really secrete a poison may be readily inferred from the effect of their bite upon insects and other small forms. Moreover, the presence of definite and well-developed poison glands can easily be shown. They occur as a pair of pouches (fig. 1) lying within the cephalothorax and connected by a delicate duct with a pore on the claw of the chelicera, or so-called "mandible" on the convex surface of the claw in such a position that it is not plugged and closed by the flesh of the victim.

The glands may be demonstrated by slowly and carefully twisting off a chelicera and pushing aside the stumps of muscles at its base. By exercising care, the chitinous wall of the chelicera and its claw may be broken away and the duct traced from the gland to its outlet. The inner lining of the sac is constituted by a highly developed glandular epithelium, supported by a basement membrane of connective tissue and covered by a muscular layer, (fig. 2). The muscles, which are striated, are spirally arranged (fig. 1), and are doubtless under control of the spider, so that the amount of poison to be injected into a wound may be varied.

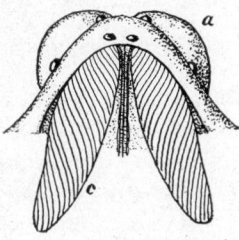

1. Head of a spider showing poison gland (*c*) and its relation to the chelicera (*a*).

The poison itself, according to Kobert (1901), is a clear, colorless fluid, of oily consistency, acid reaction, and very bitter taste. After the spider has bitten two or three times, its supply is exhausted and therefore, as in the case of snakes, the poison of the bite decreases quickly with use, until it is null. To what extent the content of the poison sacs may contain blood serum or, at least, active principles of serum, in addition to a specific poison formed by the poison glands themselves, Kobert regards as an open question. He believes that the acid part of the poison, if really present, is formed by the glands and that, in the case of some spiders, the ferment-like, or better, active toxine, comes from the blood.

But there is a wide difference between a poison which may kill an insect and one which is harmful to men. Certain it is that there is no lack of popular belief and newspaper records of fatal cases, but the evidence regarding the possibility of fatal or even very serious results for man is most contradictory. For some years, we have attempted to trace the more circumstantial newspaper

3. Chelicera of a spider.

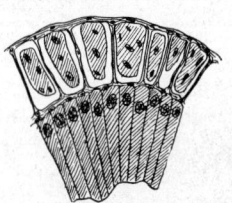

2. Section through a venom gland of Latrodectus 13-guttatus showing the peritoneal, muscular and epithelial layers. After Bordas.

accounts, which have come to our notice, of injury by North American species. The results have served, mainly, to emphasize the straits to which reporters are sometimes driven when there is a dearth of news. The accounts are usually vague and lacking in any definite clue for locating the supposed victim. In the comparatively few cases where the patient, or his physician, could be located, there was either no claim that the injury was due to spider venom, or there was no evidence to support the belief. Rarely, there was evidence that a secondary blood poisoning, such as might be brought about by the prick of a pin, or by any mechanical injury, had followed the bite of a spider. Such instances have no bearing on the question of the venomous nature of these forms.

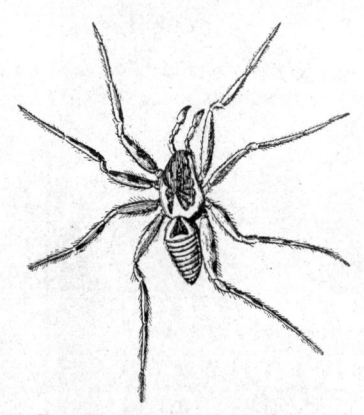

The extreme to which unreasonable fear of the bites of spiders influenced the popular mind was evidenced by the accepted explanation of the remarkable dancing mania, or tarantism, of Italy during the Middle Ages. This was a nervous disorder, supposed to be due to the bite of a spider, the European tarantula (fig. 4), though it was also, at times, attributed to the bite of the scorpion. In its typical form, it was characterized by so great a sensibility to music that under its influence the victims indulged in the wildest and most frenzied dancing, until they sank to the ground utterly exhausted and almost lifeless. The profuse perspiring resulting from these exertions was supposed to be the only efficacious remedy for the disease. Certain forms of music were regarded as of especial value in treating this tarantism, and hence the name of "tarantella" was applied to them. Our frontispiece, taken from Athanasius Kircher's *Magnes sive de Arte Magnetica*, 1643 ed., represents the most commonly implicated spider and illustrates some of what Fabre has aptly designated as "medical choreography."

4. The Italian tarantula (Lycosa tarantula). After Kobert.

The disease was, in reality, a form of hysteria, spreading by sympathy until whole communities were involved, and was paralleled by the outbreaks of the so-called St. Vitus's or St. John's dance, which swept Germany at about the same time (fig. 5). The evidence that the spider was the cause of the first is about as conclusive as is that of the demoniacal origin of the latter. The true explanation of the outbreaks is doubtless to be found in the depleted physical and mental condition of the people, resulting from the wars and the frightful plagues which devastated all Europe previous to, and during these times. An interesting discussion of these aspects of the question is to be found in Hecker.

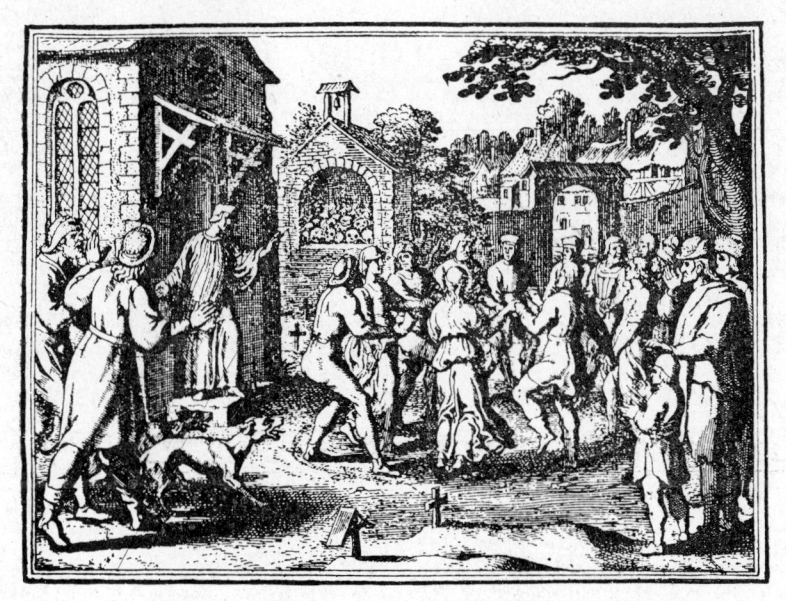

5. Dancing mania. Illustration from Johann Ludwig Gottfried's Chronik. 1632.

So gross has been the exaggeration and so baseless the popular fear regarding spiders that entomologists have been inclined to discredit all accounts of serious injury from their bites. Not only have the most circumstantial of newspaper accounts proved to be without foundation but there are on record a number of cases where the bite of many of the commoner species have been intentionally provoked and where the effect has been insignificant. Some years ago the senior author personally experimented with a number of the largest of our northern species, and with unexpected results. The first surprise was that the spiders were very unwilling to bite and that it required a considerable effort to get them to attempt to do so. In the second place, most of those experimented with were unable to pierce the skin of the palm or the back of the hand, but had to be applied to the thin skin between the fingers before they were able to draw blood. Unfortunately, no special attempt was made to determine, at the time, the species experimented with, but among them were *Theridion tepidariorum, Miranda aurantia (Argiopa), Metargiope trifasciata, Marxia stellata, Aranea trifolium, Misumena vatia,* and *Agelena nævia.* In no case was the bite more severe than a pin prick and though in some cases the sensation seemed to last longer, it was probably due to the fact that the mind was intent upon the experiment.

Similar experiments were carried out by Blackwell (1855), who believed that in the case of insects bitten, death did not result any

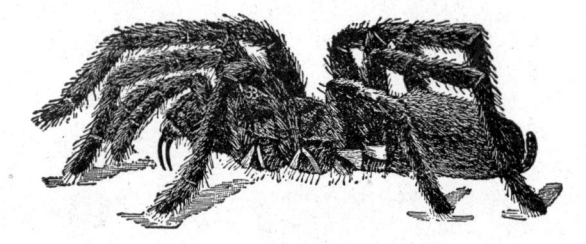

6. An American tarantula (Eurypelma hentzii). Natural size. After Comstock.

more promptly than it would have from a purely mechanical injury of equal extent. He was inclined to regard all accounts of serious injury to man as baseless. The question cannot be so summarily dismissed, and we shall now consider some of the groups which have been more explicitly implicated.

**The Tarantulas.**—In popular usage, the term " tarantula " is loosely applied to any one of a number of large spiders. The famous tarantulas of southern Europe, whose bites were supposed to cause the dancing mania, were Lycosidæ, or wolf-spiders. Though various species of this group were doubtless so designated, the one which seems to have been most implicated was *Lycosa tarantula* (L.), (fig. 4). On the other hand, in this country, though there are many Lycosidæ, the term "tarantula" has been applied to members of the superfamily Avicularoidea (fig. 6), including the bird-spiders.

Of the Old World Lycosidæ there is no doubt that several species were implicated as the supposed cause of the tarantism. In fact, as we have already noted, the blame was sometimes attached to a scorpion. However, there seems to be no doubt that most of the accounts refer to the spider known as *Lycosa tarantula*.

There is no need to enter into further details here regarding the supposed virulence of these forms, popular and the older medical literature abound in circumstantial accounts of the terrible effects of the bite. Fortunately, there is direct experimental evidence which bears on the question.

Fabre induced a common south European wolf-spider, *Lycosa narbonensis*, to bite the leg of a young sparrow, ready to leave the nest. The leg seemed paralyzed as a result of the bite, and though the bird seemed lively and clamored for food the next day, on the third day it died. A mole, bitten on the nose, succumbed after thirty-six hours. From these experiments Fabre seemed justified in his conclusion that the bite of this spider is not an accident which man can afford to treat lightly. Unfortunately, there is nothing in the experiments, or in the symptoms detailed, to exclude the probability that the death of the animals was the result of secondary infection.

As far back as 1693, as we learn from the valuable account of Kobert, (1901), the Italian physician, Sanguinetti allowed himself to be bitten on the arm by two tarantulas, in the presence of witnesses. The sensation was equivalent to that from an ant or a mosquito bite and there were no other phenomena the first day. On the second day the wound was inflamed and there was slight ulceration. It is clear that these later symptoms were due to a secondary infection. These experiments have been repeated by various observers, among whom may be mentioned Leon Dufour, Josef Erker and Heinzel, and with the similar conclusion that the bite of the Italian tarantula ordinarily causes no severe symptoms. In this conclusion, Kobert, though firmly convinced of the poisonous nature of some spiders, coincides. He also believes that striking symptoms may be simulated or artificially induced by patients in order to attract interest, or because they have been assured that the bite, under all circumstances, caused tarantism.

The so-called Russian tarantula, *Trochosa singoriensis* (fig. 7), is much larger than the Italian species, and is much feared. Kobert carried out a series of careful experiments with this species and his results have such an important bearing on the question of the venomous nature of the tarantula that we quote his summary. Experimenting first on nearly a hundred living specimens of *Trochosa singoriensis* from Crimea he says that:

"The tarantulas, no matter how often they were placed on the skin, handled, and irritated, could not be induced to bite either myself, the janitor, or the ordinary experimental animals. The objection that the tarantulas were weak and indifferent cannot stand, for as soon as I placed two of them on the shaved skin of a rabbit, instead of an attack on the animal, there began a furious battle between the two spiders, which did not cease until one of the two was killed."

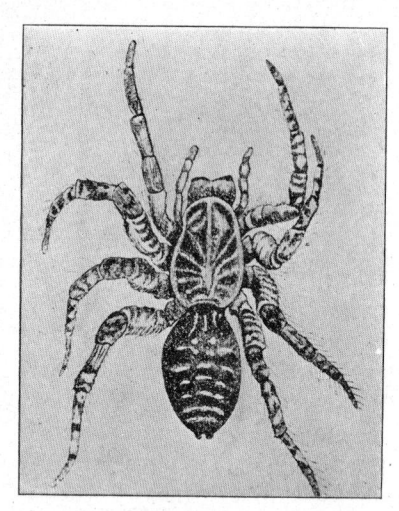

"Since the spiders would not bite, I carefully ground up the fresh animals in physiological salt solution, preparing an extract which must have contained, in solution, all of the poisonous substance of their bodies. While in the case of *Latrodectus*, as we shall see, less than one specimen sufficed to yield an active extract, I have injected the filtered extract of six fresh Russian tarantulas, of which each one was much heavier than an average *Latrodectus*, subcutaneously and into the jugular vein of various cats without the animals dying or showing any special symptoms. On the basis of my experiments I can therefore only say that the quantity of the poison soluble in physiological salt solution, even when the spiders are perfectly fresh and well nourished, is very insignificant. That the poison of the Russian tarantula is not soluble in physiological salt solution, is exceedingly improbable. Moreover, I have prepared alcoholic extracts and was unable to find them active. Since the Russian spider exceeds the Italian in size and in intensity of the bite, it seems very improbable to me that the pharmacological test of the Italian tarantula would yield essentially other results than those from the Russian species."

7. Trochosa singoriensis. After Kobert.

To the **Avicularoidea** belong the largest and most formidable appearing of the spiders and it is not strange that in the New World they have fallen heir to the bad reputation, as well as to the name of the tarantula of Europe. In this country they occur only in the South or in the far West, but occasionally living specimens are brought to our northern ports in shipments of bananas and other tropical produce, and are the source of much alarm. It should be mentioned, however, that the large spider most frequently found under such circumstances is not a tarantula at all, but one of the Heteropodidæ, or giant crab-spiders, (fig. 8).

In spite of their prominence and the fear which they arouse there are few accurate data regarding these American tarantulas. It has

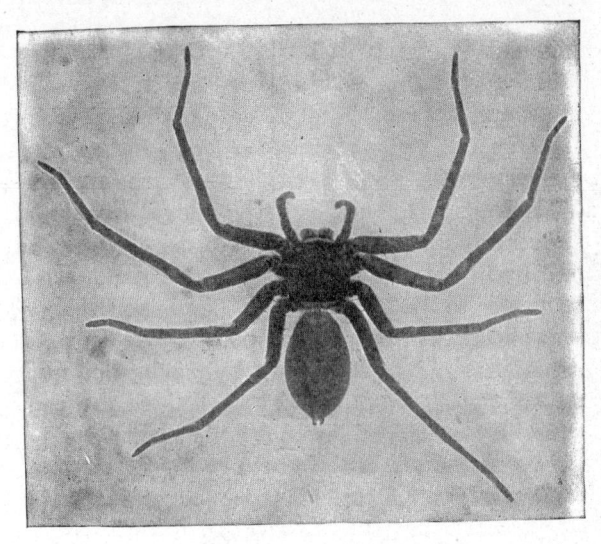

8. The giant crab-spider or banana spider (Heteropoda venatoria). Natural size. After Comstock.

often been shown experimentally that they can kill small birds and mammals, though it is doubtful if these form the normal prey of any of the species, as has been claimed. There is no question but that the mere mechanical injury which they may inflict, and the consequent chances of secondary infection, justify, in part, their bad reputation. In addition to the injury from their bite, it is claimed that the body hairs of several of the South American species are readily detached and are urticating.

Recently, Phisalix (1912) has made a study of the physiological effects of the venom of two Avicularoidea, *Phormictopus carcerides* Pocock, from Haiti and *Cteniza sauvagei* Rossi, from Corsica. The glands were removed aseptically and ground up with fine, sterilized sand in distilled water. The resultant liquid was somewhat viscid, colorless, and feebly alkaline. Injected into sparrows and mice the extract of *Phormictopus* proved very actively poisonous, that from a single spider being sufficient to kill ten sparrows or twenty mice. It manifested itself first and, above all, as a narcotic, slightly lowering the temperature and paralyzing the respiration. Muscular and cardiac weakening, loss of general sensibility, and the disappearance of reflexes did not occur until near the end. The extract from *Cteniza* was less active and, curiously enough, the comparative effect on sparrows and on mice was just reversed.

**Spiders of the Genus Latrodectus.**—While most of the popular accounts of evil effects from the bites of spiders will not stand investigation, it is a significant fact that, the world over, the best authenticated records refer to a group of small and comparatively insignificant spiders belonging to the genus *Latrodectus*, of the family Theridiidæ. The dread "Malmigniatte" of Corsica and South Europe, the "Karakurte" of southeastern Russia, the "Katipo" of New Zealand, the "Mena-vodi" and "Vancoho" of Madagascar, and our own *Latrodectus mactans*, all belong to this genus, and concerning all of these the most circumstantial accounts of their venomous nature are given. These accounts are not mere fantastic stories by uneducated natives but in many cases are reports from thoroughly trained medical men.

The symptoms produced are general, rather than local. As summarized by Kobert (1901) from a study of twenty-two cases treated in 1888, in the Kherson (Russia) Government Hospital and Berislaw (Kherson) District Hospital the typical case, aside from complications, exhibits the following symptoms. The victim suddenly feels the bite, like the sting of a bee. Swelling of the barely reddened spot seldom follows. The shooting pains, which quickly set in, are not manifested at the point of injury but localized at the joints of the lower limb and in the region of the hip. The severity of the pain forces the victim to the hospital, in spite of the fact that they otherwise have a great abhorrence of it. The patient is unable to reach the hospital afoot, or, at least, not without help, for there is usually inability to walk. The patient, even if he has ridden, reaches the hospital covered with cold sweat and continues to perspire for a considerable period. His expression indicates great suffering. The respiration may be somewhat dyspnœic, and a feeling of oppression in the region of the heart is common. There is great aversion to solid food, but increasing thirst for milk and tea. Retention of urine, and constipation occur. Cathartics and, at night, strong narcotics are desired. Warm baths give great relief. After three days, there is marked improvement and usually the patient is dismissed after the fifth. This summary of symptoms agrees well with other trustworthy records.

It would seem, then, that Riley and Howard (1889), who discussed a number of accounts in the entomological literature, were fully justified in their statement that "It must be admitted that certain spiders of the genus *Latrodectus* have the power to inflict poisonous bites, which may (probably exceptionally and depending upon exceptional conditions) bring about the death of a human being."

And yet, until recently the evidence bearing on the question has been most conflicting. The eminent arachnologist, Lucas, (1843) states that he himself, had been repeatedly bitten by the Malmigniatte without any bad effects. Dr. Marx, in 1890, gave before the Entomological Society of Washington, an account of a series of experiments to determine whether the bite of *Latrodectus mactans* is poisonous or not. He described the poison glands as remarkably small* and stated that he had introduced the poison in various ways into guinea-pigs and rabbits without obtaining any satisfactory results. Obviously, carefully conducted experiments with the supposed venom were needed and fortunately they have been carried out in the greatest detail by Kobert (1901).

This investigator pointed out that there were two factors which might account for the discrepancies in the earlier experiments. In the first place, the poison of spiders, as of snakes, might be so exhausted after two or three bites that further bites, following directly, might be without visible effect. Secondly, the application of the poison by means of the bite, is exceedingly inexact, since even after the most careful selection of the point of application, the poison might in one instance enter a little vein or lymph vessel, and in another case fail to do so. Besides, there would always remain an incalculable and very large amount externally, in the nonabsorptive epithelium. While all of these factors enter into the question of the effect of the bite in specific instances, they must be as nearly as possible obviated in considering the question of whether the spiders really secrete a venom harmful to man.

---

*This is diametrically opposed to the findings of Bordas (1905) in the case of the European *Latrodectus 13-guttatus*, whose glands are "much larger than those of other spiders." From a considerable comparative study, we should also unhesitatingly make this statement regarding the glands of our American species, *L. mactans*.

Kobert therefore sought to prepare extracts which would contain the active principles of the poison and which could be injected in definite quantities directly into the blood of the experimental animal. For this purpose various parts of the spiders were rubbed up in a mortar with distilled water, or physiological salt solution, allowed to stand for an hour, filtered, and then carefully washed, by adding water drop by drop for twenty-four hours. The filtrate and the wash-water were then united, well mixed and, if necessary, cleared by centrifuging or by exposure to cold. The mixture was again filtered, measured, and used, in part, for injection and, in part, for the determination of the organic materials.

Such an extract was prepared from the cephalothoraces of eight dried specimens of the Russian *Latrodectus* and three cubic centimeters of this, containing 4.29 mg. of organic material, were injected into the jugular vein of a cat weighing 2450 grams. The previously very active animal was paralyzed and lay in whatever position it was placed. The sensibility of the skin of the extremities and the rump was so reduced that there was no reaction from cutting or sticking. There quickly followed dyspnœa, convulsions, paralysis of the respiratory muscles and of the heart. In twenty-eight minutes the cat was dead, after having exhibited exactly the symptoms observed in severe cases of poisoning of man from the bite of this spider.

These experiments were continued on cats, dogs, guinea pigs and various other animals. Not only extracts from the cephalothorax, but from other parts of the body, from newly hatched spiders, and from the eggs were used and all showed a similar virulence. Every effort was made to avoid sources of error and the experiments, conducted by such a recognized authority in the field of toxicology, must be accepted as conclusively showing that this spider and, presumably, other species of the genus *Latrodectus* against which the clinical evidence is quite parallel, possess a poison which paralyzes the heart and central nervous system, with or without preliminary stimulus of the motor center. If the quantity of the poison which comes into direct contact with the blood is large, there may occur hæmolysis and thrombosis of the vessels.

On the other hand, check experiments were carried out, using similar extracts of many common European spiders of the genera *Tegenaria, Drassus, Agelena, Eucharia* and *Argyroneta*, as well as the Russian tarantula, *Lycosa singoriensis*. In no other case was the effect on experimental animals comparable to the *Latrodectus* extract.

Kobert concludes that in its chemical nature the poison is neither an alkaloid, nor a glycoside, nor an acid, but a toxalbumen, or poisonous enzyme which is very similar to certain other animal poisons, notably that of the scorpion.

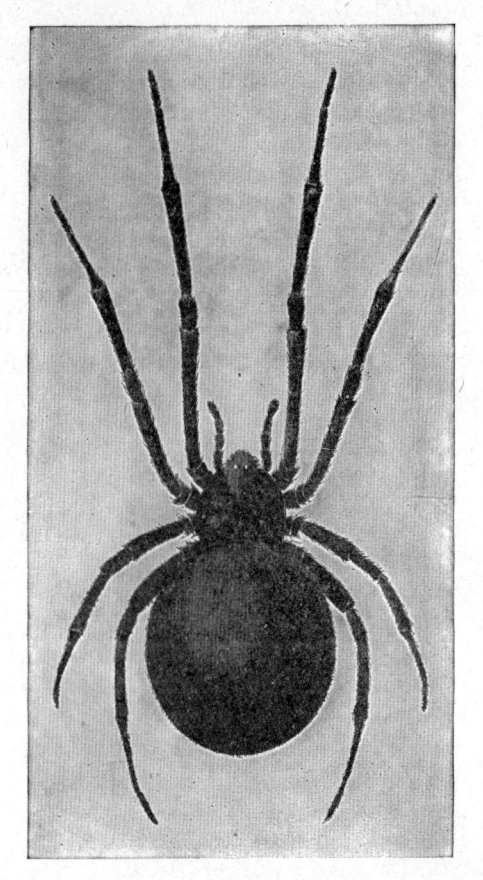

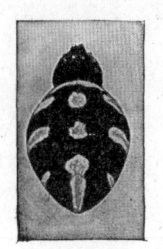

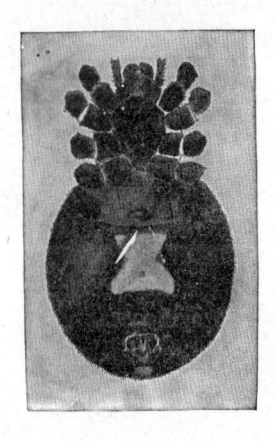

9. Latrodectus mactans; (*a*) female, x 3; (*b*) venter of female; (*c*) dorsum of male. After Comstock.

The genus *Latrodectus* is represented in the United States by at least two species, *L. mactans* and *L. geometricus*. Concerning *L. mactans* there are very circumstantial accounts of serious injury and even death in man*. *Latrodectus mactans* is coal black, marked with red or yellow or both. It has eight eyes, which are dissimilar in

*Dr. E. H. Coleman (Kellogg, 1915) has demonstrated its virulence by a series of experiments comparable with those of Kobert.

color and are distinctly in front of the middle of the thorax, the lateral eyes of each side widely separate. The tarsi of the fourth pair of legs has a number of curved setæ in a single series. It has on the ventral side of its abdomen an hour-glass shaped spot. The full-grown female is about half an inch in length. Its globose abdomen is usually marked with one or more red spots dorsally along the middle line. The male is about half as long but has in addition to the dorsal spots, four pairs of stripes along the sides. Immature females resemble the male in coloring (fig. 9).

Regarding the distribution of *Latrodectus mactans*, Comstock states that: "Although it is essentially a Southern species, it occurs in Indiana, Ohio, Pennsylvania, New Hampshire, and doubtless other of the Northern States." *L. geometricus* has been reported from California.

**Other Venomous Spiders**—While conclusive evidence regarding the venomous nature of spiders is meager and relates almost wholly to that of the genus *Latrodectus*, the group is a large one and we are not justified in dismissing arbitrarily, all accounts of injury from their bites. Several species stand out as especially needing more detailed investigation.

*Chiracanthium nutrix* is a common European species of the family Clubionidæ, concerning which there is much conflicting testimony. Among the reports are two by distinguished scientists whose accounts of personal experiences cannot be ignored. A. Forel allowed a spider of this species to bite him and not only was the pain extreme, but the general symptoms were so severe that he had to be helped to his house. The distinguished arachnologist, Bertkau reports that he, himself, was bitten and that an extreme, burning pain spread almost instantaneously over the arm and into the breast. There were slight chills the same day and throbbing pain at the wound lasted for days. While this particular species is not found in the United States, there are two other representatives of the genus and it is possible that they possess the same properties. We are unaware of any direct experimental work on the poison.

*Epeira diadema*, of Europe, belongs to a wholly different group, that of the orb-weavers, but has long been reputed venomous. Kobert was able to prepare from it an extract whose effects were very similar to that prepared from *Latrodectus*, though feebler in its action. Under ordinary circumstances this spider is unable to pierce the skin of man and though Kobert's results seem conclusive, the spider is little to be feared.

*Phidippus audax* (*P. tripunctatus*) is one of our largest Attids, or jumping spiders. The late Dr. O. Lugger describes a case of severe poisoning from the bite of this spider and though details are lacking, it is quite possible that this and other large species of the same group, which stalk their prey, may possess a more active poison than that of web-building species.

**Summary**—It is clearly established that our common spiders are not to be feared and that the stories regarding their virulence are almost wholly without foundation. On the other hand, the chances of secondary infection from the bites of some of the more powerful species are not to be ignored.

Probably all species possess a toxin secreted by the poison gland, virulent for insects and other normal prey of the spiders, but with little or no effect on man.

There are a very few species, notably of the genus *Latrodectus*, and possibly including the European *Chiracanthium nutrix* and *Epeira diadema*, which possess, in addition, a toxalbumen derived from the general body tissue, which is of great virulence and may even cause death in man and the higher animals.

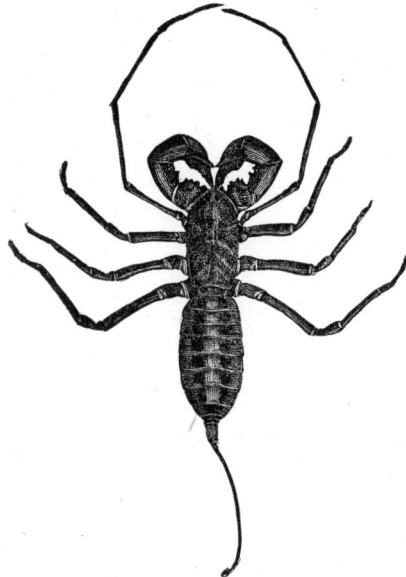

10. A whip-scorpion (Mastigoproctus giganteus). Half natural size. After Comstock.

## THE PEDIPALPIDA OR WHIP-SCORPIONS

The tailed whip-scorpions, belonging to the family Thelyphonidæ, are represented in the United States by the giant whip-scorpion *Mastigoproctus giganteus* (fig. 10), which is common in Florida, Texas and some other parts of the South. In Florida, it is locally known as the "grampus" or "mule-killer" and is very greatly feared. There is no evidence that these fears have any foundation, and Dr. Marx states that there is neither a poison gland nor a pore in the claw of the chelicera.

## THE SCORPIONIDA, OR TRUE SCORPIONS

The true scorpions are widely distributed throughout warm countries and everywhere bear an evil reputation. According to Comstock (1912), about a score of species occur in the Southern United States. These are comparatively small forms but in the tropics members of this group may reach a length of seven or eight inches. They are pre-eminently predaceous forms, which lie hidden during the day and seek their prey by night.

The scorpions (fig. 11) possess large pedipalpi, terminated by strongly developed claws, or chelæ. They may be distinguished from all other Arachnids by the fact that the distinctly segmented abdomen is divided into a broad basal region of seven segments and a terminal, slender, tail-like division of five distinct segments.

The last segment of the abdomen, or telson, terminates in a ventrally-directed, sharp spine, and contains a pair of highly developed poison glands. These glands open by two small pores near the tip of the spine. Most of the species when running carry the tip of the abdomen bent upward over the back, and the prey, caught and held by the pedipalpi, is stung by inserting the spine of the telson and allowing it to remain for a time in the wound.

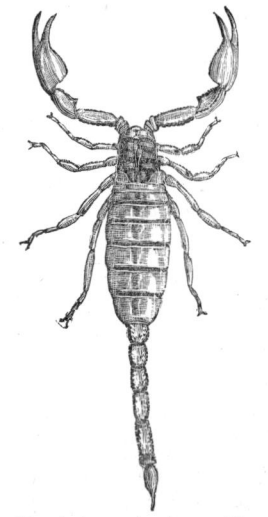

11. A true scorpion. After Comstock.

The glands themselves have been studied in *Prionurus citrinus* by Wilson (1904). He found that each gland is covered by a sheet of muscle on its mesal and dorsal aspects, which may be described as the *compressor muscle*. The muscle of each side is inserted by its edge along the ventral inner surface of the chitinous wall of the telson, close to the middle line, and by a broader insertion laterally. A layer of fine connective tissue completely envelops each gland and forms the basis upon which the secreting cells rest. The secreting epithelium is columnar; and apparently of three different types of cells.

1. The most numerous have the appearance of mucous cells, resembling the goblet cells of columnar mucous membranes. The nucleus, surrounded by a small quantity of protoplasm staining with hæmatoxylin, lies close to the base of the cell.

2. Cells present in considerable numbers, the peripheral portions of which are filled with very numerous fine granules, staining with acid dyes such as methyl orange.

3. Cells few in number, filled with very large granules, or irregular masses of a substance staining with hæmatoxylin.

The poison, according to Kobert (1893), is a limpid, acid-reacting fluid, soluble in water but insoluble in absolute alcohol and ether. There are few data relative to its chemical nature. Wilson (1901) states that a common Egyptian species, *Buthus quinquestriatus*, has a specific gravity of 1.092, and contains 20.3% of solids and 8.4% ash.

The venom of different species appears to differ not only quantitatively but qualitatively. The effects of the bite of the smaller species of the Southern United States may be painful but there is no satisfactory evidence that it is ever fatal. On the other hand, certain tropical species are exceedingly virulent and cases of death of man from the bite are common.

In the case of *Buthus quinquestriatus*, Wilson (1904) found the symptoms in animals to be hypersecretion, salivation and lachrymation, especially marked, convulsions followed by prolonged muscular spasm; death from asphyxia. The temperature shows a slight, rarely considerable, rise. Rapid and considerable increase of blood-pressure (observed in dogs) is followed by a gradual fall with slowing of the heart-beat. The coagulability of the blood is not affected.

An interesting phase of Wilson's work was the experiments on desert mammals. The condition under which these animals exist must frequently bring them in contact with scorpions, and he found that they possess a degree of immunity to the venom sufficient at least to protect them from the fatal effects of the sting.

As far as concerns its effect on man, Wilson found that much depended upon the age. As high as 60 per cent of the cases of children under five, resulted fatally. Caroroz (1865), states that in a Mexican state of 15,000 inhabitants, the scorpions were so abundant and so much feared that the authorities offered a bounty for their destruction. A result was a large number of fatalities, over two hundred per year. Most of the victims were children who had attempted to collect the scorpions.

The treatment usually employed in the case of bites by the more poisonous forms is similar to that for the bite of venomous snakes. First, a tight ligature is applied above the wound so as to stop the flow of blood and lymph from that region. The wound is then freely excised and treated with a strong solution of permanganate of potash, or with lead and opium lotion.

In recent years there have been many attempts to prepare an antivenom, or antiserum comparable to what has been used so effectively in the case of snake bites. The most promising of these is that of Todd (1909), produced by the immunization of suitable animals. This antivenom proved capable of neutralizing the venom when mixed *in vitro* and also acts both prophylactically and curatively in animals. Employed curatively in man, it appears to have a very marked effect on the intense pain following the sting, and the evidence so far indicates that its prompt use greatly reduces the chance of fatal results.

## THE SOLPUGIDA, OR SOLPUGIDS

The **Solpugida** are peculiar spider-like forms which are distinguished from nearly all other arachnids by the fact that they possess no true cephalothorax, the last two leg-bearing segments being distinct, resembling those of the abdomen in this respect. The first pair of legs is not used in locomotion but seemingly functions as a second pair of pedipalpi. Figure 12 illustrates the striking peculiarities of the group. They are primarily desert forms and occur in the warm zones of all countries. Of the two hundred or more species, Comstock lists twelve as occurring in our fauna. These occur primarily in the southwest.

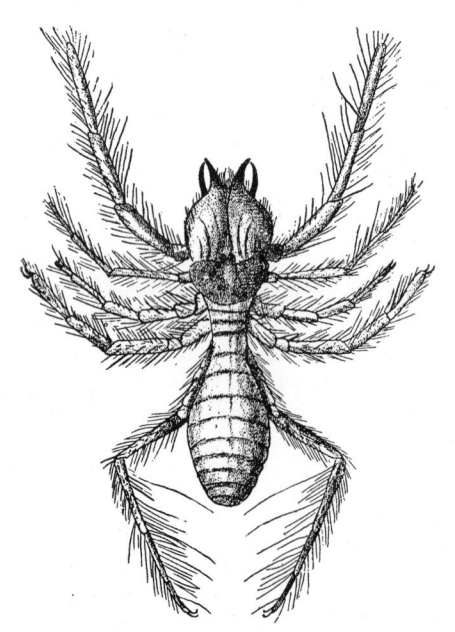

12. A solpugid (Eremobates cinerea). After Comstock.

The Solpugida have long borne a bad reputation and regarding virulence, have been classed with the scorpions. Among the effects of their bites have been described painful swelling, gangrene, loss of speech, cramps, delirium, unconsciousness and even death. Opposed to the numerous loose accounts of poisoning, there are a number of careful records by physicians and zoölogists which indicate clearly that the effects are local and though they may be severe, they show not the slightest symptom of direct poisoning.

More important in the consideration of the question is the fact that there are neither poison glands nor pores in the fangs for the exit of any poisonous secretion. This is the testimony of a number of prominent zoölogists, among whom is Dr. A. Walter, who wrote to Kobert at length on the subject and whose conclusions are presented by him.

However, it should be noted that the fangs are very powerful and are used in such a manner that they may inflict especially severe wounds. Thus, there may be more opportunity for secondary infection than is usual in the case of insect wounds.

The treatment of the bite of the Solpugida is, therefore, a matter of preventing infection. The wound should be allowed to bleed freely and then washed out with a 1:3000 solution of corrosive sublimate, and, if severe, a wet dressing of this should be applied. If infection takes place, it should be treated in the usual manner, regardless of its origin.

## THE ACARINA, OR MITES AND TICKS

A number of the parasitic Acarina evidently secrete a specific poison, presumably carried by the saliva, but in most cases its effect on man is insignificant. There is an abundant literature dealing with the poisonous effect of the bite of these forms, especially the ticks, but until recently it has been confused by failure to recognize that various species may transmit diseases of man, rather than produce injury through direct poisoning. We shall therefore discuss the Acarina more especially in subsequent chapters, dealing with parasitism and with disease transmission.

Nevertheless, after the evidence is sifted, there can be no doubt that the bites of certain ticks may occasionally be followed by a direct poisoning, which may be either local or general in its effects. Nuttall (1908) was unable to determine the cause of the toxic effect, for, in *Argas persicus*, the species most often implicated, he failed to get the slightest local or general effect on experimental animals, from the injection of an emulsion prepared by crushing three of the ticks.

It seems clearly established that the bite of certain ticks may cause a temporary paralysis, or even complete paralysis, involving the organs of respiration or the heart, and causing death. In 1912, Dr. I. U. Temple, of Pendleton, Oregon, reported several cases of what he called "acute ascending paralysis" associated with the occurrence of ticks on the head or the back of the neck. A typical severe case was that of a six year old child, who had retired in her usual normal health. The following morning upon arising she was unable to stand on her feet. She exhibited paralysis extending to the knees, slight temperature, no pain, sensory nerves normal, motor nerves completely paralyzed, reflexes absent. The following day the paralysis had extended to the upper limbs, and before night of the third day the nerves of the throat (hypoglossal) were affected. The thorax and larynx were involved, breathing was labored, she was unable to swallow liquids, phonation was impossible and she could only make low, gutteral sounds. At this stage, two ticks, fully distended with blood, were found over the junction of the spinal column with the occipital bones in the hollow depression. They were removed by the application of undiluted creoline. Though the child's life was despaired of, by the following morning she was very much improved. By evening she was able to speak. The paralysis gradually receded, remaining longest in the feet, and at the end of one week the patient was able to go home.

There was some doubt as to the exact species of tick implicated in the cases which Dr. Temple reported, although the evidence pointed strongly to *Dermacentor venustus*.* Somewhat later, Hadwen (1913) reported that "tick paralysis" occurs in British Columbia, where it affects not only man, but sheep and probably other animals. It is caused by the bites of *Dermacentor venustus* and was experimentally produced in lambs and a dog (Hadwen and Nuttall, 1913). It is only when the tick begins to engorge or feed rapidly, some days after it has become attached, that its saliva produces pathogenic effects.

Ulceration following tick bite is not uncommon. In many of the instances it is due to the file-like hypostome, with its recurved teeth, being left in the wound when the tick is forcibly pulled off.

---

*According to Stiles, the species occurring in the Northwest which is commonly identified as *D. venustus* should be called *D. andersonii* (see footnote, chapter 12).

## THE MYRIAPODA, OR CENTIPEDES AND MILLIPEDES

The old class, Myriapoda includes the **Diplopoda,** or millipedes, and the **Chilopoda,** or centipedes. The present tendency is to raise these groups to the rank of classes.

### The Diplopoda

The **Diplopoda,** or millipedes (fig. 13), are characterized by the presence of two pairs of legs to a segment. The largest of our local myriapods belong to this group. They live in moist places, feeding primarily on decaying vegetable matter, though a few species occasionally attack growing plants.

The millipedes are inoffensive and harmless. *Julus terrestris,* and related species, when irritated pour out over the entire body a yellowish secretion which escapes from cutaneous glands. It is volatile, with a pungent odor, and Phisalix (1900) has shown that it is an active poison when injected into the blood of experimental animals. This, however, does not entitle them to be considered as poisonous arthropods, in the sense of this chapter, any more than the toad can be considered poisonous to man because it secretes a venom from its cutaneous glands.

13. A millipede. After Comstock

### The Chilopoda

The **Chilopoda,** or centipedes (fig. 14), unlike the millipedes, are predaceous forms, and possess well developed poison glands for killing their prey. These

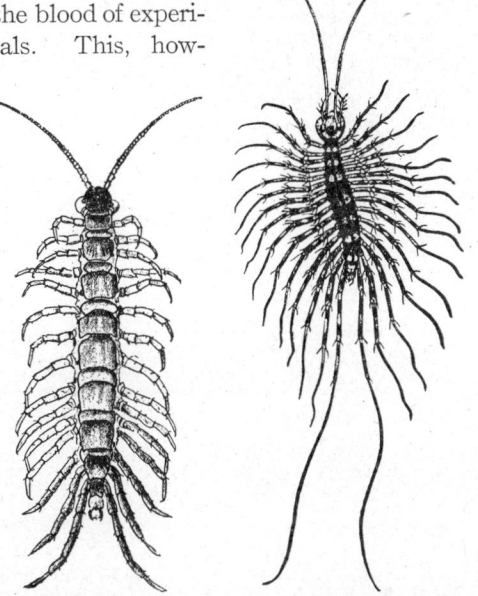

14. Two common centipedes. (*a*) Lithobius forficatus. After Comstock. (*b*) Scutigera forceps. Natural size; after Howard.

glands are at the base of the first pair of legs (fig. 15), which are bent forward so as to be used in holding their prey. The legs terminate in a powerful claw, at the tip of which is the outlet of the poison glands.

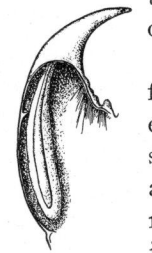

The poison is a limpid, homogeneous, slightly acid fluid, which precipitates in distilled water. Briot (1904) extracted it from the glands of *Scolopendra morsitans*, a species common in central France, and found that it was actively venomous for the ordinary experimental animals. A rabbit of two kilograms weight received an injection of three cubic centimeters in the vein of the ear and died in a minute. A white rat, weighing forty-eight grams, received one and a half cubic centimeters in the hind leg. There was an almost immediate paralysis of the leg and marked necrosis of the tissues.

15. Mandible of Scolopendra cingulata showing venom gland. After Dubosq.

As for the effect on man, there is little foundation for the fear with which centipedes are regarded. Our native species produce, at most, local symptoms,—sometimes severe local pain and swelling,—but there is no authentic record of fatal results. In the tropics, some of the species attain a large size, *Scolopendra gigantea* reaching a length of nearly a foot. These forms are justly feared, and there is good evidence that death sometimes, though rarely, results from their bite.

One of the most careful accounts of death from the sting of the scorpion is that of Linnell, (1914), which relates to a comparatively small Malayan species, unfortunately undetermined. The patient, a coolie, aged twenty, was admitted to a hospital after having been stung two days previously on the left heel. For cure, the other coolies had made him eat the head of the scorpion. On admission, the patient complained of "things creeping all over the body". Temp. 102.8°. On the fourth day he had paralysis of the legs, and on the fifth day motor paralysis to the umbilicus, sensation being unaltered. On the sixth day there was retention of the urine and on the ninth day (first test after third day) sugar was present. On the thirteenth day the patient became comatose, but could be roused to eat and drink. The temperature on the following day fell below 95° and the patient was still comatose. Death fifteenth day.

Examination of the spinal (lumbar) cord showed acute disseminated myelitis. In one part there was an acute destruction of the anterior horn and an infiltration of round cells. In another portion

Clarke's column had been destroyed. The perivascular sheaths were crowded with small round cells and the meninges were congested. Some of the cells of the anterior horn were swollen and the nuclei eccentric; chromatolysis had occurred in many of them.

As for treatment, Castellani and Chalmers (1910), recommend bathing the part well with a solution of ammonia (one in five, or one in ten). After bathing, apply a dressing of the same alkali or, if there is much swelling and redness, an ice-bag. If necessary, hypodermic injections of morphine may be given to relieve the pain. At a later period fomentations may be required to reduce the local inflammation.

## THE HEXAPODA OR TRUE INSECTS

There are a number of **Hexapoda,** or true insects, which are, in one way or another, poisonous to man. These belong primarily to the orders Hemiptera, or true bugs; Lepidoptera, or butterflies and moths (larval forms); Diptera, or flies; Coleoptera, or beetles; and Hymenoptera, or ants, bees, and wasps. There are various ways in which they may be poisonous.

1. *Piercing* or *biting* forms may inject an irritating or poisonous saliva into the wound caused by their mouth-parts.

2. *Stinging forms* may inject a poison, from glands at the caudal end of the abdomen, into wounds produced by a specially modified ovipositer, the *sting*.

3. *Nettling* properties may be possessed by the hairs of the insect.

4. *Vescicating,* or *poisonous blood plasma,* or *body fluids* are known to exist in a large number of species and may, under exceptional circumstances, affect man.

For convenience of discussion, we shall consider poisonous insects under these various headings. In this, as in the preceding discussion, no attempt will be made to give an exhaustive list of the poisonous forms. Typical instances will be selected and these will be chosen largely from North American species.

### PIERCING OR BITING INSECTS POISONOUS TO MAN

#### Hemiptera

Several families of the true bugs include forms which, while normally inoffensive, are capable of inflicting painful wounds on man. In these, as in all of the Hemiptera, the mouth-parts are modified

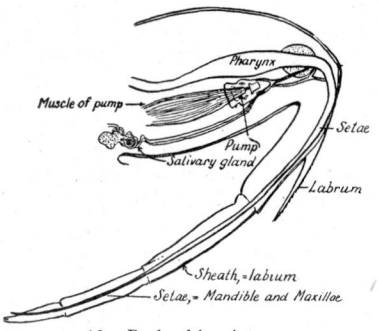

**16. Beak of hemipteron.**

to form an organ for piercing and sucking. This is well shown by the accompanying illustration (fig. 16).

The upper lip, or *labrum*, is much reduced and immovable, the lower lip, or *labium*, is elongated to form a jointed sheath, within which the lance-like mandibles and maxillae are enclosed. The mandibles are more or less deeply serrate, depending on the species concerned.

The poison is elaborated by the salivary glands, excepting, possibly, in *Belostoma* where Locy is inclined to believe that it is secreted by the maxillary glands. The salivary glands of the Hemiptera have been the subject of much study but the most recent, comprehensive work has been done by Bugnion and Popoff, (1908 and 1910) to whose text the reader is referred for details.

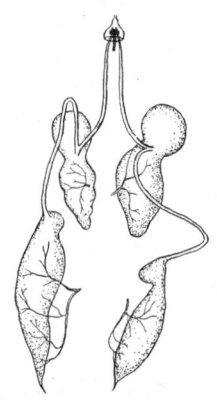

The Hemiptera have two pairs of salivary glands: the *primary gland*, of which the efferent duct leads to the salivary syringe, and the *accessory gland*, of which the very long and flexuous duct empties into the primary duct at its point of insertion. Thus, when one observes the isolated primary gland it appears as though it had efferent ducts inserted at the same point. In *Nepa* and the *Fulgoridæ* there are two accessory glands and therefore apparently three ducts at the same point on the primary gland. The *ensemble* differs greatly in appearance in different species but we shall show here Bugnion and Popoff's figure of the apparatus of *Notonecta maculata*, a species capable of inflicting a painful bite on man (fig. 17).

**17. Salivary glands of Notonecta maculata. After Bugnion and Popoff.**

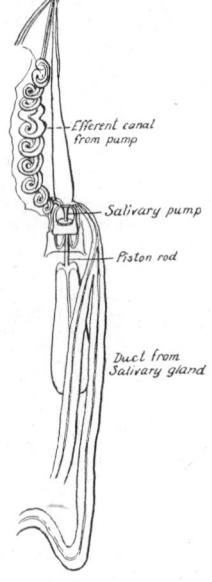

**18. Pharyngeal syringe or salivary pump of Fulgora maculata. After Bugnion and Popoff.**

## Hemiptera, or True Bugs

Accessory to the salivary apparatus there is on the ventral side of the head, underneath the pharynx, a peculiar organ which the

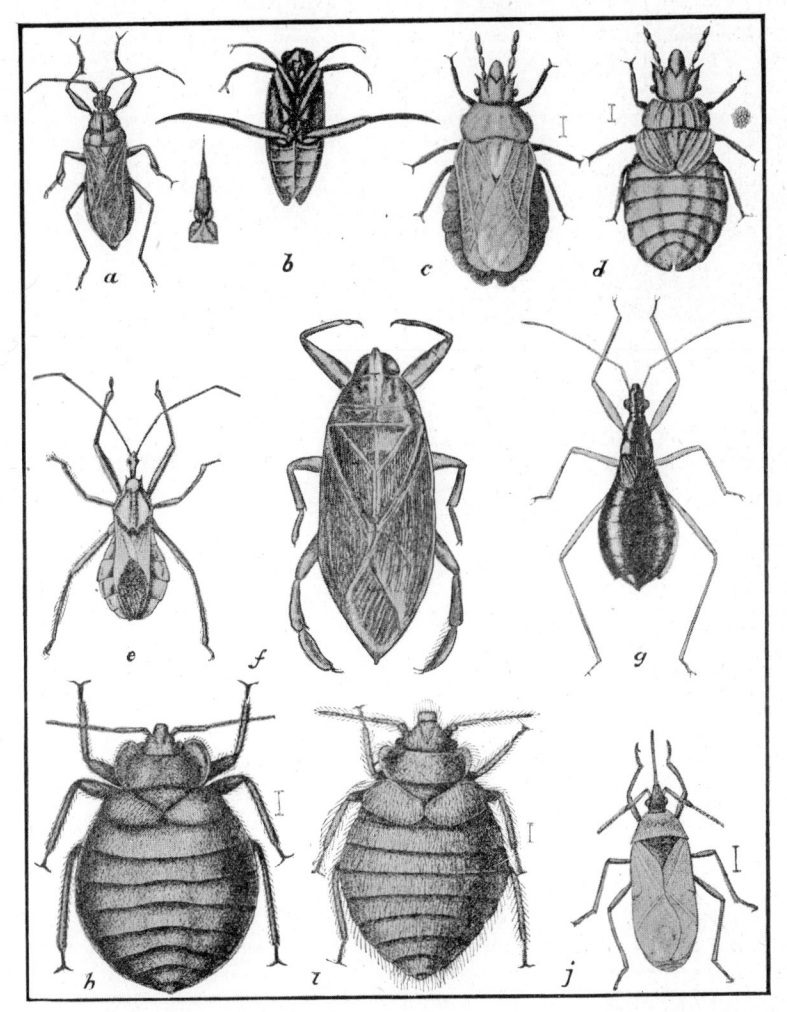

19. Heteroptera, (*a*) Melanolestes picipes; (*b*) Notonecta undulata; (*c, d*) Aradus robustus (*c*) adult, (*d*) nymph, much enlarged; (*e*) Arilus cristatus; (*f*) Belostoma americana; (*g*) Nabis (Coriscus) subcoleoptratus, enlarged; (*h*) Cimex lectularius; (*i*) Oeciacus vicarius, much enlarged; (*j*) Lyctocoris fitchii, much enlarged   After Lugger.

Germans have called the "Wanzenspritze," or syringe. The accompanying figure of the structure in *Fulgora maculata* (fig. 18) shows its relation to the ducts of the salivary glands and to the beak. It is made up of a dilatation forming the body of the pump, in which there is a chitinous piston. Attached to the piston is a strong retractor muscle. The function of the salivary pump is to suck up the saliva from the salivary ducts and to force it out through the beak.

Of the Hemiptera reported as attacking man, we shall consider briefly the forms most frequently noted.

The **Notonectidæ,** or *back swimmers*, (fig. 19*b*) are small, aquatic bugs that differ from all others in that they always swim on their backs. They are predaceous, feeding on insects and other small forms. When handled carelessly they are able to inflict a painful bite, which is sometimes as severe as the sting of a bee. In fact, they are known in Germany as "Wasserbienen."

The **Belostomatidæ,** or *giant water bugs*, (fig. 19*f*) include the largest living Hemiptera. They are attracted to lights and on account of the large numbers which swarm about the electric street lamps in some localities they have received the popular name "electric light bugs." Our largest representatives in the northern United States belong to the two genera *Belostoma* and *Banacus*, distinguished from each other by the fact that *Belostoma* has a groove on the under side of the femur of the front leg, for the reception of the tibia.

The salivary glands of Belostoma were figured by Leidy (1847) and later were studied in more detail by Locy (1884). There are two pairs of the glands, those of one pair being long and extending back as far as the beginning of the abdomen, while the others are about one-fourth as long. They lie on either side of the œsophagus. On each side of the œsophagus there is a slender tube with a sigmoid swelling which may serve as a poison reservoir. In addition to this salivary system, there is a pair of very prominent glands on the ventral side of the head, opening just above the base of the beak. These Locy has called the "cephalic glands" and he suggests that they are the source of the poison. They are the homologues of the maxillary glands described for other Hemiptera, and it is by no means clear that they are concerned with the production of venom. It seems more probable that in *Belostoma*, as in other Hemiptera, it is produced by the salivary glands, though the question is an open one.

The Belostomatidæ feed not only on insects, but on small frogs, fish, salamanders and the like. Matheson (1907) has recorded the killing of a good-sized bird by *Belostoma americana*. A woodpecker,

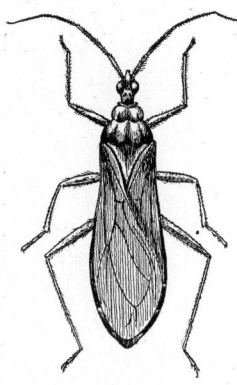

# Hemiptera, or True Bugs

or flicker, was heard to utter cries of distress, and fluttered and fell from a tree. On examination it was found that a bug of this species had inserted its beak into the back part of the skull and was apparently busily engaged in sucking the blood or brains of the bird. Various species of *Belostoma* have been cited as causing painful bites in man. We can testify from personal experience that the bite of *Belostoma americana* may almost immediately cause severe, shooting pains that may extend throughout the arm and that they may be felt for several days.

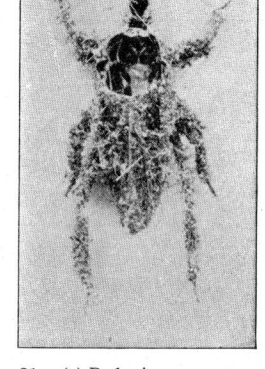

20. Reduvius (Opsicœtus) personatus. (x2).

Relief from the pain may be obtained by the use of dilute ammonia, or a menthol ointment. In the not uncommon case of secondary infection the usual treatment for that should be adopted.

The **Reduviidæ,** or *assassin-bugs* are capable of inflicting very painful wounds, as most collectors of Hemiptera know to their sorrow. Some species are frequently to be found in houses and outhouses and Dr. Howard suggests that many of the stories of painful spider bites relate to the attack of these forms.

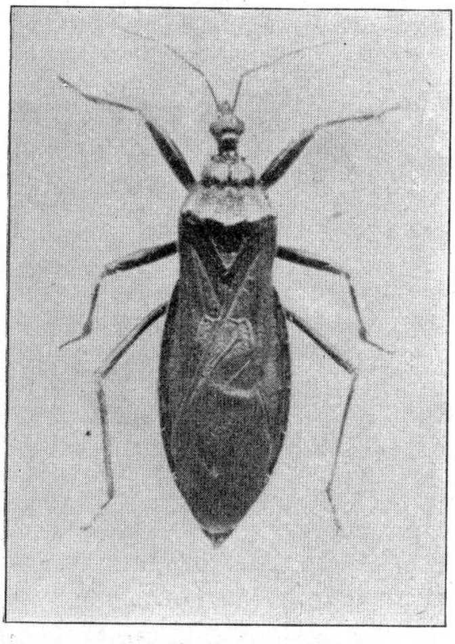

21. (*a*) Reduvius personatus, nymph. Photograph by M. V. S.

An interesting psychological study was afforded in the summer of 1899, by the "kissing-bug" scare which swept over the country. It was reported in the daily papers that a new and deadly bug had made its appearance, which had the unpleasant habit of choosing the lips or cheeks

21. (*b*) Reduvius personatus, adult (x2) Photograph by M. V. S.

for its point of attack on man. So widespread were the stories regarding this supposedly new insect that station entomologists all over the country began to receive suspected specimens for identification. At Cornell there were received, among others, specimens of stone-flies, may-flies and even small moths, with inquiries as to whether they were "kissing-bugs."

Dr. L. O. Howard has shown that the scare had its origin in newspaper reports of some instances of bites by either *Melanolestes picipes* (fig. 19a) or *Opsicoetes personatus* (fig. 20), in the vicinity of Washington, D. C. He then discusses in considerable detail the more prominent of the Reduviidæ which, with greater or less frequency pierce the skin of human beings. These are *Opsicoetes personatus*, *Melanolestes picipes*, *Coriscus subcoleoptratus* (fig. 19g), *Rasahus thoracicus*, *Rasahus biguttatus* (fig. 22), *Conorhinus sanguisugus* (fig. 71), and *C. abdominalis* (fig. 23).

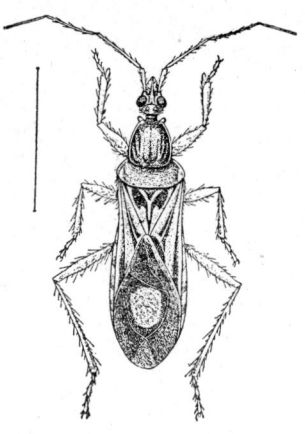

22. Rasahus biguttatus. (x2). After Howard

One of the most interesting of these species is *Reduvius personatus*, (=*Opsicœtus personatus*), which is popularly known as the "masked bed-bug hunter." It owes this name to the fact that the immature nymphs (fig. 21) have their bodies and legs completely covered by dust and lint, and that they are supposed to prey upon bedbugs. LeConte is quoted by Howard as stating that "This species is remarkable for the intense pain caused by its bite. I do not know whether it ever willingly plunges its rostrum into any person, but when caught, or unskilfully handled it always stings. In this case the pain is almost equal to the bite of a snake, and the swelling and irritation which result from it will sometimes last for a week."

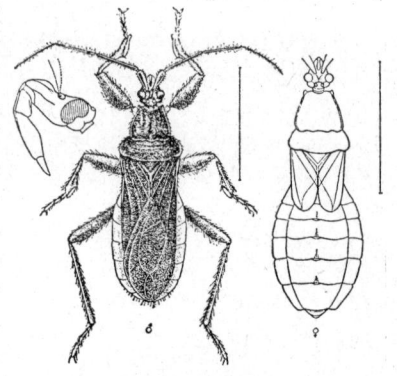

23. Conorhinus abdominalis (x2). After Marlatt.

A species which very commonly attacks man is *Conorhinus sanguisugus*, the so-called "big bed-bug" of the south and southern United States. It is frequently found in houses and is known to inflict an exceedingly painful bite. As in the case of a number of other predaceous Hemiptera, the salivary glands of these forms are highly developed. The effect of the bite on their prey and, as Marlatt has pointed out, the constant and uniform character of the symptoms in nearly all cases of bites in man, clearly indicate that their saliva contains a specific substance. No satisfactory studies of the secretions have been made. On the other hand, Dr. Howard is doubtless right in maintaining that the very serious results which sometimes follow the bite are due to the introduction of extraneous poison germs. This is borne out by the symptoms of most of the cases cited in literature and also by the fact that treatment with corrosive sublimate, locally applied to the wound, has yielded favorable results.

**Other Hemiptera Reported as Poisonous to Man**—A large number of other Hemiptera have been reported as attacking man. Of these, there are several species ot Lygæidæ, Coreidæ, and Capsidæ. Of the latter, *Lygus pratensis*, the tarnished plant-bug, is reported by Professor Crosby as sucking blood. *Orthotylus flavosparsus* is another Capsid which has been implicated. *Empoasca mali* and *Platymetopius acutus* of the Jassidæ have also been reported as having similar habits.

Whenever the periodical cicada or "seventeen-year locust" becomes abundant, the newspapers contain accounts of serious results from its bites. The senior author has made scores of attempts to induce this species to bite and only once successfully. At that time the bite was in no wise more severe than a pin-prick. A student in our department reports a similar experience. There is no case on record which bears evidence of being worthy of any credence, whatsoever.

Under the heading of poisonous Hemiptera we might consider the bed-bugs and the lice. These will be discussed later, as parasites and as carriers of disease, and therefore need only be mentioned here.

## DIPTERA

Several species of blood-sucking Diptera undoubtedly secrete a saliva possessing poisonous properties. Chief among these are the Culicidæ, or mosquitoes, and the Simuliidæ, or black-flies. As we shall consider these forms in detail under the heading of parasitic species and insects transmitting disease, we shall discuss here only the poison of the mosquitoes.

It is well known that mosquitoes, when they bite, inject into the wound a minute quantity of poison. The effect of this varies according to the species of mosquito and also depends very much on the susceptibility of the individual. Soon after the bite a sensation of itching is noticed and often a wheal, or eminence, is produced on the skin, which may increase to a considerable swelling. The scratching which is induced may cause a secondary infection and thus lead to serious results. Some people seem to acquire an immunity against the poison.

The purpose of this irritating fluid may be, as Reaumur suggested, to prevent the coagulation of the blood and thus not only to cause it to flow freely when the insect bites but to prevent its rapid coagulation in the stomach. Obviously, it is not developed as a protective fluid, and its presence subjects the group to the additional handicap of the vengeance of man.

As to the origin of the poison, there has been little question, until recent years, that it was a secretion from the salivary glands. Macloskie (1888) showed that each gland is subdivided into three lobes, the middle of which differs from the others in having evenly granulated contents and staining more deeply

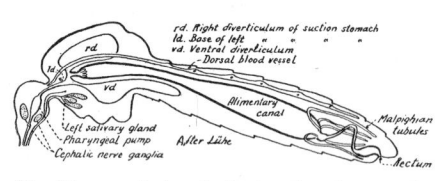

24. Diagram of a longitudinal section of a mosquito.

than the others (fig. 24). This middle lobe he regarded as the source of the poison. Bruck, (1911), by the use of water, glycerine, chloroform, and other fluids, extracted from the bodies of a large number of mosquitoes a toxine which he calls *culicin*. This he assumes comes from the salivary glands. Animal experimentation showed that this extract possessed hemolytic powers. Inoculated into the experimenter's own skin it produced lesions which behaved exactly as do those of mosquito bites.

Similarly, most writers on the subject have concurred with the view that the salivary glands are the source of the poison. However, recent work, especially that of Nuttall and Shipley (1903), and Schaudinn (1904), has shown that the evidence is by no means conclusive. Nuttall dissected out six sets (thirty-six acini) of glands from freshly killed *Culex pipiens* and placed them in a drop of salt solution.  The drop was allowed to dry, it being thought that the salt crystals would facilitate the grinding up of the glands with the end of a small glass rod, this being done under microscopic control. After grinding up, a small drop of water was added of the size of the original drop of saline, and an equal volume of human blood taken from the clean finger-tip was quickly mixed therewith, and the whole drawn up into a capillary tube.  Clotting was not prevented and no hemolysis occurred.  Salivary gland emulsion added to a dilute suspension of corpuscles did not lead to hemolysis.  This experiment was repeated a number of times, with slight modification, but with similar results.  The data obtained from the series "do not support the hypothesis that the salivary glands, at any rate in *Culex pipiens*, contain a substance which prevents coagulation."

Much more detailed, and the more important experiments made along this line, are those of Schaudinn (1904).  The results of these experiments were published in connection with a technical paper on the alternation of generations and of hosts in *Trypanosoma* and *Spirochæta*, and for this reason seem to have largely escaped the notice of entomologists.  They are so suggestive that we shall refer to them in some detail.

Schaudinn observed that the three œsophageal diverticula (commonly, but incorrectly, known as the "sucking stomach") (fig. 24) usually contain large bubbles of gas and in addition, he always found yeast cells.  On the ground of numerous observations, Schaudinn was convinced that these yeast plants are normal and constant commensals of the insect.  He regarded them as the cause of the gas bubbles to be found in diverticula.  It was found that as the insect fed, from time to time the abdomen underwent convulsive contractions which resulted in the emptying of the œsophageal diverticula and the salivary glands through blood pressure.

In order to test the supposed toxic action of the salivary glands, Schaudinn repeatedly introduced them under his skin and that of his assistant, in a drop of salt solution, and never obtained a suggestion of the irritation following a bite of the insect, even though the glands were carefully rubbed to fragments after their implantation. Like Nuttall, he failed to get satisfactory evidence that the secretion of the salivary glands retarded coagulation of the blood.

He then carefully removed the œsophageal diverticula with their content of yeast and introduced them into an opening in the skin of the hand.  Within a few seconds there was noticeable the characteristic itching irritation of the mosquito bite; and in a short time there appeared reddening and typical swelling. This was usually much more severe than after the usual mosquito bite, and the swelling persisted and itched longer. This was because by the ordinary bite of the mosquito most of the yeast cells are again sucked up, while in these experiments they remained in the wound. These experiments were repeated a number of times on himself, his assistant and others, and always with the same result. From them Schaudinn decided that the poisonous action of the mosquito bite is caused by an enzyme from a commensal fungus. These conclusions have not, as yet, been satisfactorily tested.

Relief from the effect of the mosquito bite may be obtained by bathing the swellings with weak ammonia or, according to Howard, by using moist soap. The latter is to be rubbed gently on the puncture and is said to speedily allay the irritation. Howard also quotes from the *Journal of Tropical Medicine and Hygiene* to the effect that a few drops of a solution of thirty to forty grains of iodine to an ounce of saponated petroleum rubbed into the mosquito bite, or wasp sting, allay the pain instantaneously.

Methods of mosquito control will be discussed later, in considering these insects as parasites and as carriers of disease.

## STINGING INSECTS

The stinging insects all belong to the order **Hymenoptera**. In a number of families of this group the ovipositor is modified to form a sting and is connected with poison-secreting glands. We shall consider the apparatus of the honey-bee and then make briefer reference to that of other forms.

**Apis mellifica, the honey bee**—The sting of the worker honey-bee is situated within a so-called sting chamber at the end of the abdomen. This chamber is produced by the infolding of the greatly reduced and modified eighth, ninth and tenth abdominal segments into the seventh.* From it the dart-like sting can be quickly exserted.

The sting (fig. 25) is made up of a central shaft, ventro-laterad of which are the paired *lancets*, or darts, which are provided with sharp, recurved teeth. Still further laterad lie the paired whitish, finger-

---

*It should be remembered that in all the higher Hymenoptera the first abdominal segment is fused with the thorax and that what is apparently the sixth segment is, in reality, the seventh.

like *sting palpi*. Comparative morphological as well as embryological studies have clearly established that these three parts correspond to the three pairs of gonopophyses of the ovipositor of more generalized insects.
An examination of the internal structures (fig. 26) reveals two distinct types of poison glands, the acid-secreting and the alkaline-secreting glands, and a prominent poison reservoir. In addition, there is a small pair of accessory structures which have been called lubricating glands, on account of the supposed function of their product. The acid-secreting gland empties into the distal end of the poison reservoir which in turn pours the secretion into the muscular bulb-like enlargement at the base of the shaft. The alkaline secreting gland empties into the bulb ventrad of the narrow neck of the reservoir.

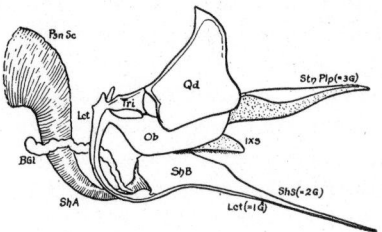

25. Sting of a honey bee. *Psn Sc*, base of acid poison gland; *B Gl*, alkaline poison gland; *Stn Plp*, sting palpi; *Sh B*, bulb of sting; *Sh A*, basal arm; *Lct*, lancets or darts; *Sh s*, shaft of sting. Modified from Snodgrass.

The poison is usually referred to as formic acid. That it is not so easily explained has been repeatedly shown and is evidenced by the presence of the two types of glands. Carlet maintains that the product of either gland is in itself innocent, —it is only when they are combined that the toxic properties appear.

The most detailed study of the poison of the honey-bee is that of Josef Langer (1897), who in the course of his work used some 25,000 bees. Various methods of obtaining the active poison for experimental purposes were used. For obtaining the pure secretion, bees were held in the fingers and compressed until the sting was exserted, when a clear drop of the poison was visible at its tip. This was then taken up in a capillary tube or dilute solutions obtained by dipping the tip of the sting into a definite amount of distilled water.

26. Poison apparatus of a honey bee. Modified from Snodgrass.

An aqueous solution of the poison was more readily obtained by pulling out the sting and poison sacs by means of forceps, and grinding them up in water. The somewhat clouded fluid was then filtered one or more times. For obtaining still greater quantities, advantage was taken of the fact that while alcohol coagulates the poison, the active principle remains soluble in water. Hence the stings with the annexed glands where collected in 96 per cent alcohol, after filtering off of the alcohol were dried at 40° C., then rubbed to a fine powder and this was repeatedly extracted with water. Through filtering of this aqueous extract there was obtained a yellowish-brown fluid which produced the typical reactions, according to concentration of the poison.

The freshly expelled drop of poison is limpid, of distinct acid reaction, tastes bitter and has a delicate aromatic odor. On evaporation, it leaves a sticky residue, which at 100 degrees becomes fissured, and suggests dried gum arabic. The poison is readily soluble in water and possesses a specific gravity of 1.1313. On drying at room temperature, it leaves a residue of 30 per cent, which has not lost in poisonous action or in solubility. In spite of extended experiments, Langer was unable to determine the nature of the active principle. He showed that it was not, as had been supposed, an albuminous body, but rather an organic base.

The pure poison, or the two per cent aqueous solution, placed on the uninjured skin showed absolutely no irritating effect, though it produced a marked reaction on the mucus membrane of the nose or eye. A single drop of one-tenth per cent aqueous solution of the poison brought about a typical irritation in the conjunctiva of the rabbit's eye. On the other hand, the application of a drop of the poison, or its solution, to the slightest break in the skin, or by means of a needle piercing the skin, produced typical effects. There is produced a local necrosis, in the neighborhood of which there is infiltration of lymphocytes, œdema, and hyperæmia.

The effect of the sting on man (fig. 27) is usually transitory but there are some individuals who are made sick for hours, by a single sting. Much depends, too, on the place struck. It is a common experience that an angry bee will attempt to reach the eye of its victim and a sting on the lid may result in severe and prolonged swelling. In the case of a man stung on the cheek, Legiehn observed complete aphonia and a breaking out of red blotches all over the body. A sting on the tongue has been known to cause such collateral œdema as to endanger life through suffocation. Cases of death of man from the attacks of bees are rare but are not unknown. Such results are usually from a number of stings but, rarely, death has been known to follow a single sting, entering a blood vessel of a particularly susceptible individual.

It is clearly established that partial immunity from the effects of the poison may be acquired. By repeated injections of the venom, mice have been rendered capable of bearing doses that certainly would have killed them at first. It is a well-known fact that most bee-keepers become gradually hardened to the stings, so that the irritation and the swelling become less and less. Some individuals

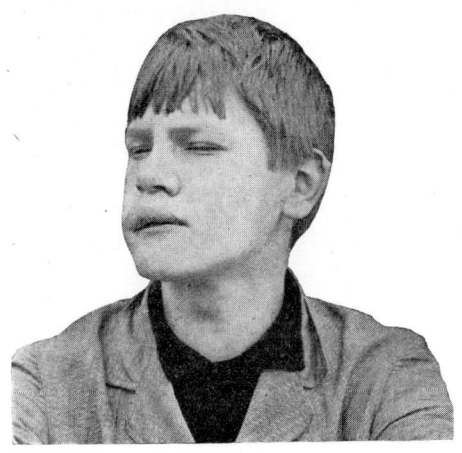

Effect of bee stings. After Root.

have found this immunity a temporary one, to be reacquired each season. A striking case of acquired immunity is related by the Roots in their "A B C and X Y Z of Bee Culture." The evidence in the case is so clear that it should be made more widely available and hence we quote it here.

A young man who was determined to become a bee-keeper, was so susceptible to the poison that he was most seriously affected by a single sting, his body breaking out with red blotches, breathing growing difficult, and his heart action being painfully accelerated. "We finally suggested taking a live bee and pressing it on the back of his hand until it merely pierced his skin with the sting, then immediately brushing off both bee and sting. This was done and since no serious effect followed, it was repeated inside of four or five days. This was continued for some three or four weeks, when the patient began to have a sort of itching sensation all over his body. The hypodermic injections of bee-sting poison were then discontinued. At the end of a month they were repeated at intervals of four or five days. Again, after two or three weeks the itching sensation came on, but it was less pronounced. The patient was given a rest of about a month, when the doses were repeated as before." By this course of treatment the young man became so thoroughly immunized that neither unpleasant results nor swelling followed the attacks of the insects and he is able to handle bees with the same freedom that any experienced bee-keeper does.

In an interesting article in the *Entomological News* for November, 1914, J. H. Lovell calls attention to the fact that "There has been a widespread belief among apiarists that a beekeeper will receive more stings when dressed in black than when wearing white clothing. A large amount of evidence has been published in the various bee journals showing beyond question that honey-bees under certain conditions discriminate against black. A few instances may be cited in illustration. Of a flock of twelve chickens running in a bee-yard seven black ones were stung to death, while five light colored ones escaped uninjured. A white dog ran among the bee-hives without attracting much attention, while at the same time a black dog was furiously assailed by the bees. Mr. J. D. Byer, a prominent Canadian beekeeper, relates that a black and white cow, tethered about forty feet from an apiary, was one afternoon attacked and badly stung by bees. On examination it was found that the black spots had five or six stings to one on the white. All noticed this fact, although no one was able to offer any explanation. A white horse is in much less danger of being stung, when driven near an apiary, than a black one. It has, indeed, been observed repeatedly that domestic animals of all kinds, if wholly or partially black, are much more liable to be attacked by bees, if they wander among the hives, than those which are entirely white.

In order to test the matter experimentally, the following series of experiments was performed. In the language of the investigator:

"On a clear, warm day in August I dressed wholly in white with the exception of a black veil. Midway on the sleeve of my right arm there was sewed a band of black cloth ten inches wide. I then entered the bee-yard and, removing the cover from one of the hives, lifted a piece of comb with both hands and gently shook it. Instantly many of the bees flew to the black band, which they continued to attack as long as they were disturbed. Not a single bee attempted to sting the left sleeve, which was of course entirely white, and very few even alighted upon it."

"This experiment was repeated a second, third and fourth time; in each instance with similar results. I estimated the number of bees on the band of black cloth at various moments was from thirty to forty; it was evident from their behavior that they were extremely irritable. To the left white sleeve and other portions of my clothing they paid very little attention; but the black veil was very frequently attacked."

"A few days later the experiments were repeated, but the band of black cloth, ten inches wide, was sewed around my left arm instead of around the right arm as before. When the bees were disturbed, after the hive cover had been removed, they fiercely attacked the band of black cloth as in the previous experiences; but the right white sleeve and the white suit were scarcely noticed. At one time a part of the black cloth was almost literally covered with furiously stinging bees, and the black veil was assailed by hundreds. The bees behaved in a similar manner when a second hive on the opposite side of the apiary was opened."

"A white veil which had been procured for this purpose, was next substituted for the black veil. The result was most surprising, for, whereas in the previous experiments hundreds of bees had attacked the black veil, so few flew against the white veil as to cause me no inconvenience. Undoubtedly beekeepers will find it greatly to their advantage to wear white clothing when working among their colonies of bees and manipulating the frames of the hives."

When a honey-bee stings, the tip of the abdomen, with the entire sting apparatus, is torn off and remains in the wound. Here the muscles continue to contract, for some minutes, forcing the barbs deeper and deeper into the skin, and forcing out additional poison from the reservoir.

Treatment, therefore, first consists in removing the sting without squeezing out additional poison. This is accomplished by lifting and scraping it out with a knife-blade or the fingernail instead of grasping and pulling it out. Local application of alkalines, such as weak ammonia, are often recommended on the assumption that the poison is an acid to be neutralized on this manner, but these are of little or no avail. They should certainly not be rubbed in, as that would only accelerate the absorption of the poison. The use of cloths wrung out in hot water and applied as hot as can be borne, affords much relief in the case of severe stings. The application of wet clay, or of the end of a freshly cut potato is sometimes helpful.

In extreme cases, where there is great susceptibility, or where there may have been many stings, a physician should be called. He may find strychnine injections or other treatment necessary, if general symptoms develop.

**Other Stinging Forms**—Of the five thousand, or more, species of bees, most possess a sting and poison apparatus and some of the larger forms are capable of inflicting a much more painful sting than

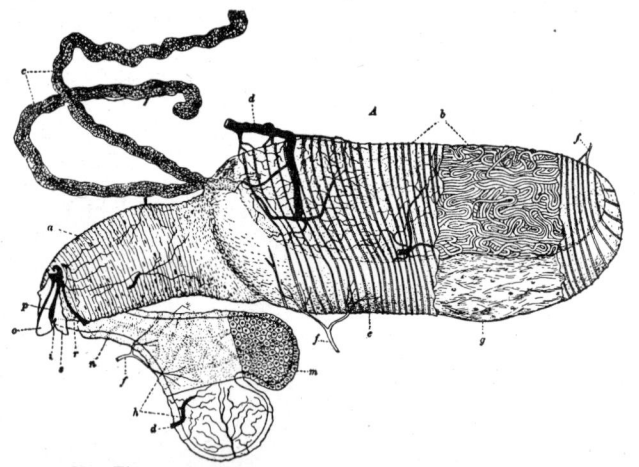

28. The poison apparatus of Formica. Wheeler, after Forel.

that of the common honey-bee. In fact, some, like the bumble bees, possess the advantage that they do not lose the sting from once using it, but are capable of driving it in repeatedly. In the tropics there are found many species of stingless bees but these are noted for their united efforts to drive away intruders by biting. Certain species possess a very irritating saliva which they inject into the wounds.

The ants are not ordinarily regarded as worthy of consideration under the heading of "stinging insects" but as a matter of fact, most of them possess well developed stings and some of them, especially in the tropics, are very justly feared. Even those which lack the sting possess well-developed poison glands and the parts of the entire stinging apparatus, in so far as it is developed in the various species, may readily be homologized with those of the honey-bee.

The ants lacking a sting are those of the subfamily **Camponotinæ**, which includes the largest of our local species. It is an interesting fact that some of these species possess the largest poison glands and reservoir (fig. 28) and it is found that when they attack an enemy they bring the tip of the abdomen forward and spray the poison in such a way that it is introduced into the wound made by the powerful mandibles.

More feared than any of the other Hymenoptera are the hornets and wasps. Of these there are many species, some of which attain

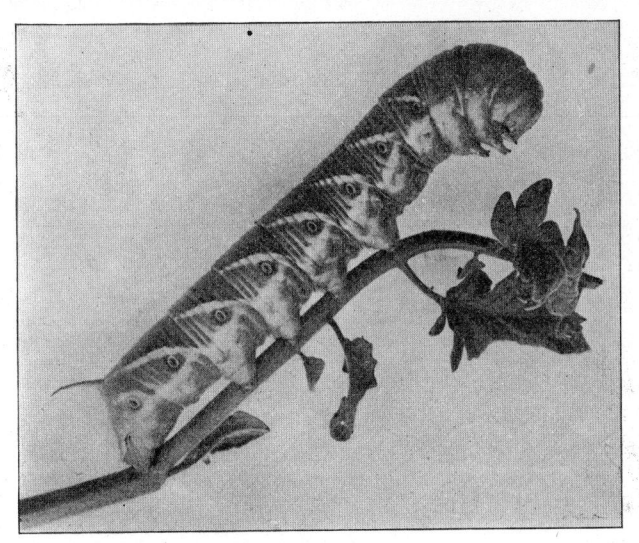

29. A harmless, but much feared larva, the "tomato worm." Natural size. Photograph by M. V. S.

a large size and are truly formidable. Phisalix (1897), has made a study of the venom of the common hornet and finds that, like the poison of the honey-bee, it is neither an albuminoid nor an alkaloid. Its toxic properties are destroyed at 120° C. Phisalix also says that the venom is soluble in alcohol. If this be true, it differs in this respect from that of the bee. An interesting phase of the work of Phisalix is that several of her experiments go to show that the venom of hornets acts as a vaccine against that of vipers.

### NETTLING INSECTS

So far, we have considered insects which possess poison glands connected with the mouth-parts or a special sting and which actively inject their poison into man. There remain to be considered those insects which possess poisonous hairs or body fluids which, under favorable circumstances, may act as poisons. To the first of these belong primarily the larvæ of certain Lepidoptera.

## LEPIDOPTERA

When we consider the reputedly poisonous larvæ of moths and butterflies, one of the first things to impress us is that we cannot

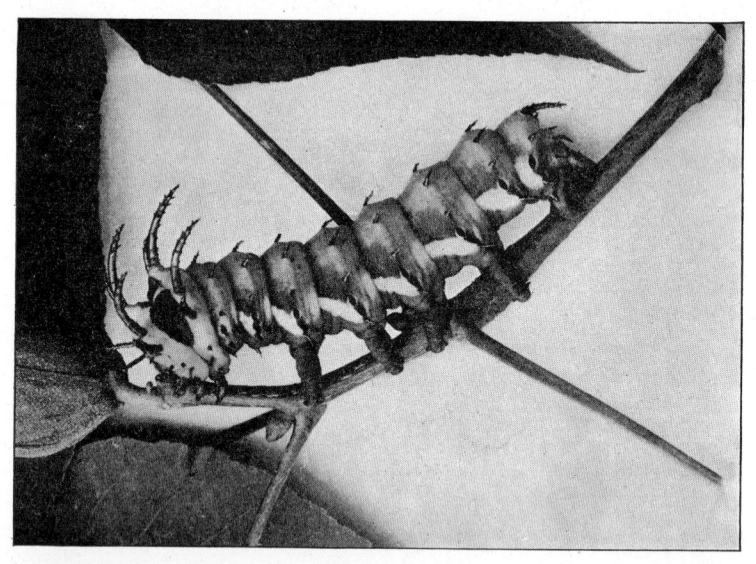

30. Another innocent but much maligned caterpillar, the larva of the Regal moth. Photograph by M. V. S.

judge by mere appearance. Various species of Sphingid, or hawk-moth larvæ, bear at the end of the body a chitinous horn, which is often referred to as a "sting" and regarded as capable of inflicting dangerous wounds. It would seem unnecessary to refer to this absurd belief if it were not that each summer the newspapers contain supposed accounts of injury from the "tomato worm" (fig. 29) and others of this group. The grotesque, spiny larva (fig. 30) of one of our largest moths, *Citheronia regalis* is much feared though perfectly harmless, and similar instances could be multiplied.

But if the larvæ are often misjudged on account of their ferocious appearance, the reverse may be true. A group of most innocent looking and attractive caterpillars is that of the flannel-moth larvæ,

## Nettling Insects

of which *Lagoa crispata* may be taken as an example. Its larva (fig. 31) has a very short and thick body, which is fleshy and com-

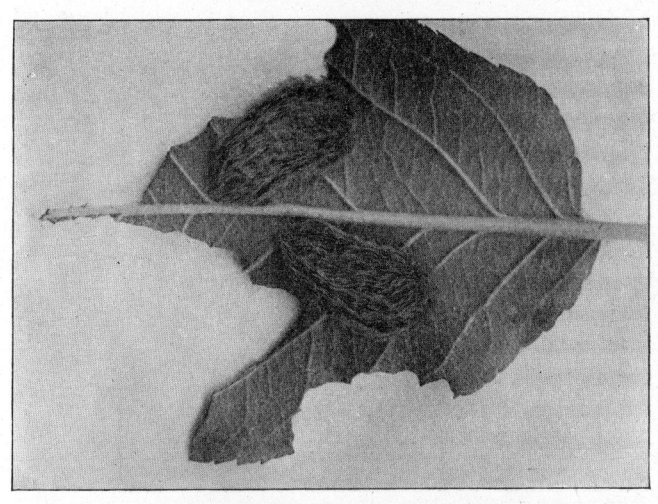

31. The flannel moth (Lagoa crispata). (*a*) Poisonous larva.

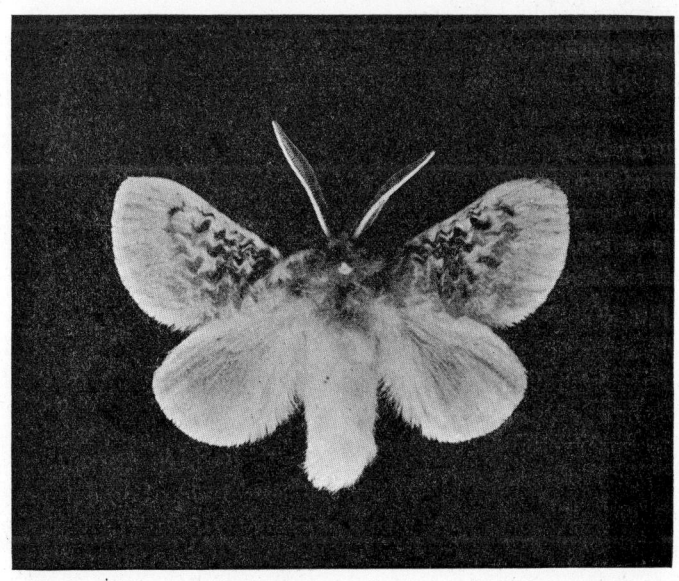

31. (*b*) Adult. Enlarged. Photographs by M. V. S.

pletely covered and hidden by long silken hairs of a tawny or brown color, giving a convex form to the upper side. Interspersed among

46      *Poisonous Arthropods*

these long hairs are numerous short spines connected with underlying hypodermal poison glands. These hairs are capable of producing a marked nettling effect when they come in contact with the skin. This species is found in our Atlantic and Southern States. Satisfactory studies of its poisonous hairs and their glands have not yet been made.

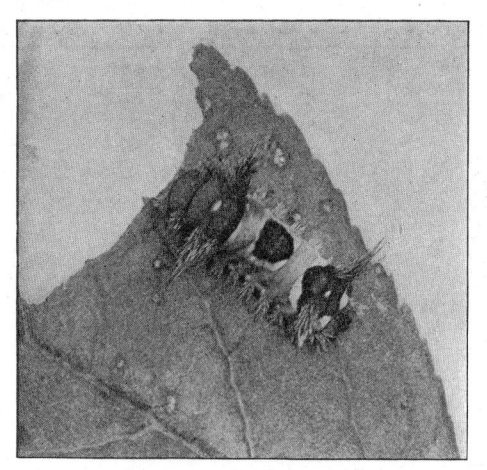

32  The poisonous saddle back caterpillar. Empretia (Sibine) stimulea. Photograph by M. V. S.

*Sibine stimulea* (*Empretia stimulea*), or the saddle-back caterpillar (fig. 32), is another which possesses nettling hairs. This species belongs to the group of Eucleidæ, or slug caterpillars. It can be readily recognized by its flattened form, lateral, bristling spines and by the large green patch on the back resembling a saddle-cloth, while the saddle is represented by an oval, purplish-brown spot. The small spines are venomous and affect some persons very painfully. The larva feeds on the leaves of a large variety of forest trees and also on cherry, plum, and

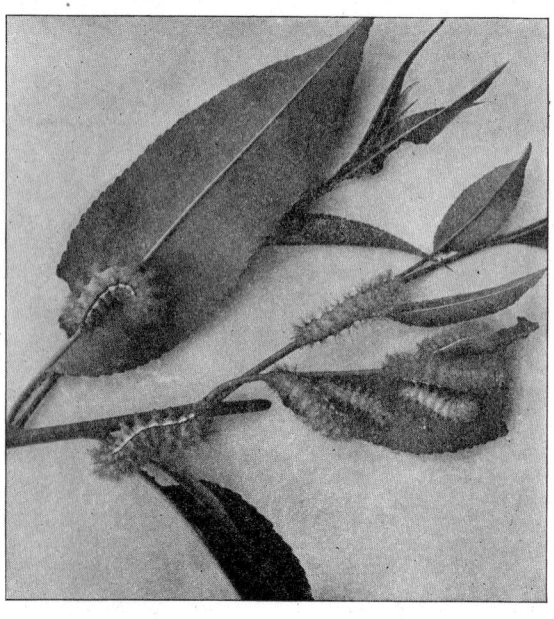

33a.  Io moth larvæ on willow. Photograph by M.V. S.

## Nettling Insects

even corn leaves. It is to be found throughout the Eastern and Southern United States.

*Automeris io* is the best known of the nettling caterpillars. It is the larva of the Io moth, one of the Saturniidæ. The mature cater-

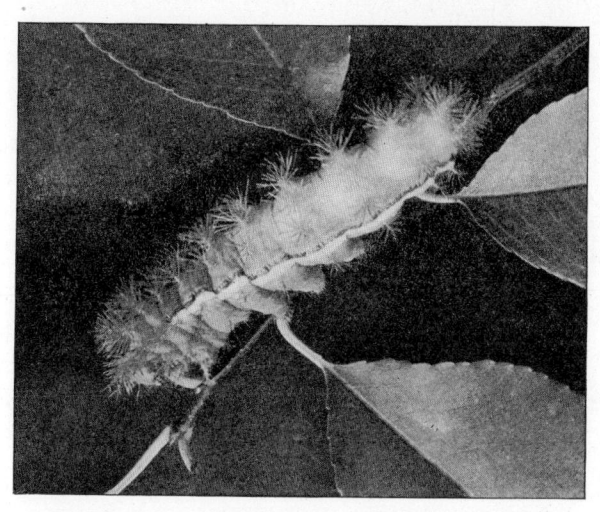

33b. Io moth. Full grown larva. Photograph by M. V. S.

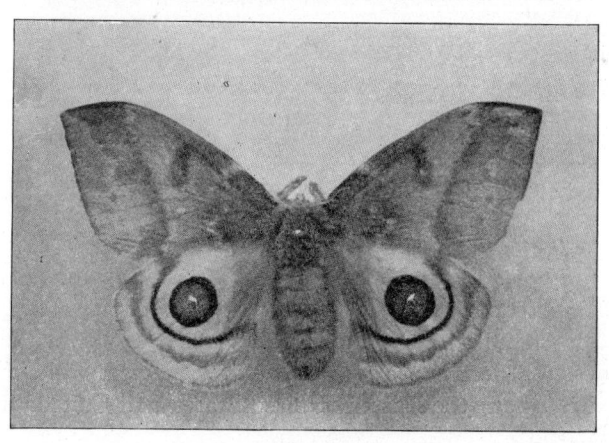

33c. Io moth. Adult. Photograph by M. V. S.

pillar, (fig. 33), which reaches a length of two and one-half inches, is of a beautiful pale green with sublateral stripes of cream and red color and a few black spines among the green ones. The green radiating spines give the body a mossy appearance. They are tipped with a slender chitinous hair whose tip is readily broken off in the skin and whose poisonous content causes great irritation. Some individuals are very susceptible to the poison, while others are able to handle the larvæ freely without any discomfort. The larvæ feed on a wide range of food plants. They are most commonly encountered on corn and on willow, because of the opportunities for coming in contact with them.

The larvæ of the brown-tail moth (*Euproctis chrysorrhœa,*) (fig. 35 and 36), where they occur in this country, are, on account of their great numbers, the most serious of all poisonous caterpillars. It is

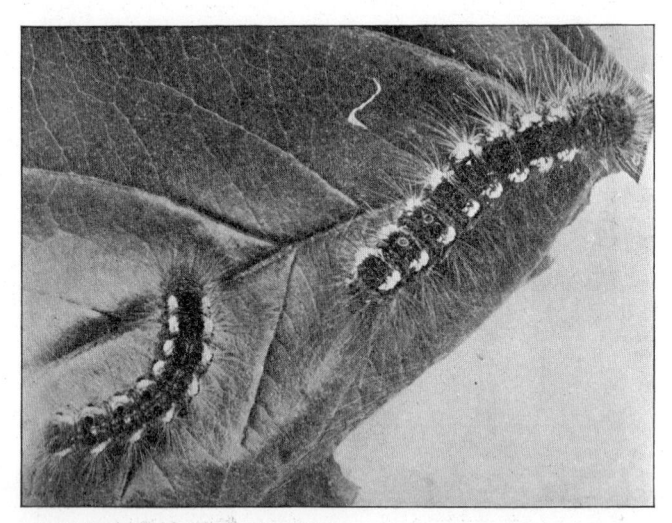

35. Larva of brown-tail moth. (Natural size). Photograph by M. V. S.

not necessary here, to go into details regarding the introduction of this species from Europe into the New England States. This is all available in the literature from the United States Bureau of Entomology and from that of the various states which are fighting the species. Suffice to say, there is every prospect that the pest will continue to spread throughout the Eastern United States and Canada and that wherever it goes it will prove a direct pest to man as well as to his plants.

Very soon after the introduction of the species there occurred in the region where it had gained a foothold, a mysterious dermatitis of man. The breaking out which usually occurred on the neck or other exposed part of the body was always accompanied by an intense itching. It was soon found that this dermatitis was caused by certain short, barbed hairs of the brown-tail caterpillars and that not only the caterpillars but their cocoons and even the adult female moths might harbor these nettling hairs and thus give rise to the irritation. In many cases the hairs were wafted to clothing on the line and when this was worn it might cause the same trouble. Still worse, it was found that very serious internal injury was often caused by breathing or swallowing the poisonous hairs.

The earlier studies seemed to indicate that the irritation was purely mechanical in origin, the result of the minute barbed hairs

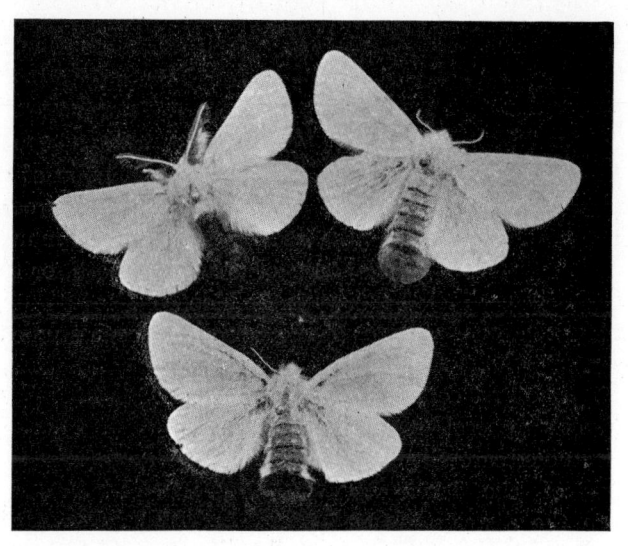

36. Browntail moths. One male and two females. Photograph by M. V. S.

working into the skin in large numbers. Subsequently, however, Dr. Tyzzer (1907) demonstrated beyond question that the trouble was due to a poison contained in the hairs. In the first place, it is only the peculiar short barbed hairs which will produce the dermatitis when rubbed on the skin, although most of the other hairs are sharply barbed. Moreover, it was found that in various ways the nettling properties could be destroyed without modifying the structure of the hairs. This was accomplished by baking for one hour at 110° C, by warming to 60° C in distilled water, or by soaking in one per cent. or in one-tenth per cent. of potassium hydrate or sodium hydrate. The most significant part of his work was the demonstration of the fact that if the nettling hairs are mingled with blood, they immediately produce a change in the red corpuscles. These at once become coarsely crenated, and the roleaux are broken up in the vicinity of the hair (fig. 37*b*). The corpuscles decrease in size, the coarse crenations are transformed into slender spines which rapidly disappear, leaving the corpuscles in the form of spheres, the light refraction of which contrasts them sharply with the normal corpuscles. The reaction always begins at the basal sharp point of the hair. It could not be produced by purely mechanical means, such as the mingling of minute particles of glass wool, the barbed hairs of a tussock moth, or the other coarser hairs of the brown-tail, with the blood.

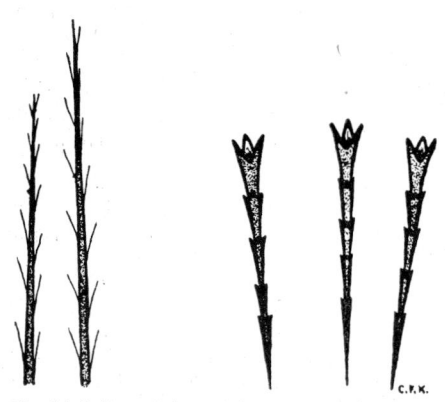

37. (*a*) Ordinary hairs and three poison hairs of subdorsal and lateral tubercles of the larva of the browntail moth. Drawing by Miss Kephart.

The question of the source of the poison has been studied in our laboratory by Miss Cornelia Kephart. She first confirmed Dr. Tyzzer's general results and then studied carefully fixed specimens of the larvæ to determine the distribution of the hairs and their relation to the underlying tissues.

The poison hairs (fig. 37), are found on the subdorsal and lateral tubercles (fig. 38), in bunches of from three to twelve on the minute papillæ with which the tubercles are thickly covered. The underlying hypodermis is very greatly thickened, the cells being three or four times the length of the ordinary hypodermal cells and being closely crowded together. Instead of a pore canal

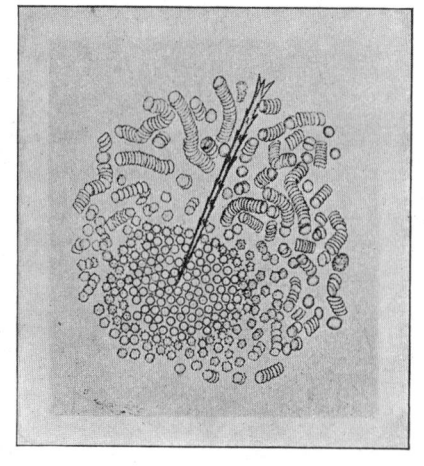

37. (*b*) Effect of the poison on the blood corpuscles of man. After Tyzzer.

through the cuticula for each individual hair, there is a single pore for each papillæ on a tubercle, all the hairs of the papilla being connected with the underlying cells through the same pore canal, (figs. 39 and 40).

The hypodermis of this region is of two distinct types of cells. First, there is a group of slender fusiform cells, one for each poison hair on the papilla, which are the trichogen, or hair-formative cells. They are crowded to one side and towards the basement membrane by a series of much larger, and more prominent cells (fig. 40), of which there is a single one for each papilla. These larger cells have a granular protoplasm with large nuclei and are obviously actively secreting. They are so characteristic in appearance as to leave no question but that they are the true poison glands.

Poisonous larvæ of many other species have been reported from Europe and especially from the tropics but the above-mentioned species are the more important of those occurring in the United States and will serve as types. It should be noted in this connection that

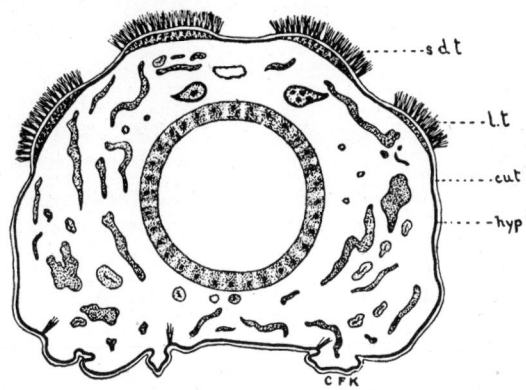

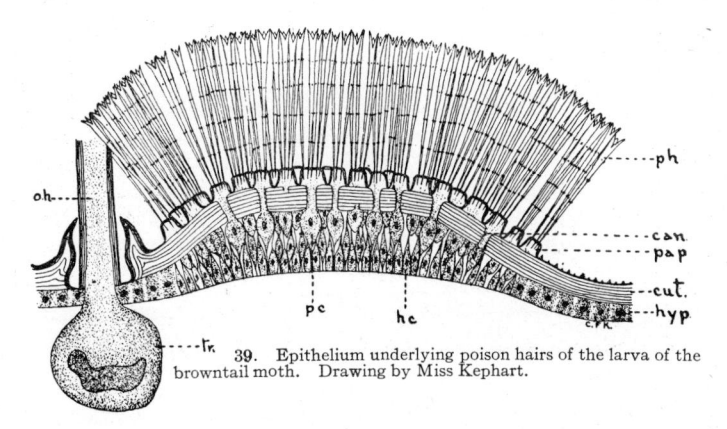

38. Cross section of the larva of the browntail moth showing the tubercles bearing the poison hairs. Drawing by Miss Kephart.

39. Epithelium underlying poison hairs of the larva of the browntail moth. Drawing by Miss Kephart.

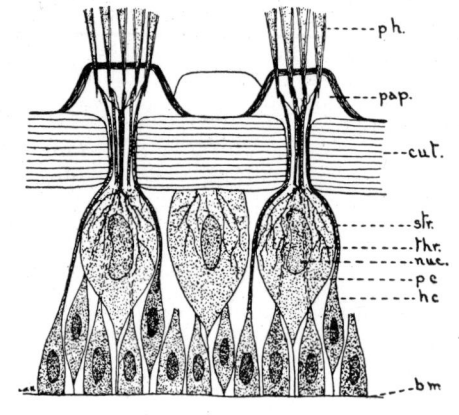

40. Same as figure 39, on larger scale.

through some curious misunderstanding Gœldi (1913) has featured the larva of *Orgyia leucostigma*, the white-marked tussock moth, as the most important of the poisonous caterpillars of this country. Though there are occasional reports of irritation from its hairs such cases are rare and there is no evidence that there is any poison present. Indeed, subcutaneous implantation of the hairs leads to no poisoning, but merely to temporary irritation.

Occasionally, the hairs of certain species of caterpillars find lodgement in the conjunctiva, cornea, or iris of the eye of man and give rise to the condition known as *opthalmia nodosa*. The essential feature of this trouble is a nodular conjunctivitis which simulates tuberculosis of the conjunctiva and hence has been called *pseudotubercular*. It may be distinguished microscopically by the presence of the hairs.

Numerous cases of opthalmia nodosa are on record. Of those from this country, one of the most interesting is reported by de Schweinitz and Shumway (1904). It is that of a child of fifteen years whose eye had become inflamed owing to the presence of some foreign body. Downward and inward on the bulbar conjunctiva were a number of flattened, grayish-yellow nodules, between which was a marked congestion of the conjunctival and

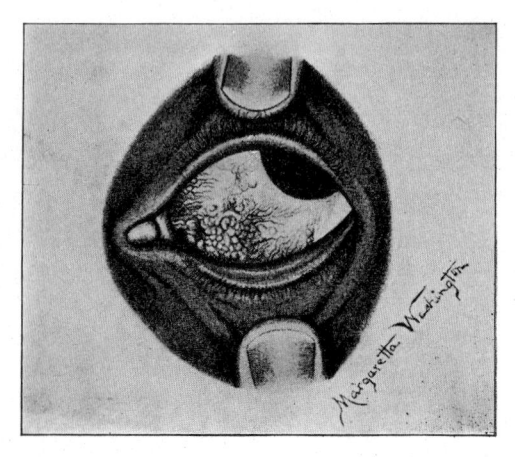

41. (*a*) Nodular conjunctivitis in the eye of a child. DeSchweinitz and Shumway.

episcleral vessels (fig. 41a). Twenty-seven nodules could be differentiated, those directly in the center of the collection being somewhat confluent and assuming a crescentic and circular appearance. The nodules were excised and, on sectioning, were found to be composed of a layer of spindle cells and round cells, outside of which the tissue was condensed into a capsule. The interior consisted of epithelioid cells, between which was a considerable intercellular substance. Directly in the center of a certain number of nodules was found the section of a hair (fig. 41b). The evidence indicated that the injury had resulted from playing with caterpillars of one of the Arctiid moths, *Spilosoma virginica*. Other reported cases have been caused by the hairs of larvæ of *Lasiocampa rubi*, *L. pini*, *Porthetria dispar*, *Psilura monacha* and *Cnethocampa processionea*.

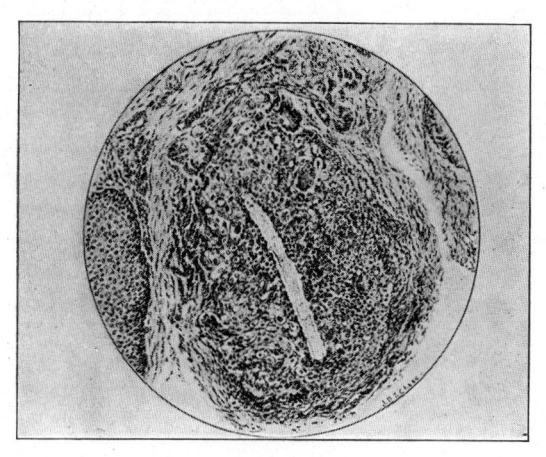

41b.  Section through one of the nodules showing the caterpillar hair.  DeSchweinitz and Shumway.

**Relief from Poisoning by Nettling Larvæ**—The irritation from nettling larvæ is often severe and, especially in regions where the brown-tail abounds, inquiries as to treatment arise. In general, it may be said that cooling lotions afford relief, and that scratching, with the possibilities of secondary infection, should be avoided, in so far as possible.

Among the remedies usually at hand, weak solutions of ammonia, or a paste of ordinary baking soda are helpful. Castellani and Chalmers recommend cleaning away the hairs by bathing the region with an alkaline lotion, such as two per cent solution of bicarbonate of soda, and then applying an ointment of ichthyol (10%).

## 54 Poisonous Arthropods

In the brown-tail district, there are many proprietary remedies of which the best ones are essentially the following, as recommended by Kirkland (1907):

| | |
|---|---|
| Carbolic acid | ½ drachm. |
| Zinc oxide | ½ oz. |
| Lime water | 8 oz. |

Shake thoroughly and rub well into the affected parts.

In some cases, and especially where there is danger of secondary infection, the use of a weak solution of creoline (one teaspoonful to a quart of water), is to be advised.

### VESICATING INSECTS AND THOSE POSSESSING OTHER POISONS IN THEIR BLOOD PLASMA

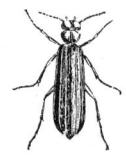

We have seen that certain forms, for example, the poisonous spiders, not only secrete a toxine in their poison glands, but that such a substance may be extracted from other parts of their body, or even their eggs. There are many insects which likewise possess a poisonous blood plasma. Such forms have been well designated by Taschenberg as *cryptotoxic* (χρυπτος = hidden). We shall consider a few representative forms.

42a. Blister beetle.

**The Blister Beetles**—Foremost among the cryptotoxic insects are the *Meloidæ* or "blister beetles," to which the well-known "Spanish fly" (fig. 42a), formerly very generally used in medical practice, belongs. The vesicating property is due to the presence in the blood plasma of a peculiar, volatile, crystalline substance known as *cantharidin*, which is especially abundant in the reproductive organs of the beetle. According to Kobert, the amount of this varies in different species from .4 or .5% to 2.57% of the dry weight of the beetle.

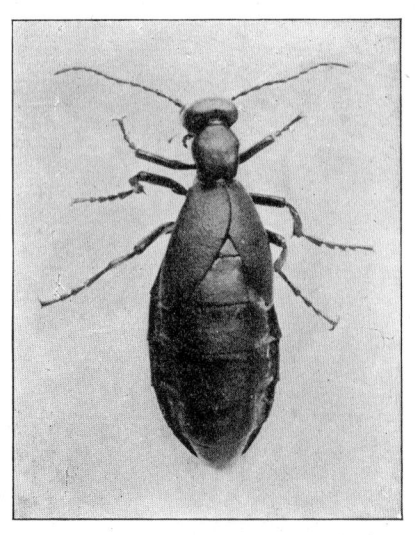

42b. An American blister beetle. Meloe angusticollis. Photograph by M. V. S.

While blister beetles have been especially used for external application, they are also at times used internally as a stimulant and a diuretic. The powder or extract was formerly much in vogue as an aphrodisiac, and formed the essential constituent of various philters, or "love powders". It is now known that its effects on the reproductive organs appear primarily after the kidneys have been affected to such an extent as to endanger life, and that many cases of fatal poison have been due to its ignorant use.

There are many cases on record of poisoning and death due to internal use, and in some instances from merely external application. There are not rarely cases of poisoning of cattle from feeding on herbage bearing a large number of the beetles and authentic cases are known of human beings who have been poisoned by eating the flesh of such cattle. Kobert states that the beetles are not poisonous to birds but that the flesh of birds which have fed on them is poisonous to man, and that if the flesh of chickens or frogs which have fed on the cantharidin be fed to cats it causes in them the same symptoms as does the cantharidin.

Treatment of cases of cantharidin poison is a matter for a skilled physician. Until he can be obtained, emetics should be administered and these should be followed by white of egg in water. Oils should be avoided, as they hasten the absorption of the poison.

**Other Cryptotoxic Insects**—Though the blister beetles are the best known of the insects with poisonous blood plasma, various others have been reported and we shall refer to a few of the best authenticated.

One of the most famous is the Chrysomelid beetle, *Diamphidia simplex*, the body fluids of whose larvæ are used by certain South African bushmen as an arrow poison. Its action is due to the presence of a toxalbumin which exerts a hæmolytic action on the blood, and produces inflammation of the subcutaneous connective tissue and mucous membranes. Death results from general paralysis. Krause (1907) has surmised that the active principle may be a bacterial toxine arising from decomposition of the tissues of the larva, but he presents no support of this view and it is opposed by all the available evidence.

In China, a bug, *Heuchis sanguinea*, belonging to the family Cicadidæ, is used like the Meloidæ, to produce blistering, and often causes poisoning. It has been assumed that its vescicating properties are due to cantharidin, but the presence of this substance has not been demonstrated.

Certain Aphididæ contain a strongly irritating substance which produces, not merely on mucous membranes but on outer skin, a characteristic inflammation.

It has been frequently reported that the larvæ of the Eurpoean cabbage butterfly, *Pieris brassicæ*, accidentally eaten by cows, horses, ducks, and other domestic animals, cause severe colic, attempts to vomit, paralysis of the hind legs, salivation, and stomatitis. On *postmortem* there are to be found hæmorrhagic gastro-enteritis, splenitis, and nephritis. Kobert has recently investigated the subject and has found a poisonous substance in the blood of not only the larvæ but also the pupæ.

# CHAPTER III

## PARASITIC ARTHROPODA AFFECTING MAN

The relation of insects to man as simple parasites has long been studied, and until very recent years the bulk of the literature of medical entomology referred to this phase of the subject. This is now completely overshadowed by the fact that so many of these parasitic forms are more than simple parasites, they are transmitters of other microscopic parasites which are pathogenic to man. Yet the importance of insects as parasites still remains and must be considered in a discussion of the relation of insects to the health of man. In taking up the subject we shall first consider some general features of the phenomenon of animal parasitism.

Parasitism is an adaptation which has originated very often among living organisms and in widely separated groups. It would seem simple to define what is meant by a "parasite" but, in reality, the term is not easily limited. It is often stated that a parasite is "An organism which lives at the expense of another," but this definition is applicable to a predatory species or, in its broadest sense, to all organisms. For our purpose we may say with Braun: "A parasite is an organism which, for the purpose of obtaining food, takes up its abode, temporarily or permanently, on or within another living organism".

Thus, parasitism is a phase of the broad biological phenomenon of *symbiosis*, or living together of organisms. It is distinguished from *mutualism*, or symbiosis in the narrow sense, by the fact that only one party to the arrangement obtains any advantage, while the other is to a greater or less extent injured.

Of parasites we may distinguish on the basis of their location on or in the host, *ecto-parasites*, which live outside of the body; and *endo-parasites*, which live within the body. On account of their method of breathing the parasitic arthropods belong almost exclusively to the first of these groups.

On the basis of relation to their host, we find *temporary parasites*, those which seek the host only occasionally, to obtain food; and the *stationary* or *permanent parasites* which, at least during certain stages, do not leave their host.

*Facultative parasites* are forms which are not normally parasitic, but which, when accidentally ingested, or otherwise brought into the body, are able to exist for a greater or less period of time in their unusual environment. These are generally called in the medical literature "pseudoparasites" but the term is an unfortunate one.

We shall now take up the different groups of arthropods, discussing the more important of the parasitic forms attacking man. The systematic relationship of these forms, and key for determining important species will be found in Chapter XII.

## ACARINA OR MITES

The **Acarina,** or *mites*, form a fairly natural group of arachnids, characterized, in general, by a sac-like, unsegmented body which is generally fused with the cephalothorax. The mouth-parts have been united to from a beak or rostrum.

The representatives of this group undergo a marked metamorphosis. Commonly, the larvæ on hatching from the egg, possess but three pairs of legs, and hence are called *hexapod larvæ*. After a molt, they transform into nymphs which, like the adult, have four pairs of legs and are called *octopod nymphs*. These after a period of growth, molt one or more times and, acquiring external sexual organs, become adult.

Most of the mites are free-living, but there are many parasitic species and as these have originated in widely separated families, the Acarina form an especially favorable group for study of the origin of parasitism. Such a study has been made by Ewing (1911), who has reached the following conclusions:

"We have strong evidence indicating that the parasitic habit has originated independently at least eleven times in the phylogeny of the Ararina. Among the zoophagous parasites, the parasitic habit has been developed from three different types of free-living Acarina: (a) predaceous forms, (b) scavengers, (c) forms living upon the juices of plants."

Ewing also showed that among the living forms of Acarina we can trace out all the stages of advancing parasitism, semiparasitism, facultative parasitism, even to the fixed and permanent type, and finally to endoparasitism.

Of the many parasitic forms, there are several species which are serious parasites of man and we shall consider the more important of these. Infestation by mites is technically known as *acariasis*.

## Acarina, or Mites 59

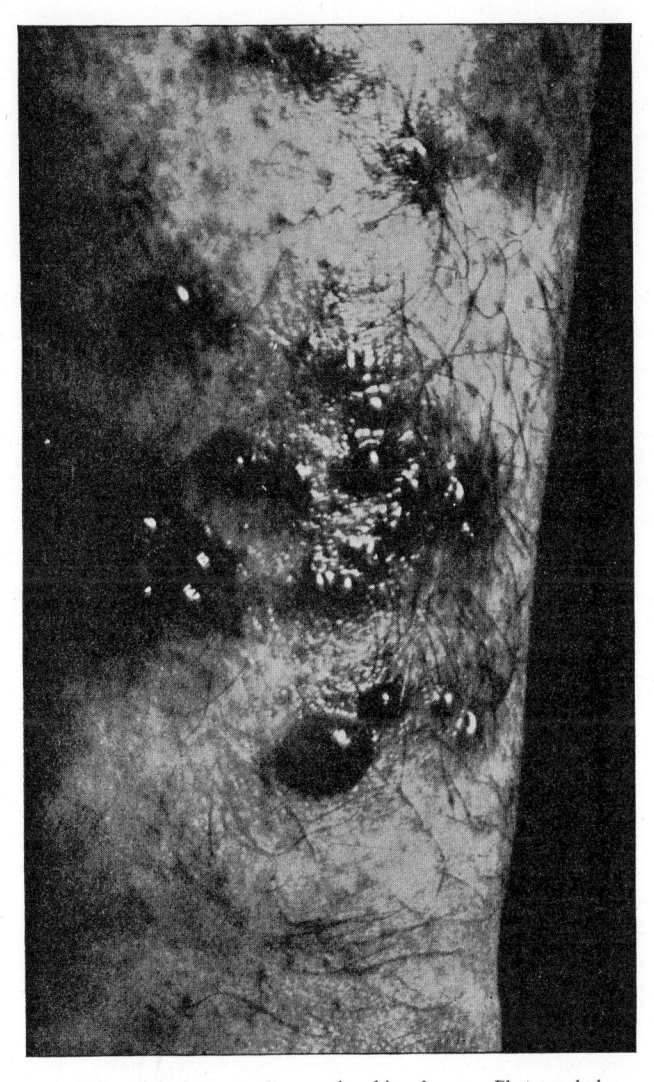

43. Effect of the harvest mites on the skin of man. Photograph by J. C. Bradley.

## The Trombidiidæ, or Harvest Mites

In many parts of this country it is impossible for a visitor to go into the fields and, particularly, into berry patches and among tall weeds and grass in the summer or early fall without being affected by an intolerable itching, which is followed, later, by a breaking out of wheals, or papules, surrounded by a bright red or violaceous aureola, (fig. 43). It is often regarded as a urticaria or eczema, produced by change of climate, an error in diet, or some condition of general health.

Sooner or later, the victim finds that it is due to none of these, but to the attacks of an almost microscopic red mite, usually called "jigger" or "chigger" in this country. As the term "chigger" is applied to one of the true fleas, *Dermatophilus penetrans*, of the tropics, these forms are more correctly known as "harvest mites." Natives of an infested region may be so immune or accustomed to its attacks as to be unaware of its presence, though such immunity is by no means possessed by all who have been long exposed to the annoyance.

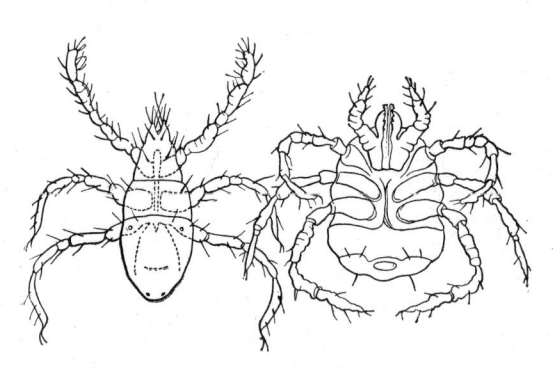

44. Harvest mites. (Larvæ of Trombidium). After C. V. Riley.

The harvest mites, or chiggers, attacking man are larval forms, possessing three pairs of legs (fig. 44). Their systematic position was at first unknown and they were classed under a special genus *Leptus*, a name which is very commonly still retained in the medical literature. It is now known that they are the larval forms of various species of the genus *Trombidium*, a group of predaceous forms, the adults of which feed primarily on insects and their eggs. In this country the species best known are those to be found late in summer, as larvæ at the base of the wings of houseflies or grasshoppers.

There is much uncertainty as to the species of the larvæ attacking man but it is clear that several are implicated. Bruyant has shown that in France the larvæ *Trombidium inapinatum* and *Trombidium holosericeum* are those most frequently found. The habit of attacking man is abnormal and the larvæ die after entering the skin. Normally they are parasitic on various insects.

Most recent writers agree that, on man, they do not bore into the skin, as is generally supposed, but enter a hair follicle or sebaceous gland and from the bottom of this, pierce the cutis with their elongate hypopharynx. According to Braun, there arises about the inserted hypopharynx a fibrous secretion—the so-called "beak" which is, in reality, a product of the host. Dr. J. C. Bradley, however, has made careful observations on their method of attack, and he assures us that the mite ordinarily remains for a long time feeding on the surface of the skin, where it produces the erythema above described. During this time it is not buried in the skin but is able to retreat rapidly into it through a hair follicle or sweat gland. The irritation from the mites ceases after a few days, but not infrequently the intolerable itching leads to so much scratching that secondary infection follows.

Relief from the irritation may be afforded by taking a warm salt bath as soon as possible after exposure or by killing the mites by application of benzine, sulphur ointment or carbolized vaseline. When they are few in number, they can be picked out with a sterile needle.

Much may be done in the way of warding off their attacks by wearing gaiters or close-woven stockings extending from ankle to the knee. Still more efficacious is the sprinkling of flowers of sulphur in the stockings and the underclothes from a little above the knee, down. The writers have known this to make it possible for persons who were especially susceptible to work with perfect comfort in badly infested regions. Powdered naphthalene is successfully used in the same way and as Chittenden (1906) points out, is a safeguard against various forms of man-infesting tropical insect pests.

The question of the destruction of the mites in the field is sometimes an important one, and under some conditions, is feasible. Chittenden states that much can be accomplished by keeping the grass, weeds, and useless herbage mowed closely, so as to expose the mites to the sun. He believes that in some cases good may be done by dusting the grass and other plants, after cutting, with flowers of sulphur or by spraying with dilute kerosene emulsion in which sulphur has been mixed. More recently (1914) he calls attention to the value of cattle, and more especially sheep, in destroying the pests by tramping on them and by keeping the grass and herbage closely cropped.

## Ixodoidea or Ticks

Until recently, the ticks attracted comparatively little attention from entomologists. Since their importance as carriers of disease has been established, interest in the group has been enormously stimulated and now they rank second only to the mosquitoes in the amount of detailed study that has been devoted to them.

The ticks are the largest of the Acarina. They are characterized by the fact that the hypostome, or "tongue" (fig. 45) is large and file-like, roughened by sharp teeth. They possess a breathing pore on each side of the body, above the third or fourth coxæ (fig. 45b).

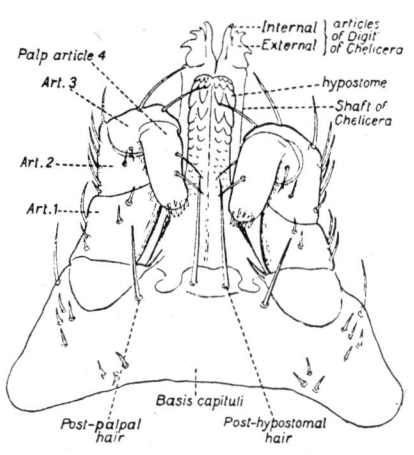

45a. Argus persicus. Capitulum of male. After Nuttall and Warburton.

There are two distinct families of the **Ixodoidea**, differing greatly in structure, life-history and habits. These are the **Argasidæ** and the **Ixodidæ**. We shall follow Nuttall (1908) in characterizing these two families and in pointing out their biological differences, and shall discuss briefly the more important species which attack man. The consideration of the ticks as carriers of disease will be reserved for a later chapter.

### Argasidæ

In the ticks belonging to the family **Argasidæ**, there is comparatively little sexual dimorphism, while this is very marked in the Ixodidæ. The capitulum, or so-called "head" is ventral, instead of terminal; the palpi are leg-like, with the segments subequal; the scutum, or dorsal shield, is absent; eyes, when present, are lateral, on supracoxal folds. The

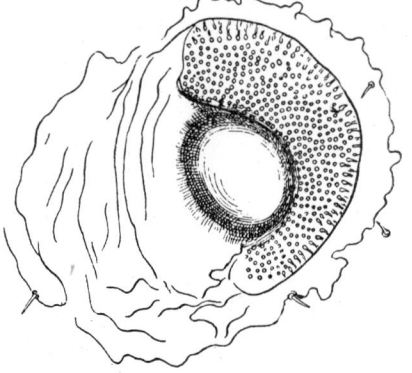

45b. Left spiracle of nymph of *Argus persicus*. After Nuttall and Warburton.

spiracles are very small; coxæ unarmed; tarsi without ventral spurs, and the pulvilli are absent or rudimentary.

In habits and life history the Argasidæ present striking characteristics. In the first place, they are long-lived, a factor which counts for much in the maintenance of the species. They are intermittent feeders, being comparable with the bed-bug in this respect. There are two or more nymphal stages, and they may molt after attaining maturity. The female lays comparatively few eggs in several small batches.

Nuttall (1911) concludes that "The Argasidæ represent the relatively primitive type of ticks because they are less constantly para-

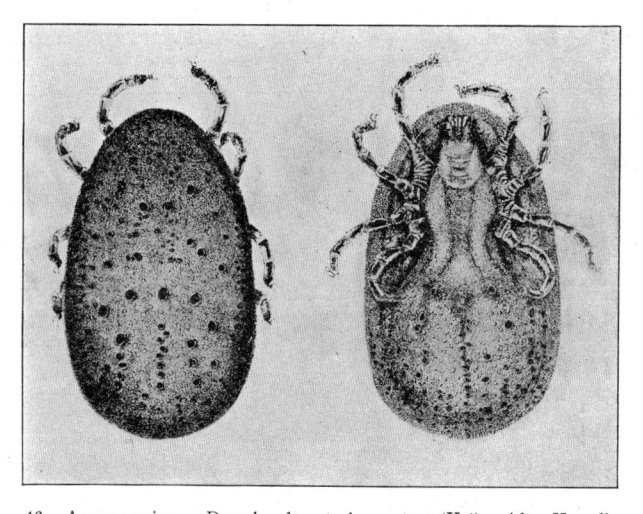

46. Argus persicus. Dorsal and ventral aspects. (X 4). After Hassell.

sitic than are the Ixodidæ. Their nymphs and adults are rapid feeders and chiefly infest the habitat of their hosts. * * * Owing to the Argasidæ infesting the habitats of their hosts, their resistance to prolonged starvation and their rapid feeding habits, they do not need to bring forth a large progeny, because there is less loss of life in the various stages, as compared with the Ixodidæ, prior to their attaining maturity."

Of the Argasidæ, we have in the United States, several species which have been reported as attacking man.

*Argas persicus*, the famous "Miana bug" (fig. 46), is a very widely distributed species, being reported from Europe, Asia, Africa, and Australia. It is everywhere preeminently a parasite of fowls.

According to Nuttall it is specifically identical with *Argas americanus* Packard or *Argas miniatus* Koch, which is commonly found on fowls in the United States, in the South and Southwest. Its habits are comparable to those of the bed-bug. It feeds intermittently, primarily at night, and instead of remaining on its host, it then retreats to cracks and crevices. Hunter and Hooker (1908) record that they have found the larva to remain attached for five or eight days before dropping. Unlike the Ixodidæ, the adults oviposit frequently.

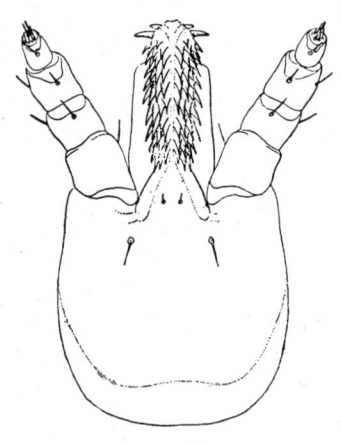

The most remarkable feature of the biology of this species is the great longevity, especially of the adult. Hunter and Hooker report keeping larvæ confined in summer in pill boxes immediately after hatching for about two months while under similar conditions those of the Ixodid, *Boophilus annulatus* lived for but two or three days.

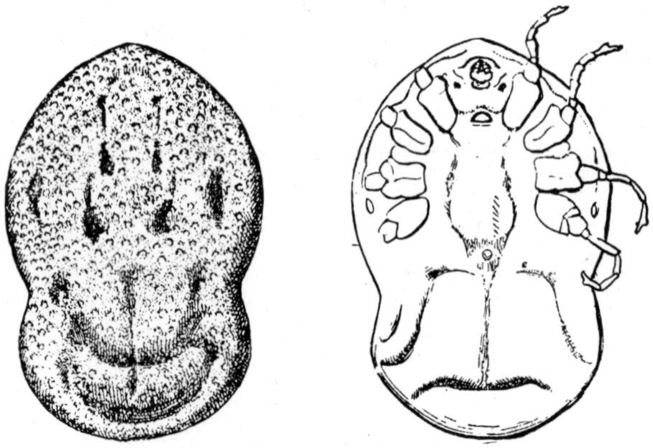

47. Otiobius (Ornithodoros) megnini, head of nymph, After Stiles.

48. Otiobius (Ornithodoros) megnini, male. (*a*) dorsal, (*b*) ventral aspect. After Nuttall and Warburton.

Many writers have recorded keeping adults for long periods without food. We have kept specimens in a tin box for over a year and a half and at the end of that time a number were still alive. Laboulliene kept unfed adults for over three years. In view of the effectiveness of sulphur in warding off the attacks of Trombidiidæ, it is astonishing to find that Lounsbury has kept adults of *Argas persicus* for three months in a box nearly filled with flowers of sulphur, with no apparent effect on them.

We have already called attention to the occasional serious effects of the bites of this species. While such reports have been frequently discredited there can be no doubt that they have foundation in fact. The readiness with which this tick attacks man, and the extent to which old huts may be infested makes it especially troublesome.

*Otiobius (Ornithodoros) megnini*, the "spinose ear-tick" (figs. 47, 48), first described from Mexico, as occurring in the ears of horses, is a common species in our Southwestern States and is recorded by Banks as occurring as far north as Iowa.

The species is remarkable for the great difference between the spiny nymph stage and the adult. The life history has been worked out by Hooker (1908). Seed ticks, having gained entrance to the ear, attach deeply down in the folds, engorge, and in about five days, molt; as nymphs with their spinose body they appear entirely unlike the larvæ. As nymphs they continue feeding sometimes for months. Finally the nymph leaves the host, molts to form the unspined adult, and without further feeding is fertilized and commences oviposition.

The common name is due to the fact that in the young stage the ticks occur in the ear of their hosts, usually horses or cattle. Not uncommonly it has been reported as occurring in the ear of man and causing very severe pain. Stiles recommends that it be removed by pouring some bland oil into the ear.

Banks (1908) reports three species of *Ornithodoros*—*O. turicata, coriaceus* and *talaje*—as occurring in the United States. All of these attack man and are capable of inflicting very painful bites.

### Ixodidæ

The ticks belonging to the family **Ixodidæ** (figs. 49 and 50) exhibit a marked sexual dimorphism. The capitulum is anterior, terminal, instead of ventral as in the Argasidæ; the palpi are relatively rigid (except in the subfamily Ixodinæ), with rudimentary fourth segment; scutum present; eyes, when present, dorsal, on side of scutum. The spiracles are generally large, situated well behind the fourth coxæ; coxæ generally with spurs; pulvilli always present.

In habits and life history the typical Ixodidæ differ greatly from the Argasidæ. They are relatively short-lived, though some recent

66                Parasitic Arthropods

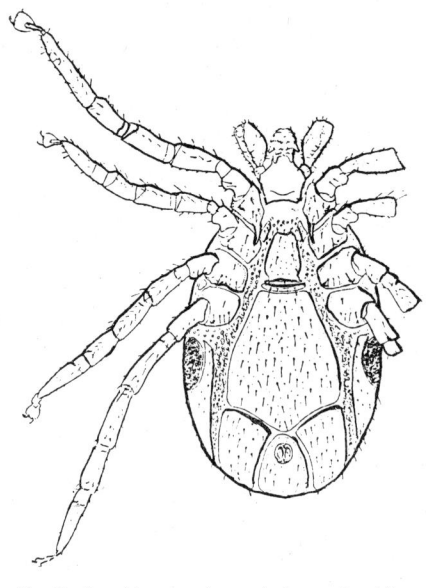

49. Ixodes ricinus; male, ventral aspect. After Braun and Luehe.

work indicates that their longevity has been considerably under-estimated. Typically, they are permanent feeders, remaining on the host, or hosts, during the greater part of their life. They molt twice only, on leaving the larval and the nymphal stages. The adult female deposits a single, large batch of eggs. Contrasting the habits of the Ixodidæ to those of the Argasidæ, Nuttall (1911) emphasizes that the Ixodidæ are more highly specialized parasites. "The majority are parasitic on hosts having no fixed habitat and consequently all stages, as a rule, occur upon the host."

As mere parasites of man, apart from their power to transmit disease, the Ixodidæ are much less important than the Argasidæ. Many are reported as occasionally attacking man and of these the following native species may be mentioned.

*Ixodes ricinus*, the European castor bean tick (figs. 49, 50), is a species which has been often reported from this country but Banks (1908) has shown that, though it does occur, practically all of the records apply to *Ixodes scapularis* or *Ixodes cookei*. In Europe, *Ixodes ricinus* is very abundant and very commonly attacks

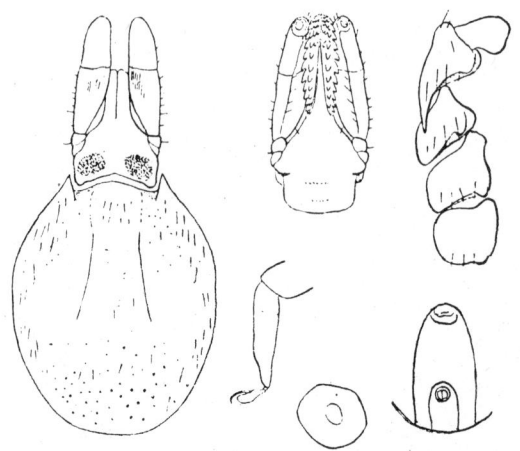

50. Ixodes ricinus, var. scapularis, female. Capitulum and scutum; ventral aspect of capitulum; coxæ; tarsus 4; spiracle; genital and anal grooves. After Nuttall and Warburton.

man. At the point of penetration of the hypostome there is more or less inflammation but serious injury does not occur unless there have been introduced pathogenic bacteria or, unless the tick has been abruptly removed, leaving the capitulum in the wound. Under the latter circumstances, there may be an abscess formed about the foreign body and occasionally, serious results have followed. Under certain conditions the tick, in various stages, may penetrate under the skin and produce a tumor, within which it may survive for a considerable period of time.

*Ixodes cookei* is given by Banks as "common on mammals in the Eastern States as far west as the Rockies." It is said to affect man severely.

*Amblyomma americanum*, (fig. 158e), the "lone star tick," is widely distributed in the United States. Its common name is derived from the single silvery spot on the scutum of the female. Hunter and Hooker regard this species as, next to *Boophilus annulatus*, the most important tick in the United States. Though more common on cattle, it appears to attack mammals generally, and "in portions of Louisiana and Texas it becomes a pest of considerable importance to moss gatherers and other persons who spend much time in the forests."

*Amblyomma cajennense*, noted as a pest of man in central and tropical America, is reported from various places in the south and southwestern United States.

*Dermacentor variabilis* is a common dog tick of the eastern United States. It frequently attacks man, but the direct effects of its bite are negligible.

The "Rocky Mountain spotted fever tick" (*Dermacentor andersoni* according to Stiles, *D. venustus* according to Banks) is, from the viewpoint of its effects on man, the most important of the ticks of the United States. This is because, as has been clearly established, it transmits the so-called "spotted fever" of man in our northwestern states. This phase of the subject will be discussed later and it need merely be mentioned here, that this species has been reported as causing painful injuries by its bites. Dr. Stiles states that he has seen cases of rather severe lymphangitis and various sores and swellings developing from this cause. In one case, of an individual bitten near the elbow, the arm became very much swollen and the patient was confined in bed for several days. The so-called tick paralysis produced by this species is discussed in a preceding chapter.

There are many other records of various species of ticks attacking man, but the above-mentioned will serve as typical and it is not necessary to enter into greater detail.

**Treatment of Tick Bites**—When a tick attaches to man the first thing to be done is to remove it without leaving the hypostome in the wound to fester and bring about secondary effects. This is best accomplished by applying to the tick's body some substance which will cause it to more readily loosen its hold. Gasoline or petroleum, oil or vaseline will serve. For removing the spinose ear-tick, Stiles recommends pouring some bland oil into the ear. Others have used effectively a pledget of cotton soaked in chloroform.

In general, the treatment recommended by Wellman for the bites of *Ornithodoros moubata* will prove helpful. It consists of prolonged bathing in very hot water, followed by the application of a strong solution of bicarbonate

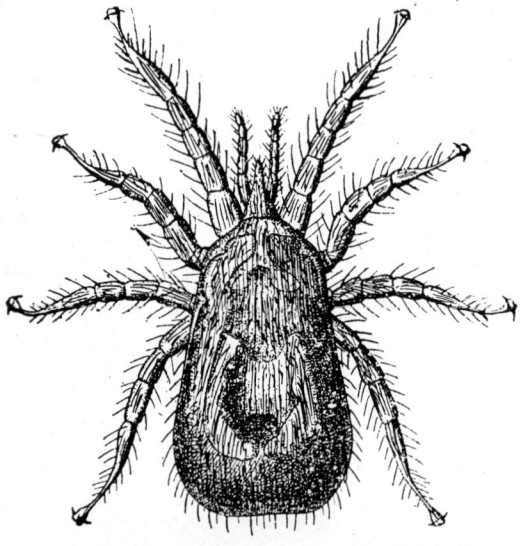

51. Dermanyssus gallinæ, female. After Delafond.

of soda, which is allowed to dry upon the skin. He states that this treatment is comforting. For severe itching he advises smearing the bites with vaseline, which is slightly impregnated with camphor or menthol. Medical aid should be sought when complications arise.

The **Dermanyssidæ** are Gamasid mites which differ from others of the group in that they are parasitic on vertebrates. None of the species normally attack man, but certain of them, especially the poultry mite, may be accidental annoyances.

*Dermanyssus gallinæ* (fig. 51), the red mite of poultry, is an exceedingly common and widespread parasite of fowls. During the day it lives in cracks and crevices of poultry houses, under supports of roosts, and in litter of the food and nests, coming out at night to feed.

They often attack people working in poultry houses or handling and plucking infested fowls. They may cause an intense pruritis, but they do not produce a true dermatosis, for they do not find conditions favorable for multiplication on the skin of man.

## Tarsonemidæ

The representatives of the family **Tarsonemidæ** are minute mites, with the body divided into cephalothorax and abdomen. There is marked sexual dimorphism. The females possess stigmata at the anterior part of the body, at the base of the rostrum, and differ from all other mites in having on each side, a prominent clavate organ between the first and second legs. The larva, when it exists, is hexapodous and resembles the adult. A number of the species are true parasites on insects, while others attack plants. Several of them may be accidental parasites of man.

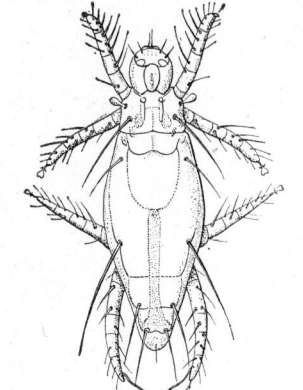

52. Pediculoides ventricosus, female. After Webster.

*Pediculoides ventricosus* (fig. 52 and 53) is, of all the Tarsonemidæ reported, the one which has proved most troublesome to man. It is a predaceous species which attacks a large number of insects but which has most commonly been met with by man through its fondness for certain grain-infesting insects, notably the Angoumois grain moth, *Sitotroga cerealella*, and the wheat straw-worm, *Isosoma grande*. In recent years it has attracted much attention in the United States and its distribution and habits have been the object of detailed study by Webster (1901).

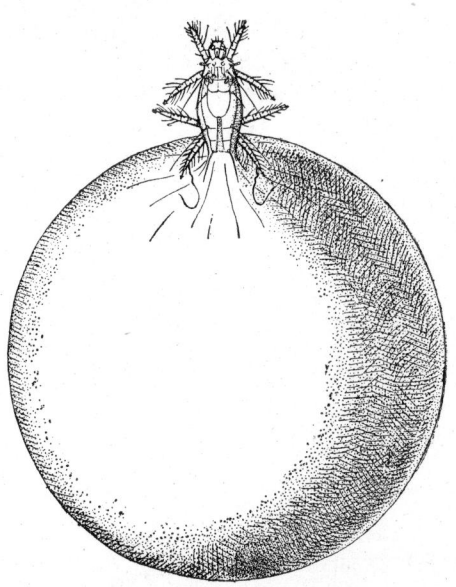

53. Pediculoides ventricosus, gravid female. (X 80). After Webster.

There is a very striking sexual dimorphism in this species. The non-gravid female is elongate, about 200μ by 70μ (fig. 52), with the abdomen slightly striated longitudinally. The gravid female (fig. 53) has the abdomen enormously swollen, so that it is from twenty to a hundred times greater than the rest of the body. The species is viviparous and the larvæ undergo their entire growth in the body of the mother. They emerge as sexually mature males and females which soon pair. The male (fig. 54) is much smaller, reaching a length of only 320μ but is relatively broad, 8cμ, and angular. Its abdomen is very greatly reduced.

As far back as 1850 it was noted as causing serious outbreaks of peculiar dermatitis among men handling infested grain. For some time the true source of the difficulty was unknown and it was even believed that the grain had been poisoned. Webster has shown that in this country (and probably in Europe as well) its attacks have been mistaken for those of the red bugs or "chiggers" (larval Trombiidæ). More recently a number of outbreaks of a mysterious "skin disease" were traced to the use of straw mattresses, which were found to be swarming with these almost microscopic forms which had turned their attentions to the occupants of the beds. Other cases cited were those of farmers running wheat through a fanning mill, and of thrashers engaged in feeding unthrashed grain into the cylinder of the machine.

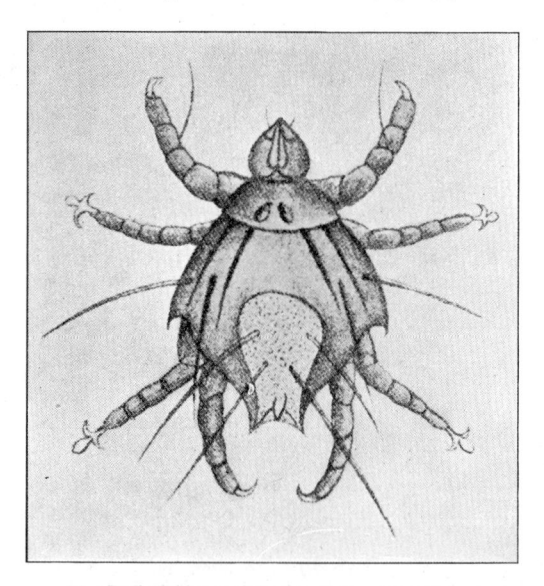

54. Pediculoides ventricosus, male. After Braun.

The medical aspects of the question have been studied especially by Schamberg and Goldberger and from the latter's summary (1910) we derive the following data. Within twelve to sixteen hours after exposure, itching appears and in severe cases, especially where exposure is continued night after night by sleeping on an infested bed, the itching may become almost intolerable. Simultaneously, there appears an eruption which characteristically consists of wheals surrounded by a vesicle (fig. 55). The vesicle as a rule does not exceed a pin head in size but may become as large as a pea. Its contents

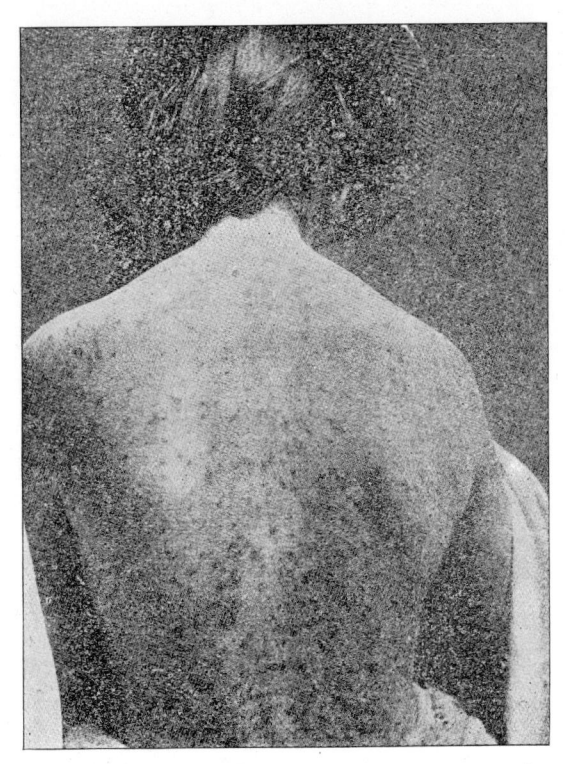

55. Lesions produced by the attacks of Pediculoides ventricosus. After Webster.

rapidly become turbid and in a few hours it is converted into a pustule. The eruption is most abundant on the trunk, slight on the face and extremities and almost absent on the feet and hands. In severe cases there may be constitutional disturbances marked, at the outset, by chilliness, nausea, and vomiting, followed for a few days by a slight elevation of temperature, with the appearance of albumin in the urine. In some cases the eruption may simulate that of chicken-pox or small-pox.

Treatment for the purpose of killing the mites is hardly necessary as they attach feebly to the surface and are readily brushed off by friction of the clothes. "Antipruritic treatment is always called for; warm, mildly alkaline baths or some soothing ointment, such as zinc oxide will be found to fulfil this indication." Of course, reinfestation must be guarded against, by discarding, or thoroughly fumigating infested mattresses, or by avoiding other sources. Goldberger suggests that farm laborers who must work with infested wheat or straw might protect themselves by anointing the body freely with some bland oil or grease, followed by a change of clothes and bath as soon as their work is done. We are not aware of any experiments to determine the effect of flowers of sulphur, but their efficiency in the case of "red bugs" suggests that they are worth a trial against *Pediculoides*.

Various species of **Tyroglyphidæ** (fig. 150f) may abound on dried fruits and other products and attacking persons handling them, may cause a severe dermatitis, comparable to that described above for *Pediculoides ventricosus*. Many instances of their occurrence as such temporary ectoparasites are on record. Thus, workers who handle vanilla pods are subject to a severe dermatitis, known as vanillism, which is due to the attacks of *Tyroglyphus siro*, or a closely related species. The so-called "grocer's itch" is similarly caused by mites infesting various products. Castellani has shown that in Ceylon, workers employed in the copra mills, where dried cocoanut is ground up for export, are much annoyed by mites, which produce the so-called "copra itch." The skin of the hands, arms and legs, and sometimes of the whole body, except the face, is covered by fairly numerous, very pruriginous papules, often covered by small, bloody crusts due to scratching. The condition is readily mistaken for scabies. It is due to the attacks of *Tyroglyphus longior castellanii* which occur in enormous numbers in some samples of the copra.

## Sarcoptidæ

The **Sarcoptidæ** are minute whitish mites, semi-globular in shape, with a delicate transversely striated cuticula. They lack eyes and tracheæ. The mouth-parts are fused at the base to form a cone which is usually designated as the head. The legs are short and stout, and composed of five segments. The tarsi may or may not possess a claw and may terminate in a pedunculated sucker, or simple long bristle, or both. The presence or absence of these structures and their distribution are much used in classification. The mites live on or under the skin of mammals and birds, where they produce the disease known as scabies, mange, or itch. Several species of the Sarcoptidæ attack man but the most important of these, and the one pre-eminent as the "itch mite" is *Sarcoptes scabiei*.

The female of *Sarcoptes scabiei*, of man, is oval and yellowish white; the male more rounded and of a somewhat reddish tinge, and much smaller. The body is marked by transverse striæ which are partly interrupted on the back. There are transverse rows of scales, or pointed spines, and scattered bristles on the dorsum.

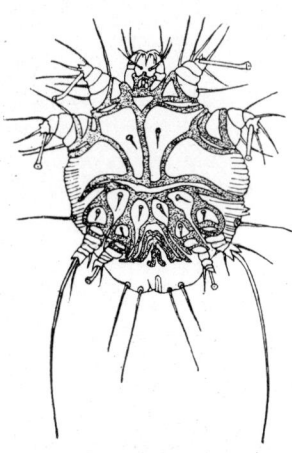

56a. Sarcoptes scabiei, male. (X 100). After Fürstenberg.

The male (fig. 56) which is from 200–240μ in length, and 150–200μ in breadth, possesses pedunculated suckers on each pair of legs except the third, which bears, instead, a long bristle. The female (fig. 56) 300–450μ in length and 250–350μ in breadth, has the pedunculated suckers on the first and second pairs of legs, only, the third and fourth terminating in bristles.

The mite lives in irregular galleries from a few millimeters to several centimeters in length, which it excavates in the epidermis (fig. 57). It works especially where the skin is thin, such as between the fingers, in the bend of the elbows and knees, and in the groin, but it is by no means restricted to these localities. The female, alone, tunnels into the skin; the males remain under the superficial epidermal scales, and seldom are found, as they die soon after mating.

As she burrows into the skin the female deposits her eggs, which measure about 150 x 100μ. Fürstenberg says that each deposits an average of twenty-two to twenty-four eggs, though Gudden reports a single burrow as containing fifty-one. From these

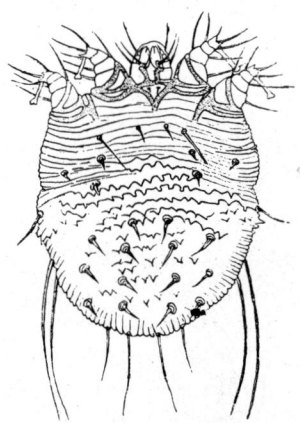

56b. Sarcoptes scabiei, female. (X 100.) After Fürstenberg.

there develop after about seven days, the hexapod larvæ. These molt on the sixteenth day to form an octopod nymph, which molts again the twenty-first day. At the end of the fourth week the nymphs molt to form the sexually mature males and the so-called pubescent females. These pair, the males die, and the females again cast their skin, and become the oviparous females. Thus the life cycle is completed in about twenty-eight days.

The external temperature exercises a great influence on the development of the mites and thus, during the winter, the areas of infestation not only do not spread, but they become restricted. As soon as the temperature rises, the mites increase and the infestation becomes much more extensive.

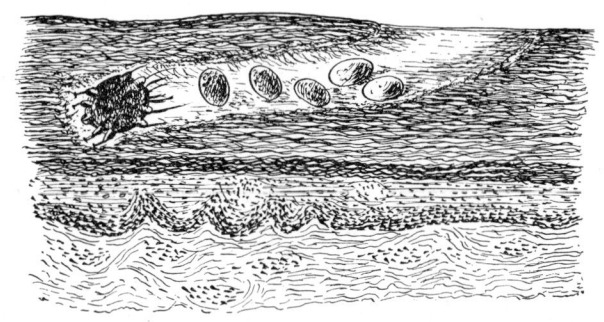

57. Sarcoptes scabiei. Diagrammatic representation of the course in the skin of man.

In considering the possible sources of infestation, and the chances of reinfestation after treatment, the question of the ability of the mite to live apart from its host is a very important one. Unfortunately, there are few reliable data on this subject. Gerlach found that, exposed in the dry, warm air of a room they became very inactive within twenty-four hours, that after two days they showed only slight movement, and that after three or four days they could not be revived by moisture and warming. The important fact was brought out that in moist air, in folded soiled underwear, they survived as long as ten days. Bourguignon found that under the most favorable conditions the mites of *Sarcoptes scabiei equi* would live for sixteen days.

The disease designated the "itch" or "scabies," in man has been known from time immemorial, but until within less than a hundred years it was almost universally attributed to malnutrition, errors of diet, or "bad blood." This was in spite of the fact that the mite was known to Mouffet and that Bonomo had figured both the adult and the egg and had declared the mite the sole cause of the disease. In 1834 the Corsican medical student, Francis Renucci, demonstrated the mite before a clinic in Saint Louis Hospital in Paris and soon thereafter there followed detailed studies of the life history of the various itch mites of man and animals.

The disease is a cosmopolitan one, being exceedingly abundant in some localities. Its spread is much favored where large numbers of people are crowded together under insanitary conditions and hence it increases greatly during wars and is widely disseminated and abundant immediately afterwards. Though more commonly to be met with among the lower classes, it not infrequently appears among those of the most cleanly, careful habits, and it is such cases that are most liable to wrong diagnosis by the physician.

58. Scabies on the hand. From portfolio of Dermochromes by permission of Rebman & Co., of New York, Publishers.

Infection occurs solely through the passage, direct or indirect, of the young fertilized females to the skin of a healthy individual. The adult, oviparous females do not quit their galleries and hence do not serve to spread the disease. The young females move about more or less at night and thus the principal source of infestation is through sleeping in the same bed with an infested person, or indirectly through bedclothes, or even towels or clothing. Diurnal infestation through contact or clothing is exceptional. Many cases are known of the disease being contracted from animals suffering from scabies, or mange.

When a person is exposed to infestation, the trouble manifests itself after eight or ten days, though there usually elapses a period of twenty to thirty days before there is a suspicion of anything serious. The first symptom is an intense itching which increases when the patient is in bed. When the point of irritation is examined the galleries may usually be seen as characteristic sinuous lines, at first whitish in color but soon becoming blackish because of the contained eggs and excrement. The galleries, which may not be very distinct in some cases, may measure as much as four centimeters in length. Little vesicles, of the size of a pin head are produced by the secretions of the feeding mite; they are firm, and projecting, and contain a limpid fluid. Figures 58 and 59 show the typical appearance of scabies on the hands, while figure 60 shows a severe general infestation. The intolerable itching induces scratching and through this various complications may arise. The lesions are not normally found on the face and scalp, and are rare on the back.

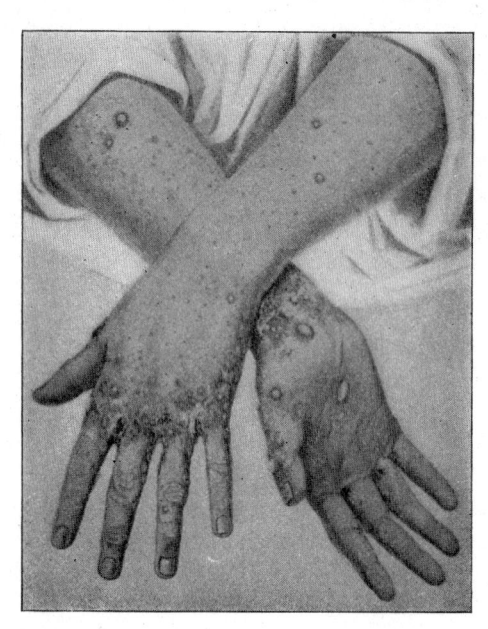

59. Scabies on the hand. After Duhring.

Formerly, scabies was considered a very serious disease, for its cause and method of treatment were unknown, and potentially it may continue indefinitely. Generation after generation of the mites may develop and finally their number become so

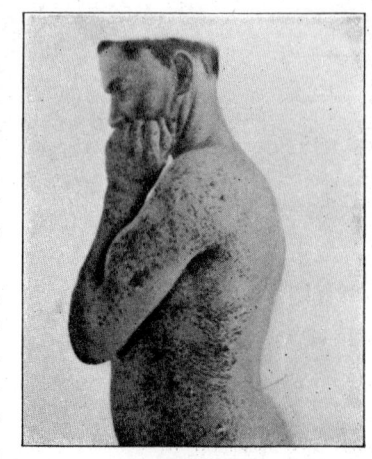

60. Generalized infection of Scabies. After Morrow.

great that the general health of the individual is seriously affected. Now that the true cause of the disease is known, it is easily controlled.

Treatment usually consists in softening the skin by friction with soap and warm water, followed by a warm bath, and then applying some substance to kill the mites. Stiles gives the following directions, modified from Bourguignon's, as "a rather radical guide, to be modified according to facilities and according to the delicacy of the skin or condition of the patient":

1. The patient, stripped naked, is energetically rubbed all over (except the head) for twenty minutes, with green soap and warm water. 2. He is then placed in a warm bath for thirty minutes, during which time the rubbing is continued. 3. The parasiticide is next rubbed in for twenty minutes and is allowed to remain on the body for four or five hours; in the meantime the patient's clothes are sterilized, to kill the eggs or mites attached to them. 4. A final bath is taken to remove the parasiticide.

The parasiticide usually relied on is the officinal sulphur ointment of the United States pharmacopœia. When infestation is severe it is necessary to repeat treatment after three or four days in order to kill mites which have hatched from the eggs.

The above treatment is too severe for some individuals and may, of itself, produce a troublesome dermatitis. We have seen cases where the treatment was persisted in and aggravated the condition because it was supposed to be due to the parasite. For delicate-skinned patients the use of balsam of Peru is very satisfactory, and usually causes no irritation whatever. Of course, sources of reinfection should be carefully guarded against.

*Sarcoptes scabiei crustosæ*, which is a distinct variety, if not species, of the human itch mite, is the cause of so-called Norwegian itch. This disease is very contagious, and is much more resistant than the ordinary scabies. Unlike the latter, it may occur on the face and scalp.

*Sarcoptes scabiei* not only attacks man but also occurs on a large number of mammals. Many species, based on choice of host, and minute differences in size and secondary characters, have been established, but most students of the subject relegate these to varietal rank. Many of them readily attack man, but they have become sufficiently adapted to their normal host so that they are usually less persistent on man.

*Notoedres cati* (usually known as *Sarcoptes minor*) is a species of itch mites which produce an often fatal disease of cats. The body is rounded and it is considerably smaller than *Sarcoptes scabiei*, the female (fig. 61) measuring 215–230μ long and 165-175μ wide; the males 145–150μ by 120-125μ. The most important character

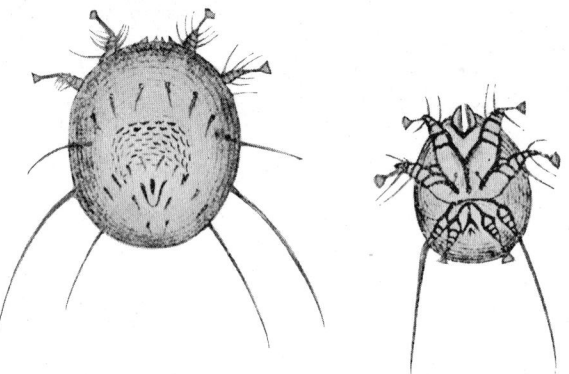

61. Notœdres cati, male and female. After Railliet.

separating *Notoedres* from *Sarcoptes* is the position of the anus, which is dorsal instead of terminal. The mite readily transfers to man but does not persist, the infestation usually disappearing spontaneously in about two weeks. Infested cats are very difficult to cure, unless treatment is begun at the very inception of the outbreak, and under ordinary circumstances it is better to kill them promptly, to avoid spread of the disease to children and others who may be exposed.

### Demodecidæ

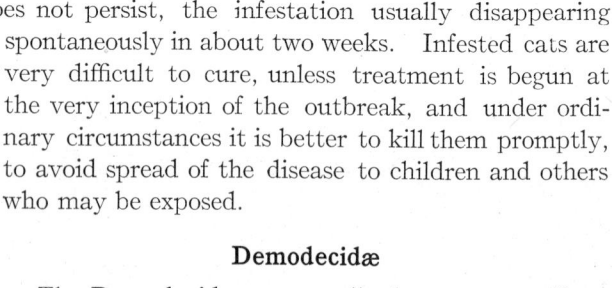

The **Demodecidæ** are small, elongate, vermiform mites which live in the hair follicles of mammals. The family characteristics will be brought out in the discussion of the species infesting man, *Demodex folliculorum*.

*Demodex folliculorum* (fig. 62) is to be found very commonly in the hair follicles and sebaceous glands of man. It is vermiform in appearance, and with the elongate abdomen transversely striated so as to give it the appearance of segmentation. The female is 380–400μ long by 45μ; the male 300μ by 40μ. The three-

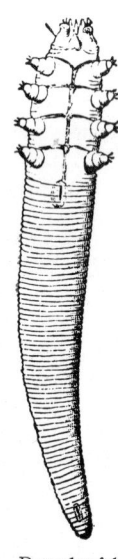

62. Demodex folliculorum. (X200) After Blanchard.

jointed legs, eight in number, are reduced to mere stubs in the adult. The larval form is hexopod. These mites thus show in their form a striking adaptation to their environment. In the sebaceous glands

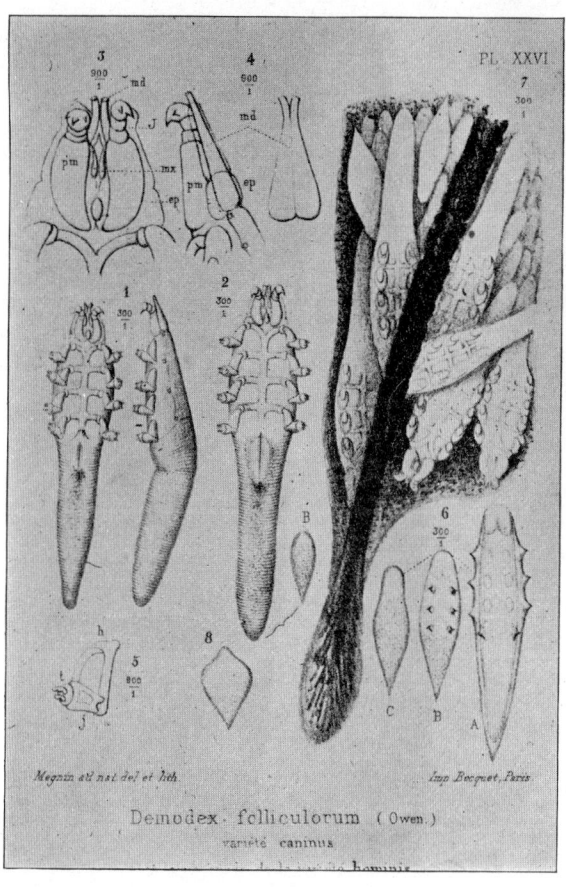

63. Demodex folliculorum. Section through skin showing the mites in situ. Magnification of Nos. 1, 2, 6 and 7, X 150; Nos. 3, 4, 5, X 450. After Megnin.

and hair follicles they lie with their heads down (fig. 63). Usually there are only a few in a gland, but Gruby has counted as many as two hundred.

The frequency with which they occur in man is surprising. According to European statistics they are found in 50 per cent to 60 per cent or even more. Gruby found them in forty out of sixty persons examined. These figures are very commonly quoted, but reliable data for the United States seem to be lacking. Our studies indicate that it is very much less common in this country than is generally assumed.

The Demodex in man does not, as a rule, cause the slightest inconvenience to its host. It is often stated that they give rise to comedons or "black-heads" but there is no clear evidence that they are ever implicated. Certain it is that they are not the usual cause. A variety of the same, or a very closely related species of *Demodex*, on the dog gives rise to the very resistant and often fatal follicular mange.

## Hexapoda or True Insects

The **Hexapoda**, or true insects, are characterized by the fact that the adult possesses three pairs of legs. The body is distinctly segmented and is divided into head, thorax, and abdomen.

The mouth-parts in a generalized form, consist of an upper lip, or *labrum*, which is a part of the head capsule, and a central unpaired *hypopharynx*, two *mandibles*, two *maxillæ* and a lower lip, or *labium*, made up of the fused pair of second maxillæ. These parts may be greatly modified, dependent upon whether they are used for biting, sucking, piercing and sucking, or a combination of biting and sucking.

Roughly speaking, insects may be grouped into those which undergo *complete metamorphosis* and those which have *incomplete metamorphosis*. They are said to undergo complete metamorphosis when the young form, as it leaves the egg, bears no resemblance to the adult. For example, the maggot changes to a quiescent pupa and from this emerges the winged active fly. They undergo incomplete metamorphosis, when the young insect, as it leaves the egg, resembles the adult to a greater or less extent, and after undergoing a certain number of molts becomes sexually mature.

Representatives of several orders have been reported as accidental or facultative parasites of man, but the true parasites are restricted to four orders. These are the Siphunculata; the Hemiptera, the Diptera and the Siphonaptera.

## Siphunculata

The order **Siphunculata** was established by Meinert to include the true sucking lice. These are small wingless insects, with reduced mouth-parts, adapted for sucking; thorax apparently a single piece due to indistinct separation of its three segments; the compound eyes reduced to a single ommatidium on each side. The short, powerful legs are terminated by a single long claw. Metamorphosis incomplete.

There has been a great deal of discussion regarding the structure of the mouth-parts, and the relationships of the sucking lice, and the questions cannot yet be regarded as settled. The conflicting views are well represented by Cholodkovsky (1904 and 1905) and by Enderlein (1904).

Following Graber, it is generally stated that the mouth-parts consist of a short tube furnished with hooks in front, which constitutes the lower lip, and that within this is a delicate sucking tube derived from the fusion of the labrum and the mandibles. Opposed to this, Cholodkvosky and, more recently, Pawlowsky, (1906), have shown that the piercing apparatus lies in a blind sac under the pharynx and opening into the mouth cavity (fig. 64). It does not form a true tube but a furrow with its open surface uppermost. Eysell has shown that, in addition, there is a pair of chitinous rods which he regards as the homologues of the maxillæ.

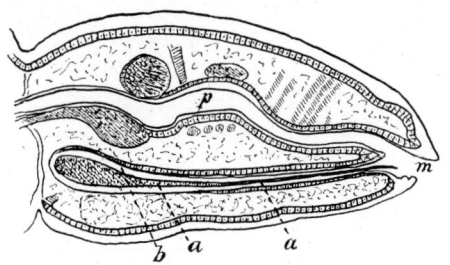

64. Pediculus showing the blind sac (*b*) containing the mouth parts (*a*) beneath the alimentary canal (*p*). After Pawlowsky.

When the louse feeds, it everts the anterior part of the mouth cavity, with its circle of hooks. The latter serve for anchoring the bug, and the piercing apparatus is then pushed out.

Most writers have classed the sucking lice as a sub-order of the Hemiptera, but the more recent anatomical and developmental studies render this grouping untenable. An important fact, bearing on the question, is that, as shown by Gross, (1905), the structure of the ovaries is radically different from that of the Hemiptera.

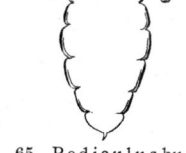

65. Pediculus humanus, ventral aspect of male. (X 10)

Lice infestation and its effects are known medically as *pediculosis*. Though their continued presence is the result of the grossest neglect and filthiness, the original infestation may be innocently obtained and by people of the most careful habits.

Three species commonly attack man. Strangely enough, there are very few accurate data regarding their life history.

*Pediculus humanus* (fig. 65), the head louse, is the most widely distributed. It is usually referred to in medical literature as *Pediculus capitis*, but the Linnean specific name has priority. In color it is of a pale gray, blackish on the margins. It is claimed by some authors that the color varies according to the color of the skin of the host. The abdomen is composed of seven distinct segments, bearing spiracles laterally. There is considerable variation in size. The males average 1.8 mm. and the females 2.7 mm. in length.

The eggs, fifty to sixty in number, stick firmly to the hairs of the host and are known as nits. They are large and conspicuous, especially on dark hair and are provided with an operculum, or cap, at the free end, where the nymphs emerge. They hatch in about six days and about the eighteenth day the young lice are sexually mature.

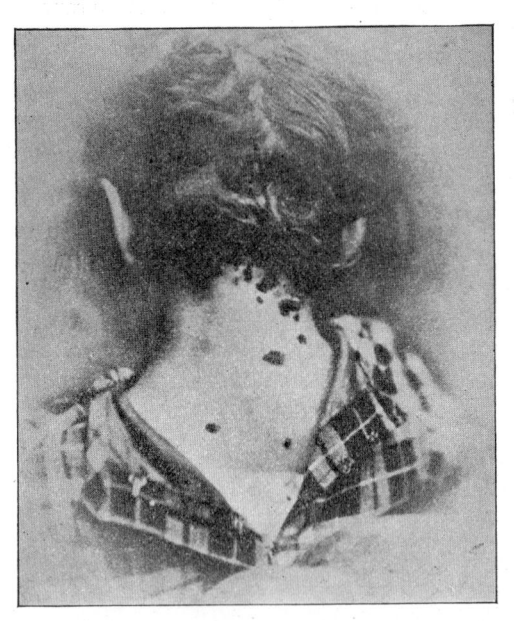

66. Pediculosis of the head. The illustration shows the characteristic indications of the presence of lice, viz: the occipital eczema gluing the hairs together, the swollen cervical glands, and the porrigo, or eruption of contagious pustules upon the neck. After Fox.

The head lice live by preference on the scalp of their host but occasionally they are found on the eyelashes and beard, or in the pubic region. They may also occur elsewhere on the body. The penetration of the rostrum into the skin and the discharge of an irritating saliva produce a severe itching, accompanied by the formation of an eczema-like eruption (fig. 66). When the infestation is severe, the discharge from the pustules mats down the hair, and scabs are formed, under which the insects swarm. "If allowed to run, a regular carapace may form, called *trichoma*, and the head exudes a fœtid odor. Various low plants may grow in the trichoma, the whole being known as *plica palonica*."—Stiles.

Sources of infestation are various. School children may obtain the lice from seatmates, by wearing the hats or caps of infested mates, or by the use, in common, of brushes and combs. They may be obtained from infested beds or sleeper berths. Stiles reports an instance in which a large number of girls in a fashionable boarding school developed lousiness a short time after traveling in a sleeping car.

Treatment is simple, for the parasites may readily be controlled by cleanliness and washing the head with a two per cent solution of carbolic acid or even kerosene. The latter is better used mixed with equal parts of olive oil, to avoid irritation. The treatment should be applied at night and followed the next morning by a shampoo with soap and warm water. It is necessary to repeat the operation in a few days. Xylol, used pure, or with the addition of five per cent of vaseline, is also very efficacious. Of course, the patient must be cautioned to stay away from a lighted lamp or fire while using either the kerosene or xylol. While these treatments will kill the eggs or nits, they will not remove them from the hairs. Pusey recommends repeated washings with vinegar or 25 per cent of acetic acid in water, for the purpose of loosening and removing the nits.

Treatment of severe infestations in females is often troublesome on account of long hair. For such cases the following method recommended by Whitfield (1912) is especially applicable:

The patient is laid on her back on the bed with her head over the edge, and beneath the head is placed a basin on a chair so that the hair lies in the basin. A solution of 1 in 40 carbolic acid is then poured over the hair into the basin and sluiced backwards and forwards until the whole of the hair is thoroughly soaked with it. It is especially necessary that care should be taken to secure thorough saturation of the hair over the ears and at the nape of the neck, since these parts are not only the sites of predilection of the parasites but they are apt to escape the solution. This sluicing is carried out for ten minutes by the clock. At the end of ten minutes the hair is lifted from the basin and allowed to drain, but is not dried or even thoroughly wrung out. The whole head is then swathed with a thick towel or better, a large piece of common house flannel, which is fastened up to form a sort of turban, and is allowed to remain thus for an hour. It can then be washed or simply allowed to dry, as the carbolic quickly disperses. At the end of this period every pediculus and what is better, every ovum is dead and no relapse will occur unless there is exposure to fresh contagion. Whitfield states that there seem to be no disadvantages in this method, which he has used for years. He has never seen carboluria result from it, but would advise first cutting the hair of children under five years of age.

*Pediculus corporis* ( = *P. vestimenti*) the body louse, is larger than the preceding species, the female measuring 3.3 mm., and the male 3 mm. in length. The color is a dirty white, or grayish. *P. corporis* has been regarded by some authorities as merely a variety of *P. humanus* but Piaget maintains there are good characters separating the two species.

The body louse lives in the folds and seams of the clothing of its host, passing to the skin only when it wishes to feed. Brumpt states that he has found enormous numbers of them in the collars of glass-ware or grains worn by certain naked tribes in Africa.

Exact data regarding the life-history of this species have been supplied, in part, by the work of Warburton (1910), cited by Nuttall. He found that *Pediculus corporis* lives longer than *P. humanus* under adverse conditions. This is doubtless due to its living habitually on the clothing, whereas *humanus* lives upon the head, where it has more frequent opportunities of feeding. He reared a single female upon his own person, keeping the louse enclosed in a cotton-plugged tube with a particle of cloth to which it could cling. The tube was kept next to his body, thus simulating the natural conditions of warmth and moisture under which the lice thrive. The specimen was fed twice daily, while it clung to the cloth upon which it rested. Under these conditions she lived for one month. Copulation commenced five days after the female had hatched and was repeated a number of times, sexual union lasting for hours. The female laid one hundred and twenty-four eggs within twenty-five days.

The eggs hatched after eight days, under favorable conditions, such as those under which the female was kept. They did not hatch in the cold. Eggs kept near the person during the day and hung in clothing by the bedside at night, during the winter, in a cold room, did not hatch until the thirty-fifth day. When the nymphs emerge from the eggs, they feed at once, if given a chance to do so. They are prone to scatter about the person and abandon the fragment of cloth to which the adult clings.

The adult stage is reached on the eleventh day, after three molts, about four days apart. Adults enter into copulation about the fifth day and as the eggs require eight days for development, the total cycle, under favorable conditions, is about twenty-four days. Warburton's data differ considerably from those commonly quoted and serve to emphasize the necessity for detailed studies of some of the commonest of parasitic insects.

Body lice are voracious feeders, producing by their bites and the irritating saliva which they inject, rosy elevations and papules which become covered with a brownish crust. The intense itching provokes scratching, and characteristic white scars (fig. 67) surrounded by brownish pigment (fig. 68) are formed. The skin may become thickened and take on a bronze tinge. This melanoderma is especially marked in the region between the shoulders but it may become generalized, a prominent characteristic of "vagabond's disease." According to Dubre and Beille, this melanoderma is due to a toxic substance secreted by the lice, which indirectly provokes the formation of pigment.

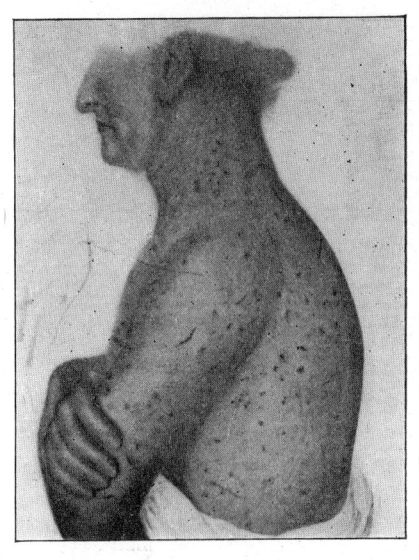

67. Pediculosis in man caused by the body louse. After Morrow.

Control measures, in the case of the body louse, consist in boiling or steaming the clothes or in some cases, sterilizing by dry heat. The dermatitis may be relieved by the use of zinc-oxide ointment, to which Pusey recommends that there be added, on account of their parasiticidal properties, sulphur and balsam of Peru, equal parts, 15 to 30 grains to the ounce.

*Phthirius pubis* (= *P. inguinalis*), the pubic louse, or so-called "crab louse," differs greatly from the preceding in appearance. It is characterized by its relatively short head which fits into a broad depression in the thorax. The latter is broad and flat and merges into the abdomen. The first pair of legs is slender and terminated by a straight claw. The second and third pairs of legs are thicker

86     *Parasitic Arthropods*

and are provided with powerful claws fitted for clinging to hairs. The females (fig. 69) measure 1.5 to 2 mm. in length by 1.5 mm. in breadth. The male averages a little over half as large. The eggs, or nits, are fixed at the base of the hairs. Only a few, ten to fifteen are deposited by a single female, and they hatch in about a week's time. The young lice mature in two weeks.

The pubic louse usually infests the hairs of the pubis and the perineal region. It may pass to the arm pits or even to the beard or moustache. Rarely, it occurs on the eyelids, and it has even been found, in a very few instances, occurring in all stages, on the scalp. Infestation may be contracted from beds or even from badly infested persons in a crowd. We have seen several cases which undoubtedly were due to the use of public water closets. It produces papular eruption and an intense pruritis. When abundant, there occurs a grayish discoloration of the skin which Duguet has shown is due to a poisonous saliva injected by the louse, as is the melanoderma caused by the body louse.

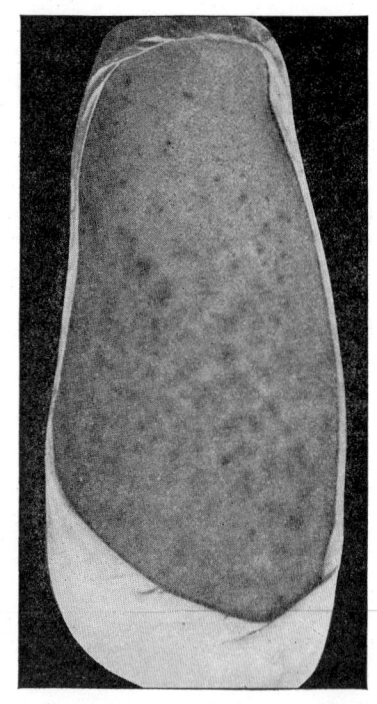

68. Melanoderma caused by the body louse. From Portfolio of Dermochromes, by permission of Rebman & Co., New York, Publishers.

The pubic louse may be exterminated by the measures recommended for the head louse, or by the use of officinal mercurial ointment.

### HEMIPTERA

Several species of **Hemiptera-Heteroptera** are habitual parasites of man, and others occur as occasional or accidental parasites. Of all these, the most important and widespread are the bed-bugs, belonging to the genus *Cimex* (= *Acanthia*).

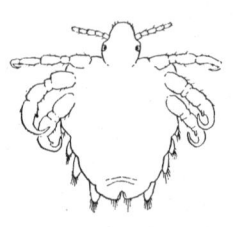

69. Phthirius pubis. Ventral aspect of female. (X 12).

## The Bed-bugs

**The Bed-bugs**—The bed-bugs are characterized by a much flattened oval body, with the short, broad head unconstricted behind, and fitting into the strongly excavated anterior margin of the thorax. The compound eyes are prominent, simple eyes lacking. Antennæ four-jointed, the first segment short, the second long and thick, and the third and fourth slender. The tarsi are short and three segmented.

It is often assumed in the literature of the subject that there is but a single species of *Cimex* attacking man, but several such species are to be recognized. These are distinguishable by the characters given in Chapter XII. We shall consider especially *Cimex lectularius*, the most common and widespread species.

*Cimex lectularius* (= *Acanthia lectularia*, *Clinocoris lectularius*), is one of the most cosmopolitan of human parasites but, like the lice, it has been comparatively little studied until recent years, when the possibility that it may be concerned with the transmission of various diseases has awakened interest in the details of its life-history and habits.

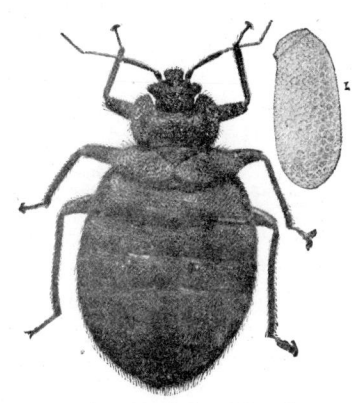

70. Cimex lectularius adult and eggs. Photograph by M. V. S.

The adult insect (fig. 70) is 4–5 mm. long by 3 mm. broad, reddish brown in color, with the beak and body appendages lighter in color. The short, broad and somewhat rectangular head has no neck-like constriction but fits into the broadly semilunar prothorax. The four segmented labium or proboscis encloses the lancet-like maxillæ and mandibles. The distal of the four antennal segments is slightly club-shaped. The prothorax is characteristic of the species, being deeply incised anteriorly and with its thin lateral margins somewhat turned up. The mesothorax is triangular, with the apex posteriorly, and bears the greatly atrophied first pair of wings. There is no trace of the metathoracic pair. The greatly flattened abdomen has eight visible segments, though in reality the first is greatly reduced and has been disregarded by most writers. The body is densely covered with short bristles and hairs, the former being peculiarly saber-shaped structures sharply toothed at the apex and along the convex side (fig. 159*b*).

The peculiar disagreeable odor of the adult bed-bug is due to the secretion of the stink glands which lie on the inner surface of the mesosternum and open by a pair of orifices in front of the metacoxæ, near the middle line. In the nymphs, the thoracic glands are not developed but in the abdomen there are to be found three unpaired dorsal stink glands, which persist until the fifth molt, when they become atrophied and replaced by the thoracic glands. The nymphal glands occupy the median dorsal portion of the abdomen, opening by paired pores at the anterior margin of the fourth, fifth and sixth segments. The secretion is a clear, oily, volatile fluid, strongly acid in reaction. Similar glands are to be found in most of the Hemiptera-Heteroptera and their secretion is doubtless protective, through being disagreeable to the birds. In the bed-bug, as Marlatt points out, "it is probably an illustration of a very common phenomenon among animals, i. e., the persistence of a characteristic which is no longer of any special value to the possessor." In fact, its possession is a distinct disadvantage to the bed-bug, as the odor frequently reveals the presence of the bugs, before they are seen.

The eggs of the bed-bug (fig. 70) are pearly white, oval in outline, about a millimeter long, and possess a small operculum or cap at one end, which is pushed off when the young hatches. They are laid intermittently, for a long period, in cracks and crevices of beds and furniture, under seams of mattresses, under loose wall paper, and similar places of concealment of the adult bugs. Girault (1905) observed a well-fed female deposit one hundred and eleven eggs during the sixty-one days that she was kept in captivity. She had apparently deposited some of her eggs before being captured.

The eggs hatch in six to ten days, the newly emerged nymphs being about 1.5 mm. in length and of a pale yellowish white color. They grow slowly, molting five times. At the last molt the mesathoracic wing pads appear, characteristic of the adult. The total length of the nymphal stage varies greatly, depending upon conditions of food supply, temperature and possibly other factors. Marlatt (1907) found under most favorable conditions a period averaging eight days between molting which, added to an equal egg period, gave a total of about seven weeks from egg to adult insect. Girault (1912) found the postembryonic period as low as twenty-nine days and as high as seventy days under apparently similar and normal conditions of food supply. Under optimum and normal conditions of food supply, beginning August 27, the average nymphal life was

69.9 days; average number of meals 8.75 and the molts 5. Under conditions allowing about half the normal food supply the average nymphal life was from 116.9 to 139 days. Nymphs starved from birth lived up to 42 days. We have kept unfed nymphs, of the first stage, alive in a bottle for 75 days. The interesting fact was brought out that under these conditions of minimum food supply there were sometimes six molts instead of the normal number.

The adults are remarkable for their longevity, a factor which is of importance in considering the spread of the insect and methods of control. Dufour (1833) (not De Geer, as often stated) kept specimens for a year, in a closed vial, without food. This ability, coupled with their willingness to feed upon mice, bats, and other small mammals, and even upon birds, accounts for the long periods that deserted houses and camps may remain infested. There is no evidence that under such conditions they are able to subsist on the starch of the wall paper, juices of moistened wood, or the moisture in the accumulations of dust, as is often stated.

There are three or four generations a year, as Girault's breeding experiments have conclusively shown. He found that the bed-bug does not hibernate where the conditions are such as to allow it to breed and that breeding is continuous unless interrupted by the lack of food or, during the winter, by low temperature.

Bed-bugs ordinarily crawl from their hiding places and attack the face and neck or uncovered parts of the legs and arms of their victims. If undisturbed, they will feed to repletion. We have found that the young nymph would glut itself in about six minutes, though some individuals fed continuously for nine minutes, while the adult required ten to fifteen minutes for a full meal. When gorged, it quickly retreats to a crack or crevice to digest its meal, a process which requires two or three days. The effect of the bite depends very greatly on the susceptibility of the individual attacked. Some persons are so little affected that they may be wholly ignorant of the presence of a large number of bugs. Usually the bite produces a small hard swelling, or wheal, whitish in color. It may even be accompanied by an edema and a disagreeable inflammation, and in such susceptible individuals the restlessness and loss of sleep due to the presence of the insects may be a matter of considerable importance. Stiles (1907) records the case of a young man who underwent treatment for neurasthenia, the diagnosis being agreed upon by several prominent physicians; all symptoms promptly disappeared, however, immediately following a thorough fumigation of his rooms, where nearly a pint of bed-bugs were collected.

It is natural to suppose that an insect which throughout its whole life is in such intimate relationship with man should play an important rôle in the transmission of disease. Yet comparatively little is definitely known regarding the importance of the bed-bug in this respect. It has been shown that it is capable of transmitting the bubonic plague, and South American trypanosomiasis. Nuttall succeeded in transmitting European relapsing fever from mouse to mouse by its bite. It has been claimed that Oriental sore, tuberculosis, and even syphilis may be so carried. These phases of the subject will be considered later.

The sources of infestation are many, and the invasion of a house is not necessarily due to neglect, though the continued presence of the pests is quite another matter. In apartments and closely placed houses they are known to invade new quarters by migration. They are frequently to be met with in boat and sleeper berths, and even the plush seats of day coaches, whence a nucleus may be carried in baggage to residences. They may be brought in the laundry or in clothes of servants.

Usually they are a great scourge in frontier settlements and it is generally believed that they live in nature under the bark of trees, in lumber, and under similar conditions. This belief is founded upon the common occurrence of bugs resembling the bed-bug, in such places. As a matter of fact, they are no relation to bed-bugs but belong to plant-feeding forms alone (fig. 19 c, d).

It is also often stated that bed-bugs live in poultry houses, in swallows nests, and on bats, and that it is from these sources that they gain access to dwellings. These bugs are specifically distinct from the true bed-bug, but any of them may, rarely, invade houses. Moreover, chicken houses are sometimes thoroughly infested with the true *Cimex lectularius*.

Control measures consist in the use of iron bedsteads and the reduction of hiding places for the bugs. If the infestation is slight they may be exterminated by a vigilant and systematic hunt, and by squirting gasoline or alcohol into cracks and crevices of the beds, and furniture. Fumigation must be resorted to in more general infestations.

The simplest and safest method of fumigation is by the use of flowers of sulphur at the rate of two pounds to each one thousand cubic feet of room space. The sulphur should be placed in a pan, a well made in the top of the pile and a little alcohol poured in, to facilitate burning. The whole should be placed in a larger pan and surrounded by water so as to avoid all danger of fire. Windows should be tightly closed, beds, closets and drawers opened, and bedding spread out over chairs in order to expose them fully to the fumes. As metal is tarnished by the sulphur fumes, ornaments, clocks, instruments, and the like should be removed. When all is ready the sulphur should be fired, the room tightly closed and left for twelve to twenty-four hours. Still more efficient in large houses, or where many hiding places favor the bugs, is fumigation with hydrocyanic acid gas. This is a deadly poison and must be used under rigid precautions. Through the courtesy of Professor Herrick, who has had much experience with this method, we give in the Appendix, the clear and detailed directions taken from his bulletin on "Household Insects."

Fumigation with formaldehyde gas, either from the liquid or "solid" formalin, so efficient in the case of contagious diseases, is useless against bed-bugs and most other insects.

**Other Bed-bugs**—*Cimex hemipterus* (= *C. rotundatus*) is a tropical and subtropical species, occurring in both the old and new world. Patton and Cragg state that it is distributed throughout India, Burma, Assam, the Malay Peninsula, Aden, the Island of Mauritius, Reunion, St. Vincent and Porto Rico. "It is widely distributed in Africa, and is probably the common species associated there with man." Brumpt also records it for Cuba, the Antilles, Brazil, and Venezuela.

This species, which is sometimes called the Indian bed-bug, differs from *C. lectularius* in being darker and in having a more elongate abdomen. The head also is shorter and narrower, and the prothorax has rounded borders.

It has the same habits and practically the same life cycle as *Cimex lectularius*. Mackie, in India, has found that it is capable of transmitting the Asiatic type of recurrent fever. Roger suggested that it was also capable of transmitting kala-azar and Patton has described in detail the developmental stages of *Leishmania*, the causative organism of Kala-azar, in the stomach of this bug, but Brumpt declares that the forms described are those of a common, non-pathogenic flagellate to be found in the bug, and have nothing to do with the human disease. Brumpt has shown experimentally that *Cimex hemipterus* may transmit *Trypanosoma cruzi* in its excrement.

*Cimex boueti*, occurring in French Guinea, is another species attacking man. Its habits and general life history are the same as for the above species. It is 3 to 4.5 mm. in length, has vestigial elytra, and much elongated antennæ and legs. The extended hind legs are about as long as the body.

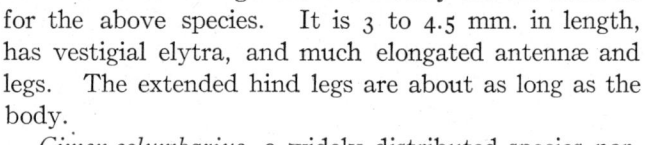

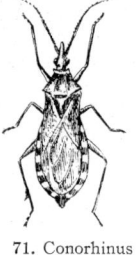

*Cimex columbarius*, a widely distributed species normally living in poultry houses and dove cotes, *C. inodorus*, infesting poultry in Mexico, *C. hirundinis*, occurring in the nests of swallows in Europe and *Oeciacus vicarius* (fig. 191) occurring in swallow's nests in this country, are species which occasionally infest houses and attack man.

71. Conorhinus sanguisugus.

*Conorhinus sanguisugus*, the cone-nosed bed-bug. We have seen in our consideration of poisonous insects, that various species of Reduviid bugs readily attack man. Certain of these are nocturnal and are so commonly found in houses that they have gained the name, of "big bed-bugs." The most noted of these, in the United States, is *Conorhinus sangiusugus* (fig. 71), which is widely distributed in our Southern States.

Like its near relatives, *Conorhinus sangiusugus* is carnivorous in habit and feeds upon insects as well as upon mammalian and human blood. It is reported as often occurring in poultry houses and as attacking horses in barns. The life history has been worked out in considerable detail by Marlatt, (1902), from whose account we extract the following.

The eggs are white, changing to yellow and pink before hatching. The young hatch within twenty days and there are four nymphal stages.

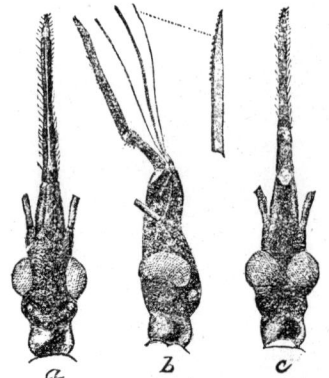

72. Beak of Conorhinus sanguisugus. After Marlatt.

In all these stages the insect is active and predaceous, the mouth-parts (fig. 72) being powerfully developed. The eggs are normally deposited, and the early stages are undoubtedly passed, out of doors, the food of the immature forms being other insects. Immature specimens are rarely found indoors. It winters both in the partly grown and adult stage, often under the bark of trees or in any similar protection, and only in its nocturnal spring and early summer flights does it attack men. Marlatt states that this insect seems to be decidedly on the increase in the region which it particularly infests,—the plains region from Texas northward and westward. In California a closely related species of similar habits is known locally as the "monitor bug."

The effect of the bite of the giant bed-bug on man is often very severe, a poisonous saliva apparently being injected into the wound. We have discussed this phase of the subject more fully under the head of poisonous insects.

*Conorhinus megistus* is a Brazilian species very commonly attacking man, and of special interest since Chagas has shown that it is the carrier of a trypanosomiasis of man. Its habits and life history have been studied in detail by Neiva, (1910).

This species is now pre-eminently a household insect, depositing its eggs in cracks and crevices in houses, though this is a relatively recent adaptation. The nymphs emerge in from twenty to forty days, depending upon the temperature. There are five nymphal stages, and as in the case of true bed-bugs, the duration of these is very greatly influenced by the availability of food and by temperature. Neiva reckons the entire life cycle, from egg to egg, as requiring a minimum of three hundred and twenty-four days.

The nymphs begin to suck blood in three to five days after hatching. They usually feed at night and in the dark, attacking especially the face of sleeping individuals. The bite occasions but little pain. The immature insects live in cracks and crevices in houses and invade the beds which are in contact with walls, but the adults are active flyers and attack people sleeping in hammocks. The males as well as the females are blood suckers.

Like many blood-sucking forms, *Conorhinus megistus* can endure for long periods without food. Neiva received a female specimen which had been for fifty-seven days alive in a tightly closed box. They rarely feed on two consecutive days, even on small quantities of blood, and were never seen to feed on three consecutive days.

Methods of control consist in screening against the adult bugs, and the elimination of crevices and such hiding places of the nymphs. Where the infestation is considerable, fumigation with sulphur is advisable.

## Parasitic Diptera or Flies

Of the **Diptera** or two-winged flies, many species occasionally attack man. Of these, a few are outstanding pests, many of them may also serve to disseminate disease, a phase of our subject which will be considered later. We shall now consider the most important of the group from the viewpoint of their direct attacks on man.

### Psychodidæ or Moth-Flies

The **Psychodidæ** or Moth-flies, include a few species which attack man, and at least one species, *Phlebotomus papatasii*, is known to transmit the so-called "three-day fever" of man. Another species is supposed to be the vector of Peruvian verruga.

The family is made up of small, sometimes very small, nematocerous Diptera, which are densely covered with hairs, giving them a moth-like appearance. The wings are relatively large, oval or lanceolate in shape, and when at rest are held in a sloping manner over the abdomen, or are held horizontally in such a way as to give the insect a triangular outline. Not only is the moth-like appearance characteristic, but the venation of the wings (fig. 163, d) is very peculiar and, according to Comstock, presents an extremely generalized form. All of the longitudinal veins separate near the base of the wing except veins $R_2$ and $R_3$ and veins $M_1$ and $M_2$. Cross veins are wanting in most cases.

Comparatively little is known regarding the life-history and habits of the Psychodidæ, but one genus, *Phlebotomus*, contains minute, blood-sucking species, commonly known as sand-flies. The family is divided into two subfamilies, the **Psychodinæ** and the **Phlebotominæ**. The second of these, the **Phlebotominæ**, is of interest to us.

**The Phlebotominæ**—The Phlebotominæ differ from the Psychodinæ in that the radical sector branches well out into the wing rather than at the base of the wing. They are usually less hairy than the Psychodinæ. The ovipositor is hidden and less strongly chitinized. The species attacking man belong to the genus *Phlebotomus*, small forms with relatively large, hairy wings which are held upright, and with elongate proboscis. The mandibles and maxillæ are serrated and fitted for biting.

According to Miss Summers (1913) there are twenty-nine known species of the genus *Phlebotomus*, five European, eleven Asiatic, seven African and six American. One species only, *Phlebotomus vexator*, has been reported for the United States. This was described by Coquillett, (1907), from species taken on Plummer's Island, Maryland. It measures only 1.5 mm. in length. As it is very probable that this species is much more widely distributed, and that other species of these minute flies will be found to occur in our fauna, we quote Coquillett's description.

*Phlebotomus vexator*, Coq.: Yellow, the mesonotum brown, hairs chiefly brown; legs in certain lights appear brown, but are covered with a white tomentum; wings hyaline, unmarked; the first vein ($R_1$) terminates opposite one-fifth of the length of the first submarginal cell (cell $R_2$); this cell is slightly over twice as long as its petiole; terminal, horny portion of male claspers slender, bearing many long hairs; the apex terminated by two curved spines which are more than one-half as long as the preceding part, and just in front of these are two similar spines, while near the middle of the length of this portion is a fifth spine similar to the others. Length 1.5 mm.

The life-history of the Phlebotomus flies has been best worked out for the European *Phlebotomus papatasii* and we shall briefly summarize the account of Dœrr and Russ (1913) based primarily on work on this species. The European Phlebotomus flies appear at the beginning of the warm season, a few weeks after the cessation of the heavy rains and storms of springtime. They gradually become more abundant until they reach their first maximum, which in Italy is near the end of July (Grassi). They then become scarcer but reach a second maximum in September. At the beginning of winter they vanish completely, hibernating individuals not being found.

After fertilization there is a period of eight to ten days before oviposition. The eggs are then deposited, the majority in a single mass covered by a slimy secretion from the sebaceous glands. The larvæ emerge in fourteen to twenty days. There is uncertainty as to the length of larval life, specimens kept in captivity remaining fifty or more days without transforming. Growth may be much more rapid in nature. The larvæ do not live in fluid media but in moist detritus in dark places. Marett believes that they live chiefly on the excrement of pill-bugs (Oniscidæ) and lizards. Pupation always occurs during the night. The remnants of the larval skin remain attached to the last two segments of the quiescent pupa and serve to attach it to the stone on which it lives. The pupal stage lasts eleven to sixteen days, the adult escaping at night.

Only the females suck blood. They attack not only man but all warm-blooded animals and, according to recent workers, also cold-blooded forms, such as frogs, lizards, and larvæ. Indeed, Townsend (1914) believes that there is an intimate relation between *Phlebotomus* and lizards, or other reptiles the world over. The Phlebotomus passes the daylight hours within the darkened recesses of the loose stone walls and piles of rock in order to escape wind and strong light. Lizards inhabit the same places, and the flies, always ready to suck blood in the absence of light and wind, have been found more prone to suck reptilian than mammalian blood.

On hot summer nights, when the wind is not stirring, the Phlebotomus flies, or sand-flies, as they are popularly called, invade houses and sleeping rooms in swarms and attack the inmates. As soon as light begins to break the flies either escape to the breeding places, or cool, dark places protected from the wind, or a part of them remain in the rooms, hiding behind pictures, under garments, and in similar places. Wherever the Phlebotomus flies occur they are an intolerable nuisance. On account of their small size they can easily pass through the meshes of ordinary screens and mosquito curtains. They attack silently and inflict a very painful, stinging bite, followed by itching. The ankles, dorsum of the feet, wrists, inner elbow, knee joint and similar places are favorite places of attack, possibly on account of their more delicate skin.

Special interest has been attracted to these little pests in recent years, since it has been shown that they transmit the European "pappataci fever" or "three day fever." More recently yet, it appears that they are the carriers of the virus of the Peruvian "verruga." This phase of the subject will be discussed later.

Control measures have not been worked out. As Newstead says, "In consideration of the facts which have so far been brought to light regarding the economy of Phlebotomus, it is clearly evident that the task of suppressing these insects is an almost insurmountable one. Had we to deal with insects as large and as accessible as mosquitoes. the adoption of prophylactic measures would be comparatively easy, but owing to the extremely minute size and almost flea-like habits of the adult insects, and the enormous area over which the breeding-places may occur, we are faced with a problem which is most difficult of solution." For these reasons, Newstead considers that the only really prophylactic measures which can at present be taken, are those which are considered as precautionary against the bites of the insects.

Of repellents, he cites as one of the best a salve composed of the following:

| | |
|---|---|
| Ol. Anisi | 3 grs. |
| Ol. Eucalypti | 3 grs. |
| Ol. Terebenth. | 3 grs. |
| Unq. Acid Borac. | |

Of sprays he recommends as the least objectionable and at the same time one of the most effective, formalin. "The dark portions and angles of sleeping apartments should be sprayed with a one per cent. solution of this substance every day during the season in which the flies are prevalent. A fine spraying apparatus is necessary for its application and an excessive amount must not be applied. It is considered an excellent plan also to spray the mosquito curtains regularly every day towards sunset; nets thus treated are claimed to repel the attacks of these insects." This effectiveness of formalin is very surprising for, as we have seen, it is almost wholly ineffective against bed-bugs, mosquitoes, house flies and other insects, where it has been tried.

A measure which promises to be very effective, where it can be adopted, is the use of electric fans so placed as to produce a current of air in the direction of the windows of sleeping apartments. On account of the inability of the Phlebotomus flies to withstand even slight breezes, it seems very probable that they would be unable to enter a room so protected.

## Culicidæ or Mosquitoes

From the medical viewpoint, probably the most interesting and important of the blood-sucking insects are the mosquitoes. Certainly this is true of temperate zones, such as those of the United States. The result is that no other group of insects has aroused such widespread interest, or has been subjected to more detailed study than have the mosquitoes, since their rôle as carriers of disease was made known. There is an enormous literature dealing with the group, but fortunately for the general student, this has been well summarized by a number of workers. The most important and helpful of the general works are those of Howard (1901), Smith (1904), Blanchard (1905), Mitchell (1907), and especially of Howard, Dyar, and Knab, whose magnificent monograph is still in course of publication.

Aside from their importance as carriers of disease, mosquitoes are notorious as pests of man, and the earlier literature on the group is largely devoted to references to their enormous numbers and their blood-thirstiness in certain regions. They are to be found in all parts of the world, from the equator to the Arctic and Antarctic regions. Linnæus, in the "Flora Lapponica," according to Howard, Dyar and Knab, "dwells at some length upon the great abundance of mosquitoes in Lapland and the torments they inflicted upon man and beast. He states that he believes that nowhere else on earth are they found in such abundance and he compares their numbers to the dust of the earth. Even in the open, you cannot draw your breath without having your mouth and nostrils filled with them; and ointments of tar and cream or of fish grease are scarcely sufficient to protect even the case-hardened cuticle of the Laplander from their bite. Even in their cabins, the natives cannot take a mouthful of food or lie down to sleep unless they are fumigated almost to suffocation." In some parts of the Northwestern and Southwestern United States it is necessary to protect horses working in the fields by the use of sheets or burlaps, against the ferocious attacks of these insects. It is a surprising fact that even in the dry deserts of the western United States they sometimes occur in enormous numbers.

Until comparatively recent years, but few species of mosquitoes were known and most of the statements regarding their life-history were based upon the classic work of Reaumur (1738) on the biology of the rain barrel mosquito, *Culex pipiens*. In 1896, Dr. Howard refers to twenty-one species in the United States, now over fifty are known; Giles, in 1900, gives a total of two hundred and forty-two for the world fauna, now over seven hundred species are known. We have found eighteen species at Ithaca, N. Y.

All of the known species of mosquitoes are aquatic in the larval stage, but in their life-histories and habits such great differences occur that we now know that it is not possible to select any one species as typical of the group. For our present purpose we shall first discuss the general characteristics and structure of mosquitoes, and shall then give the life-history of a common species, following this by a brief consideration of some of the more striking departures from what have been supposed to be the typical condition.

The **Culicidæ** are slender, nematocerous Diptera with narrow wings, antennæ plumose in the males, and usually with the proboscis much longer than the head, slender, firm and adapted for piercing in the female. The most characteristic feature is that the margins of the wings and, in most cases, the wing veins possess a fringe of scale-like hairs. These may also cover in part, or entirely, the head, thorax, abdomen and legs. The females, only, suck blood.

On account of the importance of the group in this country and the desirability of the student being able to determine material in various stages, we show in the accompanying figures the characters most used in classification.

The larvæ (fig. 73) are elongate, with the head and thorax sharply distinct. The larval antennæ are prominent, consisting of a single cylindrical and sometimes curved segment. The outer third is often narrower and bears at its base a fan-shaped tuft of hairs, the arrangement and abundance of which is of systematic importance. About the mouth are the so-called rotary mouth brushes, dense masses of long hairs borne by the labrum and having the function of sweeping food into the mouth. The form and arrangement of thoracic, abdominal, and anal tufts of hair vary in different species and present characteristics of value. On either side of the eighth abdominal segment is a patch of scales varying

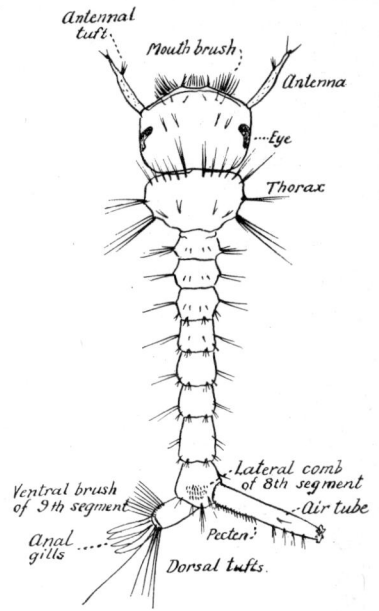

73. Culex larva showing details of external structure.

greatly in arrangement and number and of much value in separating species. Respiration is by means of tracheæ which open at the apex of the so-called anal siphon, when it is present. In addition, there are also one or two pairs of tracheal gills which vary much in appearance in different species. On the ventral side of the anal siphon is a double row of flattened, toothed spines whose number and shape are likewise of some value in separating species. They constitute the comb or pecten.

The pupa (fig. 139,b) unlike that of most insects, is active, though it takes no food. The head and thorax are not distinctly separated, but the slender flexible abdomen in sharply marked off. The antennæ, mouth-parts, legs, and wings of the future adult are now external, but enclosed in chitinous cases. On the upper surface, near the base of the wings are two trumpets, or breathing tubes, for the pupal spiracles are towards the anterior end instead of at the caudal end, as in the larva. At the tip of the abdomen is a pair of large chitinous swimming paddles.

As illustrative of the life cycle of a mosquito we shall discuss the development of a common house mosquito, *Culex pipiens*, often referred to in the Northern United States as the rain barrel mosquito. Its life cycle is often given as typical for the entire group, but, as we have already emphasized, no one species can serve this purpose.

The adults of *Culex pipiens* hibernate throughout the winter in cellars, buildings, hollow trees, or similar dark shelters. Early in the spring they emerge and deposit their eggs in a raft-like mass. The number of eggs in a single mass is in the neighborhood of two hundred, recorded counts varying considerably. A single female may deposit several masses during her life time. The duration of the egg stage is dependent upon temperature. In the warm summer time the larvæ may emerge within a day. The larvæ undergo four molts and under optimum conditions may transform into pupæ in about a week's time. Under the same favorable conditions, the pupal stage may be completed in a day's time. The total life cycle of *Culex pipiens*, under optimum conditions, may thus be completed in a week to ten days. This period may be considerably extended under less favorable conditions of temperature and food supply.

*Culex pipiens* breeds continuously throughout the summer, developing in rain barrels, horse troughs, tin cans, or indeed, in any standing water about houses, which lasts for a week or more. The catch basins of sewers furnish an abundant supply of the pests under some conditions. Such places, the tin gutters on residences, and all possible breeding places must be considered in attempts to exterminate this species.

Other species of mosquitoes may exhibit radical departures from *Culex pipiens* in life-history and habits. To control them it is essential that the biological details be thoroughly worked out for, as Howard, Dyar, and Knab have emphasized, "much useless labor and expense can be avoided by an accurate knowledge of the habits of the species." For a critical discussion of the known facts the reader is referred to their monograph. We shall confine ourselves to a few illustrations.

The majority of mosquitoes in temperate climates hibernate in the egg stage, hatching in the spring or even mild winter days in water from melting snow. It is such single-brooded species which appear in astounding numbers in the far North. Similarly, in dry regions the eggs may stand thorough dessication, and yet hatch out with great promptness when submerged by the rains. "Another provision to insure the species against destruction in such a case, exists in the fact * * * that not all the eggs hatch, a part of them lying over until again submerged by subsequent rains." In temperate North America, a few species pass the winter in the larval state. An interesting illustration of this is afforded by *Wyeomia smithii*, whose larvæ live in pitcher plants and are to be found on the coldest winter days imbedded in the solid ice. Late in the spring, the adults emerge and produce several broods during the summer.

In the United States, one of the most important facts which has been brought out by the intensive studies of recent years is that certain species are migratory and that they can travel long distances and become an intolerable pest many miles from their breeding places. This was forcibly emphasized in Dr. Smith's work in New Jersey, when he found that migratory mosquitoes, developing in the salt marshes along the coast, are the dominant species largely responsible for the fame of the New Jersey mosquito. The species concerned are *Aedes sollicitans*, *A. cantator* and *A. tæniorhynchus*. Dr. Smith decided that the first of these might migrate at least forty miles inland. It is obvious that where such species are the dominant pest, local control measures are a useless waste of time and money. Such migratory habits are rare, however, and it is probable that the majority of mosquitoes do not fly any great distance from their breeding places.

While mosquitoes are thought of primarily as a pest of man, there are many species which have never been known to feed upon human or mammalian blood, no matter how favorable the opportunity. According to Howard, Dyar, and Knab, this is true of *Culex territans*, one of the common mosquitoes in the summer months in the Northern United States. There are some species, probably many, in which the females, like the males, are plant feeders. In experimental work, both sexes are often kept alive for long periods by feeding them upon ripe banana, dried fig, raisins, and the like, and in spite of sweeping assertions that mosquitoes must have a meal of blood in order to stimulate the ovaries to development, some of the common blood-sucking species, notably *Culex pipiens*, have been bred repeatedly without opportunity to feed upon blood.

The effect of the bite varies greatly with different species and depends upon the susceptibility of the individual bitten. Some persons are driven almost frantic by the attacks of the pests when their companions seem almost unconscious of any inconvenience. Usually, irritation and some degree of inflammation appear shortly following the bite. Not infrequently a hardened wheal or even a nodule forms, and sometimes scratching leads to secondary infection and serious results.

The source of the poison is usually supposed to be the salivary glands of the insect. As we have already pointed out, (p. 34), Macloskie believed that one lobe of the gland, on each side, was specialized for forming the poison, while a radically different view is that of Schaudinn, who believed that the irritation is due to the expelled contents of the œsophageal diverticula, which contain a gas and a peculiar type of fungi or bacteria. In numerous attempts, Schaudinn was unable to produce any irritation by applying the triturated salivary glands to a wound, but obtained the typical result when he used the isolated diverticula.

The irritation of the bite may be relieved to some extent by using ammonia water, a one per cent. alcoholic solution of menthol, or preparations of cresol, or carbolic acid. Dr. Howard recommends rubbing the bite gently with a piece of moist toilet soap. Castellani and Chalmers recommend cleansing inflamed bites with one in forty carbolic lotion, followed by dressing with boracic ointment. Of course, scratching should be avoided as much as possible.

Repellents of various kinds are used, for warding off the attacks of the insects. We have often used a mixture of equal parts of oil of pennyroyal and kerosene, applied to the hands and face. Oil of citronella is much used and is less objectionable to some persons. A recommended formula is, oil of citronella one ounce, spirits of camphor one ounce, oil of cedar one-half ounce. A last resort would seem to be the following mixture recommended by Howard, Dyar, and Knab for use by hunters and fishermen in badly infested regions, against mosquitoes and blackflies.

Take 2¼ lbs. of mutton tallow and strain it. While still hot add ½ lb. black tar (Canadian tar). Stir thoroughly and pour into the receptacle in which it is to be contained. When nearly cool stir in three ounces of oil of citronella and 1¼ oz. of pennyroyal.

At night the surest protection is a good bed net. There are many types of these in use, but in order to be serviceable and at the same time comfortable it should be roomy and hung in such a way as to be stretched tightly in every direction. We prefer one suspended from a broad, square frame, supported by a right-angled standard which is fastened to the head of the bed. It must be absolutely free from rents or holes and tucked in securely under the mattress or it will serve merely as a convenient cage to retain mosquitoes which gain an entrance. While such nets are a convenience in any mosquito riden community, they are essential in regions where disease-carrying species abound. Screening of doors, windows and porches, against the pests is so commonly practiced in this country that its importance and convenience need hardly be urged.

Destruction of mosquitoes and prevention of breeding are of fundamental importance. Such measures demand first, as we have seen, the correct determination of the species which is to be dealt with, and a knowledge of its life-history and habits. If it prove to be one of the migratory forms, it is beyond mere local effort and becomes a problem demanding careful organization and state control. An excellent illustration of the importance and effectiveness of work along these lines is afforded by that in New Jersey, begun by the late Dr. John B. Smith and being pushed with vigor by his successor, Dr. Headlee.

In any case, there is necessity for community action. Even near the coast, where the migratory species are dominant, there are the local species which demand attention and which cannot be reached by any measures directed against the species of the salt marshes. The most important of local measures consist in the destruction of breeding places by filling or draining ponds and pools, clearing up of more temporary breeding places, such as cans, pails, water barrels and the like. Under conditions where complete drainage of swamps is impracticable or undesirable, judicious dredging may result in a pool or series of steep-sided pools deep enough to maintain a supply of fish, which will keep down the mosquito larvæ. Where water receptacles are needed for storage of rain water, they should be protected by careful screening or a film of kerosene over the top of the water, renewed every two weeks or so, so as to prevent mosquitoes from depositing their eggs. When kerosene is used, water drawn from the bottom of the receptacle will not be contaminated by it to any injurious extent. Where ponds cannot be drained much good will be accomplished by spraying kerosene oil on the surface of the water, or by the introduction of fish which will feed on the larvæ.

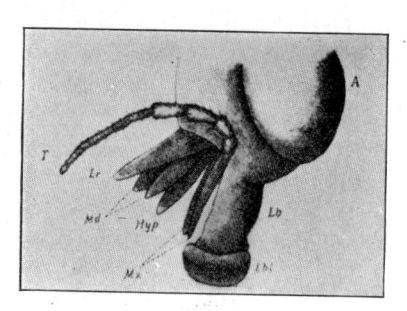

Detailed consideration of the most efficient measures for controlling mosquitoes is to be found in Dr. Howard's Bulletin No. 88 of the Bureau of Entomology, "Preventive and remedial work against mosquitoes" or, in more summarized form, in Farmers' Bulletin No. 444. One of these should be obtained by any person interested in the problems of mosquito control and public health.

74. Mouth parts of Simulium. After Grünberg.

### The Simuliidæ, or Black Flies

The **Simuliidæ,** or black flies, are small, dark, or black flies, with a stout body and a hump-back appearance. The antennæ are short but eleven-segmented, the wings broad, without scales or hairs, and with the anterior veins stout but the others very weak. The mouthparts (fig. 74) are fitted for biting.

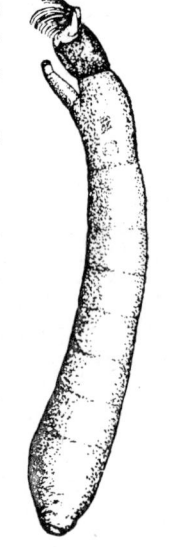

The larvæ of the Simuliidæ (fig. 75) are aquatic and, unlike those of mosquitoes, require a well ærated, or swiftly running water. Here they attach to stones, logs, or vegetation and feed upon various microorganisms. They pupate in silken cocoons open at the top. Detailed life-histories have not been worked out for most of the species. We shall consider as typical that of *Simulium pictipes*, an inoffensive species widely distributed in the Eastern United States, which has been studied especially at Ithaca, N.Y. (Johannsen, 1903).

The eggs are deposited in a compact yellowish layer on the surface of rock, on the brinks of falls and rapids where the water is flowing swiftly. They are elongate ellipsoidal in shape, about .4 by .18 mm. As myriads of females deposit in the same place the egg patches may be conspicuous coatings of a foot or much more in diameter. When first laid they are enveloped in a yellowish

75. Larva of Simulium, (x8). After Garman.

white slime, which becomes darker, until finally it becomes black just before the emerging of the larvæ. The egg stage lasts a week.

The larvæ (fig. 75) are black, soft skinned, somewhat cylindrical in shape, enlarged at both ends and attenuated in the middle. The posterior half is much stouter than the anterior part and almost club-shaped. The head bears two large fan-shaped organs which aid in procuring food. Respiration is accomplished by means of three so-called blood gills which are pushed out from the dorsal part of the rectum. The larvæ occur in enormous numbers, in moss-like patches. If removed from their natural habitat and placed in quiet water they die within three or four hours. Fastened to the rock by means of a disk-like sucker at the caudal end of the body, they ordinarily assume an erect position. They move about on the surface of the rocks, to a limited extent, with a looping gait similar to that of a measuring worm, and a web is secreted which prevents their being washed away by the swiftly flowing water. They feed chiefly upon algæ and diatoms.

The complete larval stage during the summer months occupies about four weeks, varying somewhat with the temperature and velocity of the water. At the end of this period they spin from cephalic glands, boot-shaped

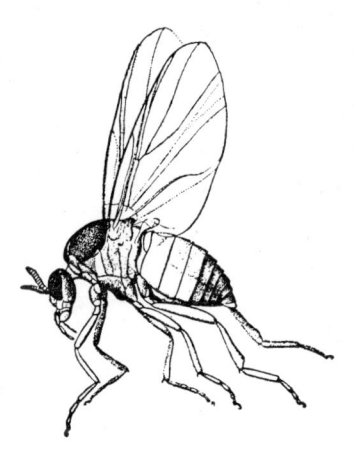

76. Simulium venustum, (x8). After Garman.

silken cocoons within which they pupate. The cocoon when spun is firmly attached to the rock and also to adjacent cocoons. Clustered continuously over a large area and sometimes one above another, they form a compact, carpet-like covering on the rocks, the reddish-brown color of which is easily distinguishable from the jet-black appearance of the larvæ. The pupal stage lasts about three weeks. The adult fly, surrounded by a bubble of air, quickly rises to the surface of the water and escapes. The adults (fig. 76) are apparently short lived and thus the entire life cycle, from egg to egg is completed in approximately eight weeks.

In the case of *Simulium pictipes* at Ithaca, N. Y., the first brood of adults emerges early in May and successive generations are produced throughout the summer and early autumn. This species winters in the larval condition. Most of the other species of *Simulium* which have been studied seem to be single brooded.

While *Simulium pictipes* does not attack man, there are a number of the species which are blood-sucking and in some regions they are a veritable scourge. In recent years the greatest interest in the group has been aroused by Sambon's hypothesis that they transmit pellagra from man to man. This has not been established, and, indeed, seems very doubtful, but the importance of these insects as pests and the possibility that they may carry disease make it urgent that detailed life-histories of the hominoxious species be worked out.

As pests a vivid account of their attacks is in Agassiz's "Lake Superior" (p. 61), quoted by Forbes (1912).

"Neither the love of the picturesque, however, nor the interests of science, could tempt us into the woods, so terrible were the black flies. This pest of flies which all the way hither had confined our ramblings on shore pretty closely to the rocks and the beach, and had been growing constantly worse, here reached its climax. Although detained nearly two days, * * * we could only sit with folded hands, or employ ourselves in arranging specimens, and such other operations as could be pursued in camp, and under the protection of a 'smudge.' One, whom scientific ardor tempted a little way up the river in a canoe, after water plants, came back a frightful spectacle, with blood-red rings round his eyes, his face bloody, and covered with punctures. The next morning his head and neck were swollen as if from an attack of erysipelas."

There are even well authenticated accounts on record of death of humans from the attacks of large swarms of these gnats. In some regions, and especially in the Mississippi Valley in this country, certain species of black flies have been the cause of enormous losses to farmers and stockmen, through their attacks on poultry and domestic animals. C. V. Riley states that in 1874 the loss occasioned in one county in Tennessee was estimated at $500,000.

The measures of prevention and protection against these insects have been well summarized by Forbes (1912). They are of two kinds: "the use of repellents intended to drive away the winged flies, and measures for the local destruction of the aquatic larvæ. The repellents used are either smudges, or surface applications made to keep the flies from biting. The black-fly will not endure a dense smoke, and the well-known mosquito smudge seems to be ordinarily sufficient for the protection of man. In the South, leather, cloth, and other materials which will make the densest and most stifling smoke, are often preserved for this use in the spring. Smudges are built in pastures for the protection of stock, and are kept burning before the doors of barns and stables. As the black-flies do not readily enter a dark room, light is excluded from stables as much as possible during the gnat season. If teams must be used in the open field while gnats are abroad, they may be protected against the attacks of the gnats by applying cotton-seed oil or axle grease to the surface, especially to the less hairy parts of the animals, at least twice a day. A mixture of oil and tar and, indeed, several other preventives, are of practical use in badly infested regions; but no definite test or exact comparison has been made with any of them in a way to give a record of the precise results."

"It is easy to drive the flies from houses or tents by burning pyrethrum powder inside; this either kills the flies or stupifies them so that they do not bite for some time thereafter." * * * "Oil of tar is commonly applied to the exposed parts of the body for the purpose of repelling the insects, and this preparation is supplied by the Hudson Bay Company to its employees. Minnesota fishermen frequently grease their faces and hands with a mixture of kerosene and mutton tallow for the same purpose." We have found a mixture of equal parts of kerosene and oil of pennyroyal efficient.

Under most circumstances very little can be done to destroy this insect in its early stage, but occasionally conditions are such that a larvicide can be used effectively. Weed (1904), and Sanderson (1910) both report excellent results from the use of phinotas oil, a proprietary compound. The first-mentioned also found that in some places the larvæ could be removed by sweeping them loose in masses with stiff stable brooms and then catching them downstream on wire netting stretched in the water.

## Chironomidæ or Midges

The flies of this family, commonly known as midges, resemble mosquitoes in form and size but are usually more delicate, and the wing-veins, though sometimes hairy, are not fringed with scales. The venation is simpler than in the mosquitoes and the veins are usually less distinct.

These midges, especially in spring or autumn, are often seen in immense swarms arising like smoke over swamps and producing a humming noise which can be heard for a considerable distance. At these seasons they are frequently to be found upon the windows of dwellings, where they are often mistaken for mosquitoes.

The larvæ are worm-like, but vary somewhat in form in the different genera. Most of them are aquatic, but a few live in the earth, in manure, decaying wood, under bark, or in the sap of trees, especially in the sap which collects in wounds.

Of the many species of **Chironomidæ,** (over eight hundred known), the vast majority are inoffensive. The sub-family Ceratopogoninæ, however, forms an exception, for some of the members of this group,

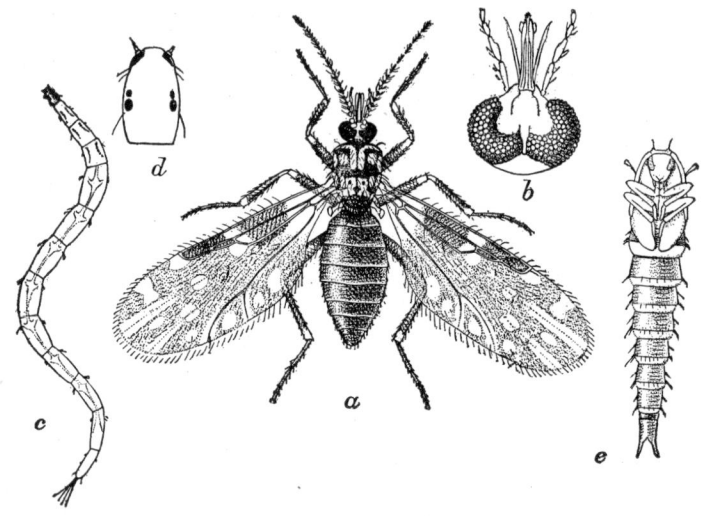

77. Culicoides guttipennis; (*a*) adult, (x 15); (*b*) head of same; (*c*) larva; (*d*) head; (*e*) pupa. After Pratt.

known as sandflies, or punkies, suck blood and are particularly troublesome in the mountains, along streams, and at the seashore. Most of these have been classed under the genus *Ceratopogon*, but the group has been broken up into a number of genera and *Ceratopogon*, in the strict sense, is not known to contain any species which sucks the blood of vertebrates.

**The Ceratopogoninæ**—The Ceratopogoninæ are among the smallest of the Diptera, many of them being hardly a millimeter long and some not even so large. They are Chironomidæ in which the thorax is not prolonged over the head. The antennæ are filiform with fourteen (rarely thirteen) segments in both sexes, those of the male being brush-like. The basal segment is enlarged, the last segment never longer than the two preceding combined, while the last five are sub-equal to, or longer than the preceding segment. The legs are relatively stouter than in the other Chironomidæ. The following three genera of this subfamily are best known as blood suckers in this country.

Of the genus *Culicoides* there are many species occurring in various parts of the world. A number are known to bite man and animals and it is probable that all are capable of inflicting injury. In some localities they are called punkies, in others, sand-flies, a name sometimes also applied to the species of *Simulium* and *Phlebotomus*. Owing to their very small size they are known by some tribes of Indians as No-see-ums. The larvæ are found in ponds, pools, water standing in hollow tree stumps, and the like. Though probably living chiefly in fresh water, we have found a species occurring in salt water. The larvæ are small, slender, legless, worm-like creatures (fig. 77c) with small brown head and twelve body segments. The pupæ (fig. 77e) are slender, more swollen at the anterior end and terminating in a forked process. They float nearly motionless in a vertical position, the respiratory tubes in contact with the surface film. The adults are all small, rarely exceeding 2¼ mm. in length. The wings are more or less covered with erect setulæ or hairs and in many species variously spotted and marked with iridescent blotches. The antennæ have fourteen segments, the palpi usually five. The wing venation and mouth-parts are shown in figures 77 and 78. Of the twenty or more species of this genus occurring in the United States the following are known to bite: *C. cinctus, C. guttipennis, C. sanguisuga, C. stellifer, C. variipennis, C. unicolor*.

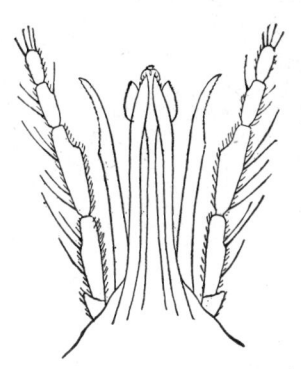

78. Culicoides guttipennis; mouth parts of adult. After Pratt.

One of the most widely distributed and commonest species in the Eastern States is *C. guttipennis* (fig. 77a). It is black with brown legs, a whitish ring before the apex of each femur and both ends of each tibia; tarsi yellow, knobs of halteres yellow. Mesonotum opaque, brown, two vittæ in the middle, enlarging into a large spot on the posterior half, also a curved row of three spots in front of each wing, and the narrow lateral margins, light gray pruinose. Wings nearly wholly covered with brown hairs, gray, with markings as shown in the figure. Length one mm.

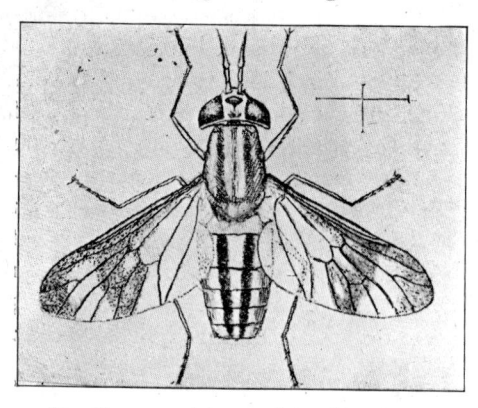

*Johannseniella* Will. is a wide-spread genus related to the foregoing. Its mouth-parts are well adapted for piercing and it is said to be a persistent blood sucker, particularly in Greenland. This genus is distinguished from *Culicoides* by its bare wings, the venation (fig. 163,c), and the longer tarsal claws. There are over twenty North American species.

79. Chrysops univittatus, (x4). After Osborn

In the Southwestern United States, *Tersesthes torrens* Towns. occurs, a little gnat which annoys horses, and perhaps man also, by its bite. It is related to *Culicoides* but differs in the number of antennal segments and in its wing venation (fig. 163,e). The fly measures but two mm. in length and is blackish in color. The antennæ of the female have thirteen segments, the palpi but three, of which the second is enlarged and swollen.

## Tabanidæ or Horse-Flies

The **Tabanidæ**,—horse-flies, ear-flies, and deer-flies,—are well-known pests of cattle and horses and are often extremely annoying to man. The characteristics of the family and of the principal North American genera are given in the keys of Chapter XII. There are over 2500 recorded species. As in the mosquitoes, the females alone are blood suckers. The males are flower feeders or live on plant juices. This is apparently true also of the females of some of the genera.

The eggs are deposited in masses on water plants or grasses and sedges growing in marshy or wet ground. Those of a common species of *Tabanus* are illustrated in figure 80, *a*. They are placed in masses of several hundred, light colored when first deposited but turning black. In a week or so the cylindrical larvæ, tapering at both ends (fig. 80, *b*), escape to the water, or damp earth, and lead

## Tabanidæ, or Horse-flies

an active, carnivorous life, feeding mainly on insect larvæ, and worms. In the forms which have been best studied the larval life is a long one, lasting for months or even for more than a year. Until recently, little was known concerning the life-histories of this group, but the studies of Hart (1895), and Hine (1903 +) have added greatly to the knowledge concerning North American forms.

Many of the species attack man with avidity and are able to inflict painful bites, which may smart for hours. In some instances the wound is so considerable that blood will continue to flow after the fly has left. We have seen several cases of secondary infection following such bites.

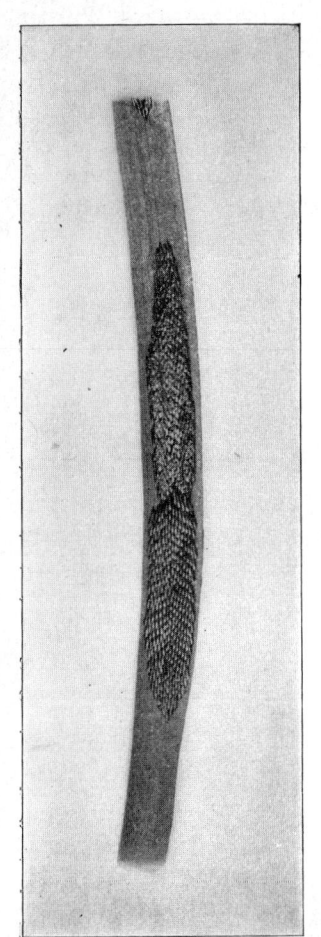

80. (a) Eggs of Tabanus. Photograph by J. T. Lloyd.

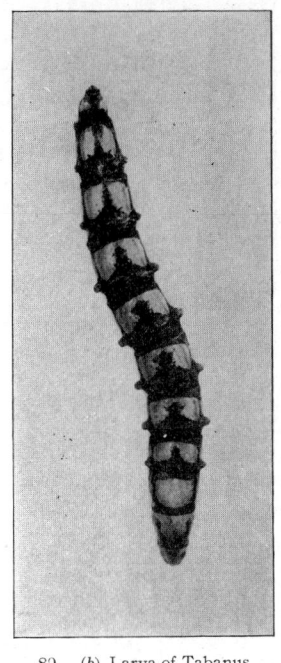

80. (b) Larva of Tabanus. Photograph by M. V. S.

The horse-flies have been definitely convicted of transferring the trypanosome of surra from diseased to healthy animals and there is good evidence that they transfer anthrax. The possibility of their being important agents in the conveyal of human diseases should not be overlooked. Indeed, Leiper has recently determined that a species of *Chrysops* transfers the blood parasite *Filaria diurna*.

## Leptidæ or Snipe-Flies

The family **Leptidæ** is made up of moderate or large sized flies, predaceous in habit. They are sufficiently characterized in the keys of Chapter XII. Four blood-sucking species belonging to three genera have been reported. Of these *Symphoromyia pachyceras* is a western species. Dr. J. C. Bradley, from personal experience, reports it as a vicious biter.

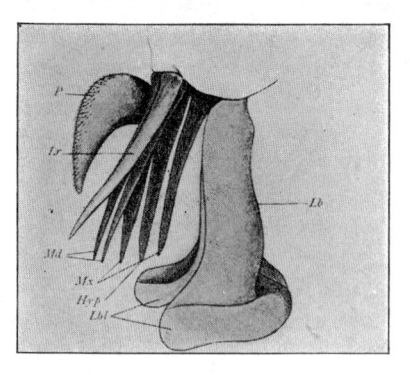

80. (c) Mouth parts of Tabanus. After Grünberg.

## Oestridæ or Bot-flies

To the family **Oestridæ** belong the bot and warble-flies so frequently injurious to animals. The adults are large, or of medium size, heavy bodied, rather hairy, and usually resemble bees in appearance.

The larvæ live parasitically in various parts of the body of mammals, such as the stomach (horse bot-fly), the subcutaneous connective tissue (warble-fly of cattle), or the nasal passage (sheep botfly or head maggot).

There are on record many cases of the occurrence of the larvæ of Oestridæ as occasional parasites of man. A number of these have been collected and reviewed in a thesis by Mme. Pètrovskaia (1910). The majority of them relate to the following species.

*Gastrophilus hæmorrhoidalis*, the red tailed bot-fly, is one of the species whose larvæ are most commonly found in the stomach of the horse. Schoch (1877) cites the case of a woman who suffered from a severe case of chronic catarrh of the stomach, and who vomited, and also passed from the anus, larvæ which apparently belonged to this species. Such cases are exceedingly rare but instances of subcutaneous infestation are fairly numerous. In the latter type these larvæ are sometimes the cause of the peculiar "creeping myasis." This is characterized at its beginning by a very painful swelling which gradually migrates, producing a narrow raised line four to twenty-five millimeters broad. When the larva is mature, sometimes after several months, it becomes stationary and a tumor is formed which opens and discharges the larva along with pus and serum.

*Gastrophilus equi* is the most widespread and common of the horse bot-flies. Portschinsky reports it as commonly causing subcutaneous myasis of man in Russia.

*Hypoderma bovis* (=*Oestrus bovis*), and *Hypoderma lineata* are the so-called warble-flies of cattle. The latter species is the more common in North America but Dr. C. G. Hewitt has recently shown that *H. bovis* also occurs. Though warbles are very common in cattle in this country, the adult flies are very rarely seen. They are about half an inch in length, very hairy, dark, and closely resemble common honey-bees.

They deposit their eggs on the hairs of cattle and the animals in licking themselves take in the young larvæ. These pass out through the walls of the œsophagus and migrate through the tissues of the animal, to finally settle down in the subcutaneous tissue of the back. The possibility of their entering directly through the skin, especially in case of infestation of man, is not absolutely precluded, although it is doubtful.

For both species of *Hypoderma* there are numerous cases on record of their occurrence in man. Hamilton (1893) saw a boy, six years of age, who had been suffering for some months from the glands on one side of his neck being swollen and from a fetid ulceration around the back teeth of the lower jaw of the same side. Three months' treatment was of no avail and the end seemed near; one day a white object, which was seen to move, was observed in the ulcer at the root of the tongue, and on being extracted was recognized as a full grown larva of *Hypoderma*. It was of usual tawny color, about half an inch long when contracted, about one third that thickness, and quite lively. The case resulted fatally. The boy had been on a dairy farm the previous fall, where probably the egg (or *larva*) was in some way taken into his mouth, and the larva found between the base of the tongue and the jaw suitable tissue in which to develop.

Topsent (1901) reports a case of "creeping myasis" caused by *H. lineata* in the skin of the neck and shoulders of a girl eight years of age. The larva travelled a distance of nearly six and a half inches. The little patient suffered excruciating pain in the place occupied by the larva.

*Hypoderma diana* infests deer, and has been known to occur in man.

*Oestris ovis*, the sheep bot-fly, or head maggot, is widely distributed in all parts of the world. In mid-summer the flies deposit living maggots in the nostrils of sheep. These larvæ promptly pass up the nasal passages into the frontal and maxillary sinuses, where they feed on the mucous to be found there. In their migrations they cause great irritation to their host, and when present in numbers may cause vertigo, paroxysms, and even death. Portschinsky in an important monograph on this species, has discussed in detail its relation to man. He shows that it is not uncommon for the fly to attack man and that the minute living larvæ are deposited in the eyes, nostrils, lips, or mouth. A typical case in which the larvæ were deposited in the eye was described by a German oculist Kayser, in 1905. A woman brought her six year old daughter to him and said that the day before, about noontime, a flying insect struck the eye of the child and that since then she had felt a pain which increased towards evening. In the morning the pain ceased but the eye was very red. She was examined at about noon, at which time she was quiet and felt no pain. She was not sensitive to light, and the only thing noticed was a slight congestion and accumulation of secretion in the corner of the right eye. A careful examination of the eye disclosed small, active, white larvæ that crawled out from the folds of the conjunctiva and then back and disappeared. Five of these larvæ were removed and although an uncomfortable feeling persisted for a while, the eye became normal in about three weeks.

Some of the other recorded cases have not resulted so favorably, for the eyesight has been seriously affected or even lost.

According to Edmund and Etienne Sergent (1907), myasis caused by the larvæ of *Oestris ovis* is very common among the shepherds in Algeria. The natives say that the fly deposits its larvæ quickly, while on the wing, without pause. The greatest pain is caused when these larvæ establish themselves in the nasal cavities. They then produce severe frontal headaches, making sleep impossible. This is accompanied by continuous secretion from the nasal cavities and itching pains in the sinuses. If the larvæ happen to get into the mouth, the throat becomes inflamed, swallowing is painful, and sometimes vomiting results. The diseased condition may last for from three to ten days or in the case of nasal infection, longer, but recovery always follows. The natives remove the larvæ from the eye mechanically by means of a small rag. When the nose is infested, tobacco fumigations are applied, and in case of throat infestation gargles of pepper, onion, or garlic extracts are used.

*Rhinœstrus nasalis*, the Russian gad-fly, parasitizes the nasopharyngeal region of the horse. According to Portschinsky, it not infrequently attacks man and then, in all the known cases deposits its larvæ in the eye, only. This is generally done while the person is quiet, but not during sleep. The fly strikes without stopping and deposits its larva instantaneously. Immediately after, the victim experiences lancinating pains which without intermission increase in violence. There is an intense conjunctivitis and if the larvæ are not removed promptly the envelopes of the eye are gradually destroyed and the organ lost.

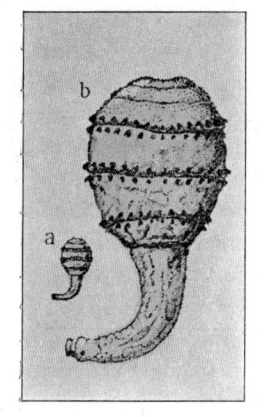

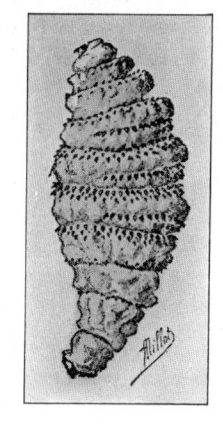

81. Larvæ of Dermatobia cyaniventris. After Blanchard.

*Dermatobia cyaniventris*—This fly (fig. 83) is widely distributed throughout tropical America, and in its larval stage is well known as a parasite of man. The larvæ (figs. 81 and 82) which are known as the "ver macaque," "torcel," "ver moyocuil" or by several other local names, enter the skin and give rise to a boil-like swelling, open at the top, and comparable with the swelling produced by the warble fly larvæ, in cattle. They cause itching and occasional excruciating pain. When mature, nearly an inch in length, they voluntarily leave their host, drop to the ground and complete their development. The adult female is about 12 mm. in length. The face is yellow, the frons black with a grayish bloom; antennæ yellow, the third segment four times as long as the second, the arista pectinate. The thorax is bluish black with grayish bloom; the abdomen depressed, brilliant metallescent blue with violet tinge. The legs are yellowish, the squamæ and wings brownish.

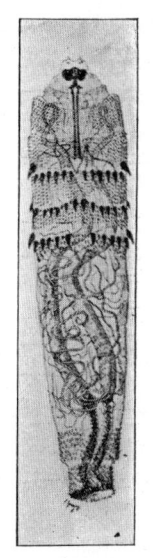

82. Young larva of Dermatobia cyaniventris. After Surcouf.

The different types of larvæ represented in figure 81 were formerly supposed to belong to different species but Blanchard regards them as merely various stages of the same species. It is only very recently that the early stage and the method by which man becomes infested were made known.

About 1900, Blanchard observed the presence of packets of large-sized eggs under the abdomen of certain mosquitoes from Central America; and in 1910, Dr. Moralès, of Costa Rica, declared that the Dermatobia deposited its eggs directly under the abdomen of the mosquito and that they were thus carried to vertebrates.

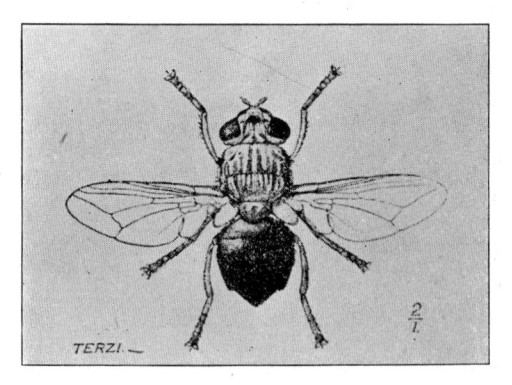

83. Dermatobia cyaniventris (x1¾). After Graham-Smith.

Dr. Nunez Tovar observed the mosquito carriers of the eggs and placing larvæ from this source on animals, produced typical tumors and reared the adult flies. It remained for Surcouf (1913) to work out the full details. He found that the Dermatobia deposits its eggs in packets covered by a very viscid substance, on leaves. These become attached to mosquitoes of the species *Janthinosoma lutzi* (fig. 84) which walk over the leaves. The eggs which adhere to the abdomen, remain attached and are thus transported. The embryo develops, but the young larva (fig. 82) remains in the egg until it has opportunity to drop upon a vertebrate fed upon by the mosquito.

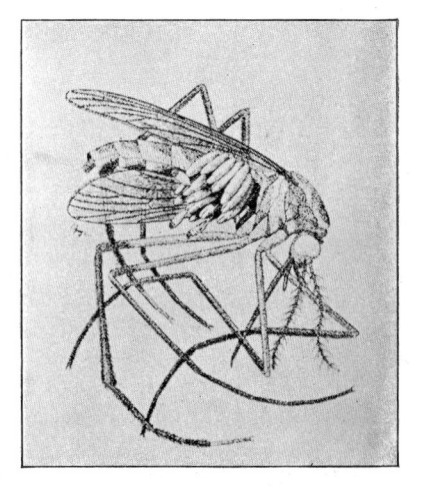

84. Mosquito carrying eggs of Dermatobia cyaniventris. After Surcouf.

## Muscidæ

The following **Muscidæ,** characterized elsewhere, deserve special mention under our present grouping of parasitic species. Other important species will be considered as facultative parasites.

*Stomoxys calcitrans*, the stable-fly, or the biting house-fly, is often confused with *Musca domestica* and therefore is discussed especially in our consideration of the latter species as an accidental carrier of disease. Its possible relation to the spread of infantile paralysis is also considered later.

The *tsetse flies*, belonging to the genus *Glossina*, are African species of blood-sucking Muscidæ which have attracted much attention because of their rôle in transmitting various trypanosome diseases of man and animals. They are characterized in Chapter XII and are also discussed in connection with the diseases which they convey.

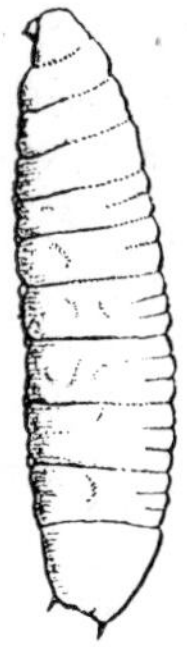

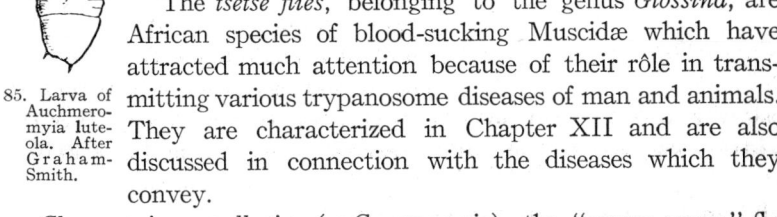

85. Larva of Auchmeromyia luteola. After Graham-Smith.

*Chrysomyia macellaria*, (= *Compsomyia*), the "screw worm"-fly is one of the most important species of flies directly affecting man, in North America. It is not normally parasitic, however, and hence will be considered with other facultative parasites in Chapter IV.

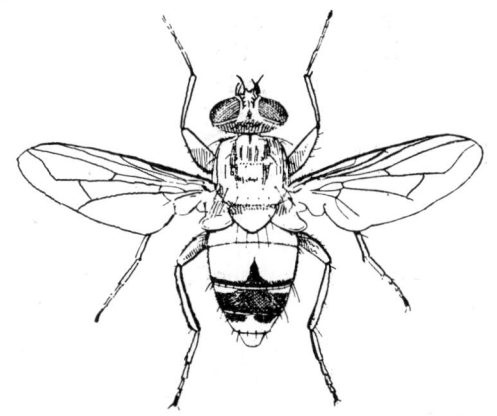

*Auchmeromyia luteola*, the Congo floor maggot. This is a muscid of grewsome habits, which has a wide distribution throughout Africa. The fly (fig. 86) deposits its eggs on the ground of the huts of the natives. The whitish larvæ (fig. 85) on hatching are slightly flattened ventrally, and each segment bears posteriorly three foot-pads transversely arranged.

86. Auchmeromyia luteola (x4). After Graham-Smith.

At night the larvæ find their way into the low beds or couches of the natives and suck their blood. The adult flies do not bite man and, as far as known, the larvæ do not play any rôle in the transmission of sleeping sickness or other diseases.

This habit of blood-sucking by muscid larvæ is usually referred to as peculiar to *Aucheromyia luteola* but it should be noted that the larvæ of *Protocalliphora* frequent the nests of birds and feed upon the young. Mr. A. F. Coutant has studied especially the life-history and habits of *P. azurea*, whose larvæ he found attacking young crows at Ithaca, N. Y. He was unable to induce the larvæ to feed on man.

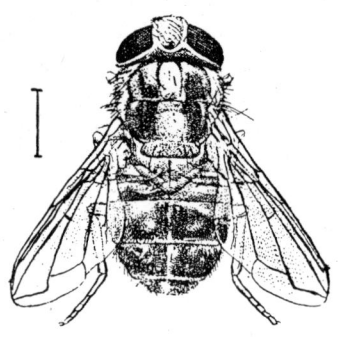

*Cordylobia anthropophaga*, (*Ochromyia anthropophaga*), or Tumbu-fly (fig. 87) is an African species whose larvæ affect man much as do those of *Dermatobia cyniventris*, of Central and South America. The larva (fig. 88), which is known as "ver du Cayor" because it was first observed in Cayor, in Senegambia, develops in the skin of man and of various animals, such as dogs, cats, and monkeys. It is about 12 mm. in length, and of the form of the larvæ of other muscids. Upon the intermediate segments are minute, brownish recurved spines which give to the larva its characteristic appearance. The life-history is not satisfactorily worked out, but Fuller (1914), after reviewing the evidence believes that, as a rule, it deposits its young in the sleeping places of man and animals, whether such be a bed, a board, the floor, or the bare ground. In the case of babies, the maggots may be deposited on the scalp. The minute maggots bore their way painlessly into the skin. As many as forty parasites have been found in one individual and one author has reported finding more than three hundred in a spaniel puppy. Though their attacks are at times extremely painful, it is seldom that any serious results follow.

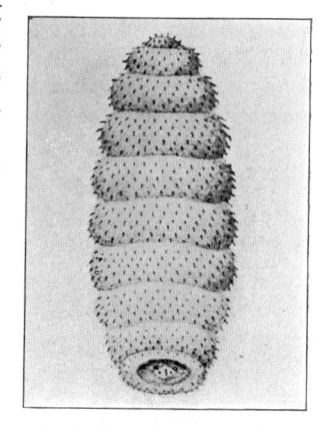

87. Cordylobia anthropophaga (x3). After Fülleborn.

88. Larva of Cordylobia anthropophaga. After Blanchard.

## The Siphonaptera or Fleas

The **Siphonaptera**, or fleas (fig. 89) are wingless insects, with highly chitinized and laterally compressed bodies. The mouth-parts are formed for piercing and sucking. Compound eyes are lacking but some species possess ocelli. The metamorphosis is complete.

This group of parasites, concerning which little was known until recently, has assumed a very great importance since it was learned

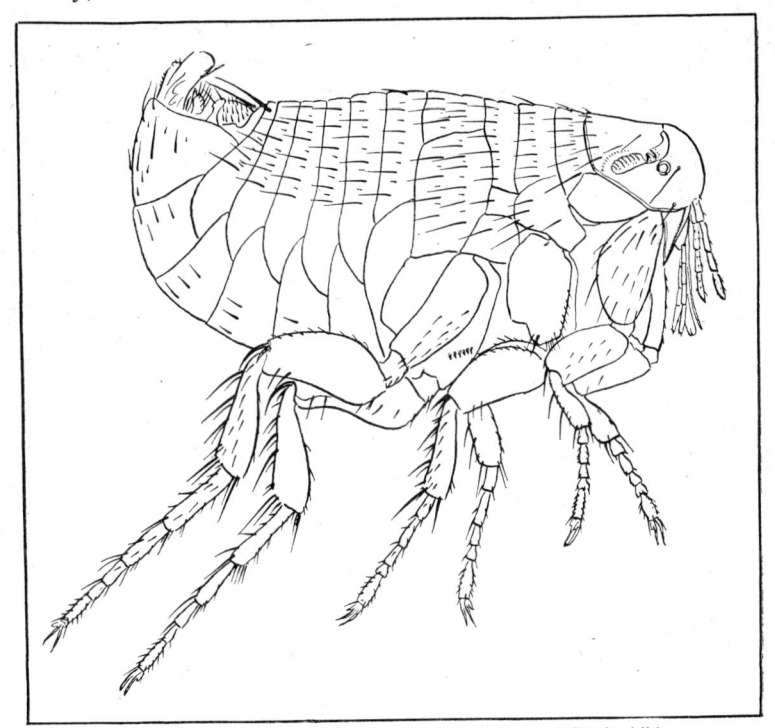

89. Xenopsylla cheopis, male (x25). After Jordan and Rothschild.

that fleas are the carriers of bubonic plague. Now over four hundred species are known. Of these, several species commonly attack man. The most common hominoxious species are *Pulex irritans*, *Xenopsylla cheopis*, *Ctenocephalus canis*, *Ctenocephalus felis*, *Ceratophyllus fasciatus* and *Dermatophilus penetrans*, but many others will feed readily on human blood if occasion arises.

We shall treat in this place of the general biology and habits of the hominoxious forms and reserve for the systematic section the discussion of the characteristics of the different genera.

The most common fleas infesting houses in the Eastern United States are the cosmopolitan dog and cat fleas, *Ctenocephalus canis* (fig. 90) and *C. felis*. Their life cycles will serve as typical. These two species have until recently been considered as one, under the name *Pulex serraticeps*. See figure 92.

The eggs are oval, slightly translucent or pearly white, and measure about .5 mm. in their long diameter. They are deposited loosely in the hairs of the host and readily drop off as the animal moves around. Howard found that these eggs hatch in one to two days. The larvæ are elongate, legless, white, worm-like creatures. They are exceedingly active, and avoid the light in every way possible. They cast their first skin in from three to seven days and their second in from three to four days. They commenced spinning in from seven to fourteen days after hatching and the imago appeared five days later. Thus in summer, at Washington, the entire life cycle may be completed in about two weeks. (cf. fig. 91, 92).

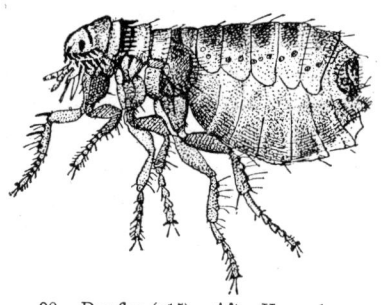

90. Dog flea (x15). After Howard.

Strickland's (1914) studies on the biology of the rat flea, *Ceratophyllus fasciatus*, have so important a general bearing that we shall cite them in considerable detail.

He found, to begin with, that there is a marked inherent range in the rate of development. Thus, of a batch of seventy-three eggs, all laid in the same day and kept together under the same condi-

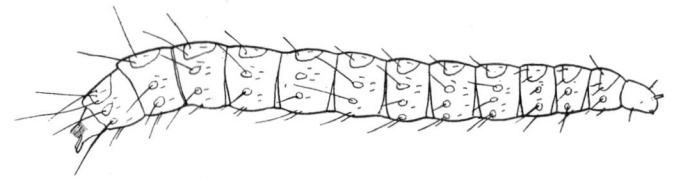

91. Larva of Xenopsylla cheopis. After Bacot and Ridewood.

tions, one hatched in ten days; four in eleven days; twenty-five in twelve days; thirty-one in thirteen days; ten in fourteen days; one in fifteen days; and one in sixteen days. Within these limits the duration of the egg period seems to depend mainly on the degree of humidity. The incubation period is never abnormally prolonged as in the case of lice, (Warburton) and varying conditions of temperature and humidity have practically no effect on the percentage of eggs which ultimately hatch.

The same investigator found that the most favorable condition for the larva is a low temperature, combined with a high degree of humidity; and that the presence of rubbish in which the larva may bury itself is essential to its successful development. When larvæ are placed in a bottle containing either wood-wool soiled by excrement, or with feathers or filter paper covered with dried blood they

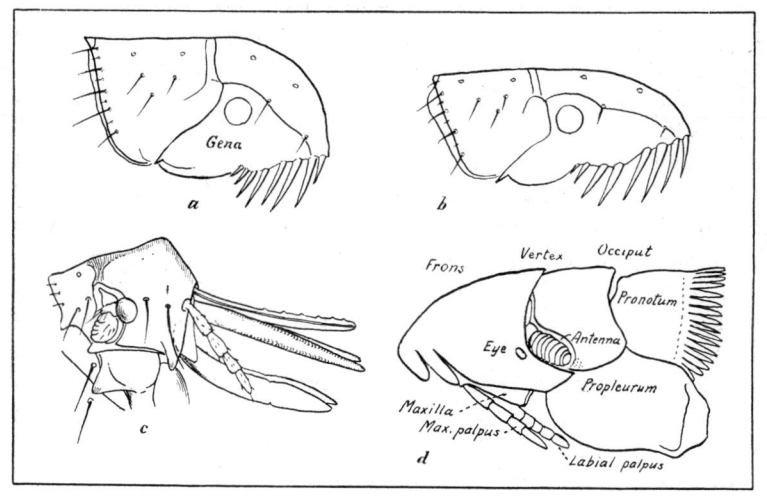

92. Head and pronotum of (*a*) dog flea; (*b*) of cat flea; (*c*) of hen flea. After Rothschild. (*d*) Nycteridiphilus (Ishnopsyllus) hexactenus. After Oudemans.

will thrive readily and pupate. They seem to have no choice between dried blood and powdered rat feces for food, and also feed readily on flea excrement. They possess the curious habit of always devouring their molted skins.

An important part of Strickland's experiments dealt with the question of duration of the pupal stage under the influence of temperature and with the longevity and habits of the adult. In October, he placed a batch of freshly formed cocoons in a small dish that was kept near a white rat in a deep glass jar in the laboratory. Two months later one small and feeble flea had emerged, but no more until February, four months after the beginning of the experiment. Eight cocoons were then dissected and seven more found to contain the imago fully formed but in a resting state. The remainder of the batch was then placed at 70° F. for one night, near a white rat. The next day all the cocoons were empty and the fleas were found on the white rat.

Thus, temperature greatly influences the duration of the pupal period, which in *Ceratophyllus fasciatus* averages seventeen days. Moreover, when metamorphosis is complete a low temperature will cause the imago to remain within the cocoon.

Sexually mature and ovipositing fleas, he fed at intervals and kept alive for two months, when the experiment was discontinued. In the presence of rubbish in which they could bury themselves, unfed rat fleas were kept alive for many months, whereas in the absence of any such substratum they rarely lived a month. In the former case, it was found that the length of life is influenced to some degree by the temperature and humidity. In an experiment carried out at 70° F. and 45 per cent humidity, the fleas did not live for more than four months, while in an experiment at 60° F. and 70 per cent humidity they lived for at least seventeen months. There was no indication that fleas kept under these conditions sucked moisture from surrounding objects, and those kept in bell jars, with an extract of flea-rubbish on filter paper, did not live any longer than those which were not so supplied.

Curiously enough, although the rat is the normal host of *Ceratophyllus fasciatus*, it was found that when given the choice these fleas would feed upon man in preference to rats. However, none of the fleas laid eggs unless they fed on rat blood.

The experiments of Strickland on copulation and oviposition in the rat flea showed that fleas do not copulate until they are sexually mature and that, at least in the case of *Ceratophyllus fasciatus*, the reproductive organs are imperfectly developed for some time (more than a week) after emerging from the pupa. When mature, copulation takes place soon after the fleas have fed on their true host—the rat—but not if they have fed on a facultative host only, such as man. Copulation is always followed by oviposition within a very short time.

The effect of the rat's blood on the female with regard to egg-laying, Strickland concludes, is stimulating rather than nutritive, as fleas that were without food for many months were observed to lay eggs immediately after one feed. Similarly, the male requires the stimulus of a meal of rat's blood before it displays any copulatory activity.

Mitzmain (1910) has described in detail the act of biting on man, as observed in the squirrel flea, *Ceratophyllus acutus*. "The flea when permitted to walk freely on the arm selects a suitable hairy space where it ceases abruptly in its locomotion, takes a firm hold with the tarsi, projects its proboscis, and prepares to puncture the skin. A puncture is drilled by the pricking epipharynx, the sawtooth mandibles supplementing the movement by lacerating the cavity formed. The two organs of the rostrum work alternately, the middle piece boring, while the two lateral elements execute a sawing movement. The mandibles, owing to their basal attachments, are, as is expressed by the advisory committee on plague investigations in India (*Journal of Hygiene*, vol. 6, No. 4, p. 499), 'capable of independent action, sliding up and down but maintaining their relative positions and preserving the lumen of the aspiratory channel.' The labium doubles back, the V-shaped groove of this organ guiding the mandibles on either side."

"The action of the proboscis is executed with a forward movement of the head and a lateral and downward thrust of the entire body. As the mouth-parts are sharply inserted, the abdomen rises simultaneously. The hind and middle legs are elevated, resembling oars. The forelegs are doubled under the thorax, the tibia and tarsi resting firmly on the epidermis serve as a support for the body during the feeding. The maxillary palpi are retracted beneath the head and thorax. The labium continues to bend, at first acting as a sheath for the sawing mandibles, and as these are more deeply inserted, it bends beneath the head with the elasticity of a bow, forcing the mandibles into the wound until the maxillæ are embedded in the skin of the victim. When the proboscis is fully inserted, the abdomen ceases for a time its lateral swinging."

"The acute pain of biting is first felt when the mandibles have not quite penetrated and subsequently during each distinct movement of the abdomen. The swinging of the abdomen gradually ceases as it becomes filled with blood. The sting of the biting gradually becomes duller and less sensitive as feeding progresses. The movements of the elevated abdomen grow noticeably feebler as the downward thrusts of the springy bow-like labium becomes less frequent."

"As the feeding process advances one can discern through the translucent walls of the abdomen a constant flow of blood, caudally from the pharynx, accompanied by a peristaltic movement. The end of the meal is signified in an abrupt manner. The flea shakes its entire body, and gradually withdraws its proboscis by lowering the abdomen and legs and violently twisting the head."

"When starved for several days the feeding of the rat fleas is conducted in a rather vigorous manner. As soon as the proboscis is buried to the full length the abdomen is raised and there ensues a gradual lateral swaying motion, increasing the altitude of the raised end of the abdomen until it assumes the perpendicular. The flea is observed at this point to gain a better foothold by advancing the fore tarsi, and then, gradually doubling back the abdomen, it turns with extreme agility, nearly touching with its dorsal side the skin of the hand upon which it is feeding. Meanwhile, the hungry parasite feeds ravenously."

"It is interesting to note the peculiar nervous action which the rodent fleas exhibit immediately when the feeding process is completed or when disturbed during the biting. Even while the rostrum is inserted to the fullest the parasite shakes its head spasmodically; in a twinkling the mouth is withdrawn and then the flea hops away."

A habit of fleas which we shall see is of significance in considering their agency in the spread of bubonic plague, is that of ejecting blood from the anus as they feed.

Fleas are famous for their jumping powers, and in control measures it is of importance to determine their ability along this line. It is often stated that they can jump about four inches, or, according to the Indian Plague Commission *Xenopsylla cheopis* cannot hop farther than five inches. Mitzmain (1910) conducted some careful experiments in which he found that the human flea, *Pulex irritans*, was able to jump as far as thirteen inches on a horizontal plane. The mean average of five specimens permitted to jump at will was seven and three-tenths inches. The same species was observed to jump perpendicularly to a height of at least seven and three-fourths inches. Other species were not able to equal this record.

The effect of the bite of fleas on man varies considerably according to the individual susceptibility. According to Patton and Cragg, this was borne out in a curious manner by the experiments of Chick and Martin. "In these, eight human hosts were tried; in seven, little or no irritation was produced, while in one quite severe inflammation was set up around each bite." Of two individuals, equally accustomed to the insects, going into an infested room, one may be literally tormented by them while the other will not notice them.

Indeed it is not altogether a question of susceptibility, for fleas seem to have a special predilection for certain individuals. The typical itching wheals produced by the bites are sometimes followed, especially after scratching, by inflammatory papules.

The itching can be relieved by the use of lotions of carbolic acid (2-3 per cent), camphor, menthol lotion, or carbolated vaseline. If forced to sleep in an infested room, protection from attacks can be in a large measure gained by sprinkling pyrethrum, bubach, or California insect powder between the sheets. The use of camphor, menthol, or oil of eucalyptus, or oil of pennyroyal is also said to afford protection to a certain extent.

In the Eastern United States the occurrence of fleas as household pests is usually due to infested cats and dogs which have the run of the house. We have seen that the eggs are not attached to the host but drop to the floor when they are laid. Verrill, cited by Osborn, states that on one occasion he was able to collect fully a teaspoonful of eggs from the dress of a lady in whose lap a half-grown kitten had been held for a short time. Patton and Cragg record seeing the inside of a hat in which a kitten had spent the night, so covered with flea eggs that it looked "as if it had been sprinkled with sugar from a sifter." It is no wonder that houses in which pets live become overrun with the fleas.

One of the first control measures, then, consists in keeping such animals out of the house or in rigorously keeping them free from fleas. The latter can best be accomplished by the use of strong tar soap or Armour's "Flesope," which may be obtained from most druggists. The use of a three per cent solution of creolin, approximately four teaspoonfuls to a quart of warm water, has also been recommended. While this is satisfactory in the case of dogs, it is liable to sicken cats, who will lick their fur in an effort to dry themselves. Howard recommends thoroughly rubbing into the fur a quantity of pyrethrum powder. This partially stupifies the fleas which should be promptly swept up and burned.

He also recommends providing a rug for the dog or cat to sleep on and giving this rug a frequent shaking and brushing, afterwards sweeping up and burning the dust thus removed.

Since the larvæ of fleas are very susceptible to exposure, the use of bare floors, with few rugs, instead of carpets or matting, is to be recommended. Thorough sweeping, so as to allow no accumulation of dust in cracks and crevices will prove efficient. If a house is once infested it may be necessary to thoroughly scrub the floors with hot soapsuds, or to spray them with gasoline. If the latter method is adopted, care must be taken to avoid the possibility of fire.

To clear a house of fleas Skinner recommends the use of flake naphthalene. In a badly infested house he took one room at a time, scattering on the floor five pounds of flake naphthalene, and closed it for twenty-four hours. It proved to be a perfect and effectual remedy and very inexpensive, as the naphthalene could be swept up and transferred to other rooms. Dr. Skinner adds, "so far as I am concerned, the flea question is solved and if I have further trouble I know the remedy. I intend to keep the dog and cat."

The late Professor Slingerland very effectively used hydrocyanic acid gas fumigation in exterminating fleas in houses. In one case, where failure was reported, he found on investigation that the house had become thoroughly reinfested from pet cats, which had been left untreated. Fumigation with sulphur is likewise efficient.

The fact that adult fleas are usually to be found on the floor, when not on their hosts, was ingeniously taken advantage of by Professor S. H. Gage in ridding an animal room at Cornell University of the pests. He swathed the legs of a janitor with sticky fly-paper and had him walk back and forth in the room. Large numbers of the fleas were collected in this manner.

In some parts of the southern United States hogs are commonly infested and in turn infest sheds, barns and even houses. Mr. H. E. Vick informs us that it is a common practice to turn sheep into barn-lots and sheds in the spring of the year to collect in their wool, the fleas which abound in these places after the hogs have been turned out.

It is a common belief that adult fleas are attracted to fresh meat and that advantage of this can be taken in trapping them. Various workers, notably Mitzman (1910), have shown that there is no basis for such a belief.

**The true chiggers**—The chigoes, or true chiggers, are the most completely parasitic of any of the fleas. Of the dozen or more known species, one commonly attacks man. This is *Dermatophilus penetrans*, more commonly known as *Sarcopsylla penetrans* or *Pulex penetrans*.

This species occurs in Mexico, the West Indies, Central and South America. There are no authentic records of its occurrence in the United States although, as Baker has pointed out, there is no reason why it should not become established in Florida and Texas. It is usually believed that Brazil was its original home. Sometime about the middle of the nineteenth century it was introduced into West Africa and has spread across that continent.

The males and the immature females of *Dermatophilus penetrans* (fig. 93) closely resemble those of other fleas. They are very active little brown insects about 1–1.2 mm. in size, which live in the dust of native huts and stables, and in dry, sandy soil. In such places they often occur in enormous numbers and become a veritable plague.

They attack not only man but various animals. According to Castellani and Chalmers, "Perhaps the most noted feature is the way

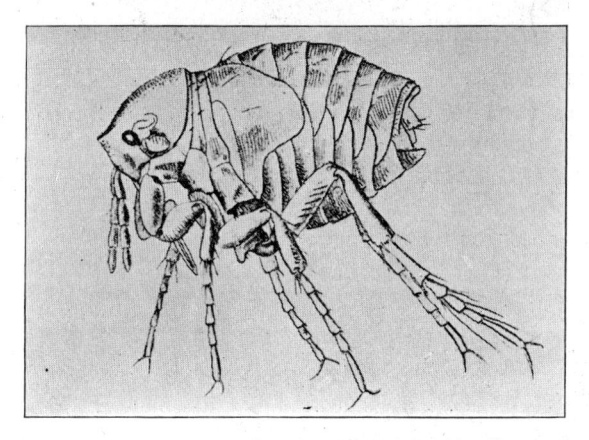

93. Dermatophilus penetrans. Much enlarged. After Karsten.

in which it attacks pigs. On the Gold Coast it appeared to be largely kept in existence by these animals. It is very easily captured in the free state by taking a little pig with a pale abdomen, and placing it on its back on the ground on which infected pigs are living. After watching a few moments, a black speck will appear on the pig's abdomen, and quickly another and another. These black specks are jiggers which can easily be transferred to a test tube. On examination they will be found to be males and females in about equal numbers."

Both the males and females suck blood. That which characterizes this species as distinguished from other fleas attacking man is that when the impregnated female attacks she burrows into the skin and there swells until in a few days she has the size and appearance of a small pea (fig. 94). Where they are abundant, hundreds of the

128    *Parasitic Arthropoda*

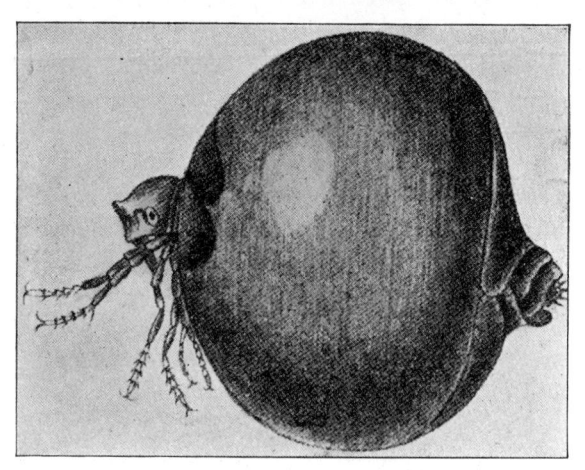

94. Dermatophilus penetrans, gravid female. After Moniez.

pests may attack a single individual (fig. 95). Here they lie with the apex of the abdomen blocking the opening. According to Fülleborn (1908) they do not penetrate beneath the epidermis. The eggs are not laid in the flesh of the victim, as is sometimes stated, but are expelled through this opening. The female then dies, withers and falls away or is expelled by ulceration. According to Brumpt, she first quits the skin and then, falling to the ground, deposits her eggs. The subsequent development in so far as known, is like that of other fleas.

The chigoe usually enters between the toes, the skin about the roots of the nails, or the soles

95. Chiggers in the sole of foot of man. Manson's Tropical Diseases. Permission of Cassell and Co.

## Siphonaptera, or Fleas

of the feet, although it may attack other parts of the body. Mense records the occurrence in folds of the epidermis, as in the neighborhood of the anus. They give rise to irritation and unless promptly and aseptically removed there often occurs pus formation and the development of a more or less serious abscess. Gangrene and even tetanus may ensue.

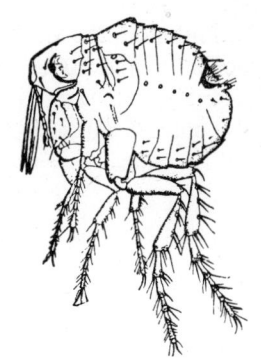

Treatment consists in the careful removal of the insect, an operation more easily accomplished a day or two after its entrance, than at first, when it is unswollen. The ulcerated point should then be treated with weak carbolic acid, or tincture of iodine, or dusted thoroughly with an antiseptic powder.

96. Echidnophaga gallinacea.

Castellani and Chalmers recommend as prophylactic measures, keeping the house clean and keeping pigs, poultry, and cattle away therefrom. "High boots should be used, and especial care should be taken not to go to a ground floor bathroom with bare feet. The feet, especially the toes, and under the nails, should be carefully examined every morning to see if any black

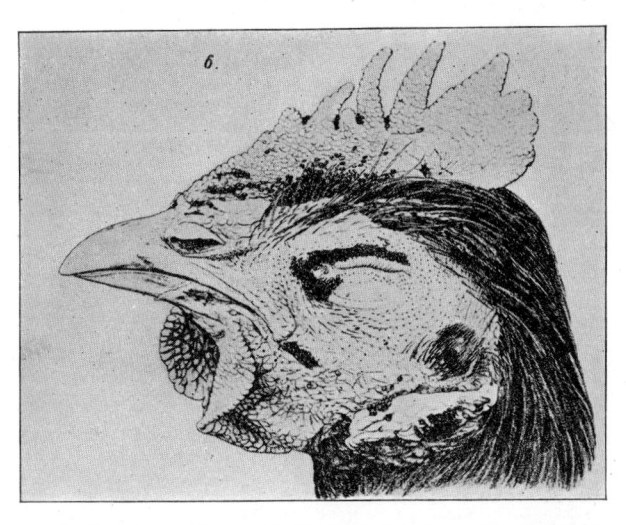

97. Echidnophaga gallinacea infesting head of chicken. After Enderlein.

dots can be discovered, when the jigger should be at once removed, and in this way suppuration will be prevented. It is advisable, also, to sprinkle the floors with carbolic lotion, Jeyes' fluid, or with pyrethrum powder, or with a strong infusion of native tobacco, as recommended by Law and Castellani."

*Echidnophaga gallinacea* (fig. 96) is a widely distributed Hectopsyllid attacking poultry (fig. 97). It occurs in the Southern and Southwestern United States and has been occasionally reported as attacking man, especially children. It is less highly specialized than *Dermatophilus penetrans*, and does not ordinarily cause serious trouble in man.

# CHAPTER IV

### ACCIDENTAL OR FACULTATIVE PARASITES

In addition to the many species of Arthropods which are normally parasitic on man and animals, there is a considerable number of those which may be classed as *accidental* or *facultative* parasites.

Accidental or facultative parasites are species which are normally free-living, but which are able to exist as parasites when accidentally introduced into the body of man or other animal. A wide range of forms is included under this grouping.

#### ACARINA

A considerable number of mites have been reported as accidental or even normal, endoparasites of man, but the authentic cases are comparatively few.

In considering such reports it is well to keep in mind von Siebold's warning that in view of the universal distribution of mites one should be on his guard. In vessels in which animal and other organic fluids and moist substances gradually dry out, mites are very abundantly found. If such vessels are used without very careful preliminary cleaning, for the reception of evacuations of the sick, or for the reception of parts removed from the body, such things may be readily contaminated by mites, which have no other relation whatever to them.

Nevertheless, there is no doubt but that certain mites, normally free-living, have occurred as accidental parasites of man. Of these the most commonly met with is *Tyroglyphus siro*, the cheese-mite.

*Tyroglyphus siro* is a small mite of a whitish color. The male measures about 500μ long by 250μ wide, the female slightly larger. They live in cheese of almost any kind, especially such as is a little decayed. "The individuals gather together in winter in groups or heaps in the hollows and chinks of the cheese and there remain motionless. As soon as the temperature rises a little, they gnaw away at the cheese and reduce it to a powder. The powder is composed of excrement having the appearance of little grayish microscopic balls; eggs, old and new, cracked and empty; larvæ, nymphs, and perfect mites, cast skins and fragments of cheese, to which must be added numerous spores of microscopic fungi."—Murray.

*Tyroglyphus siro*, and related species, have been found many times in human feces, under conditions which preclude the explanation that the contamination occurred outside of the body. They have been supposed to be the cause of dysentery, or diarrhœa, and it is probable that the *Acarus dysenteriæ* of Linnæus, and Latreille, was this species. However, there is little evidence that the mites cause any noteworthy symptoms, even when taken into the body in large numbers.

*Histiogaster spermaticus* (fig. 152) is a Tyroglyphid mite which was reported by Trouessart (1902) as having been found in a cyst in the groin, adherent to the testis. When the cyst was punctured, it yielded about two ounces of opalescent fluid containing spermatozoa and numerous mites in all stages of development. The evidence indicated that a fecundated female mite had been introduced into the urethra by means of an unclean catheter. Though Trouessart reported the case as that of a Sarcoptid, Banks places the genus *Histiogaster* with the Tyroglyphidæ. He states that our species feeds on the oyster-shell bark louse, possibly only after the latter is dead, and that in England a species feeds within decaying reeds.

*Nephrophages sanguinarius* is a peculiarly-shaped, angular mite which was found by Miyake and Scriba (1893) for eight successive days in the urine of a Japanese suffering from fibrinuria. Males, .117 mm. long by .079 mm. wide, females .36 mm. by .12 mm., and eggs were found both in the spontaneously emitted urine and in that drawn by means of a catheter. All the mites found were dead. The describers regarded this mite as a true endoparasite, but it is more probable that it should be classed as an accidental parasite.

## Myriapoda

There are on record a number of cases of myriapods occurring as accidental parasites of man. The subject has been treated in detail by Blanchard (1898 and 1902), who discussed forty cases. Since then at least eight additions have been made to the list.

Neveau-Lamaire (1908) lists thirteen species implicated, representing eight different genera. Of the *Chilognatha* there are three, *Julus terrestris*, *J. londinensis* and *Polydesmus complanatus*. The remainder are *Chilopoda*, namely, *Lithobius forficatus*, *L. malenops*, *Geophilus carpophagus*, *G. electricus*, *G. similis*, *G. cephalicus*, *Scutigera coleoptrata*, *Himantarium gervaisi*, *Chætechelyne vesuviana* and *Stigmatogaster subterraneus*.

The majority of the cases relate to infestation of the nasal fossæ, or the frontal sinus, but intestinal infestation also occurs and there is one recorded case of the presence of a species in *Julus* (fig. 13) in the auditory canal of a child.

In the nose, the myriapods have been known to live for months and according to some records, even for years. The symptoms caused by their presence are inflammation, with or without increased flow of mucus, itching, more or less intense headache, and at times general symptoms such as vertigo, delirium, convulsions, and the like. These symptoms disappear suddenly when the parasites are expelled.

In the intestine of man, myriapods give rise to obscure symptoms suggestive of infestation by parasitic worms. In a case reported by Verdun and Bruyant (1912), a child twenty months of age had been affected for fifteen days by digestive disturbances characterized by loss of appetite, nausea and vomiting. The latter had been particularly pronounced for three days, when there was discovered in the midst of the material expelled a living myriapod of the species *Chætechelyne vesuviana*. Anthelminthics had been administered without result. In some of the other cases, the administration of such drugs had resulted in the expulsion of the parasite through the anus.

One of the extreme cases on record is that reported by Shipley (1914). Specimens of *Geophilus gorizensis* (= *G. subterraneus*) 'were vomited and passed by a woman of 68 years of age. Some of the centipedes emerged through the patient's nose, and it must be mentioned that she was also suffering from a round worm. One of her doctors was of the opinion that the centipedes were certainly breeding inside the lady's intestines, and as many as seven or eight, sometimes more, were daily leaving the alimentary canal."

"According to her attendant's statements these centipedes had left the body in some hundreds during a period of twelve or eighteen months. Their presence produced vomiting and some hæmatemesis, and treatment with thymol, male-fern and turpentine had no effect in removing the creatures."

The clinical details, as supplied by Dr. Theodore Thompson were as follows:

"Examined by me July, 1912, her tongue was dry and glazed. There was bleeding taking place from the nose and I saw a living centipede she had just extracted from her nostril. Her heart, lungs and abdomen appeared normal. She was not very wasted, and did not think she had lost much flesh, nor was there any marked degree of anemia."

Shipley gives the following reasons for believing it impossible that these centipedes could have multiplied in the patient's intestine. "The breeding habits of the genus *Geophilus* are peculiar, and ill adapted for reproducing in such a habitat. The male builds a small web or nest, in which he places his sperm, and the female fertilizes herself from this nest or web, and when the eggs are fertilized they are again laid in a nest or web in which they incubate and in two or three weeks hatch out. The young *Geophilus* differ but very little from the adult, except in size. It is just possible, but improbable, that a clutch of eggs had been swallowed by the host when eating some vegetables or fruit, but against this is the fact that the *Geophilus* does not lay its eggs upon vegetables or fruit, but upon dry wood or earth. The egg-shell is very tough and if the eggs had been swallowed the egg-shells could certainly have been detected if the dejecta were examined. The specimens of the centipede showed very little signs of being digested, and it is almost impossible to reconcile the story of the patient with what one knows of the habits of the centipedes."

In none of the observed cases have there been any clear indications as to the manner of infestation. It is possible that the myriapods have been taken up in uncooked fruit or vegetables.

### LEPIDOPTEROUS LARVÆ

**Scholeciasis**—Hope (1837) brought together six records of infestation of man by lepidopterous larvæ and proposed to apply the name scholeciasis to this type of parasitism. The clearest case was that of a young boy who had repeatedly eaten raw cabbage and who vomited larvæ of the cabbage butterfly, *Pieris brassicæ*. Such cases are extremely rare, and there are few reliable data relative to the subject. In this connection it may be noted that Spuler (1906) has described a moth whose larvæ live as ectoparasites of the sloth.

### COLEOPTERA

**Canthariasis**—By this term Hope designated instances of accidental parasitism by the larvæ or adults of beetles. Reports of such cases are usually scouted by parasitologists but there seems no good basis for wholly rejecting them. Cobbold refers to a half dozen cases of accidental parasitism by the larvæ of *Blaps mortisaga*.

In one of these cases upwards of 1200 larvæ and several perfect insects were said to have been passed *per anum*. French (1905) reports the case of a man who for a considerable period voided adult living beetles of the species *Nitidula bipustulata*. Most of the other cases on record relate to the larvæ of *Dermestidæ* (larder beetles *et al.*) or *Tenebrionidæ* (meal infesting species). Infestation probably occurs through eating raw or imperfectly cooked foods containing eggs or minute larvæ of these insects.

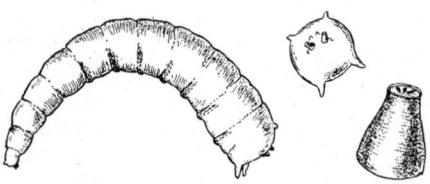

98. Larva of Piophila casei. Posterior stigmata. Caudal aspect of larva.

Brumpt cites a curious case of accidental parasitism by a coleopterous larva belonging to the genus *Necrobia*. This larva was extracted from a small tumor, several millimeters long, on the surface of the conjunctiva of the eye. The larvæ of this genus ordinarily live in decomposing flesh and cadavers.

## DIPTEROUS LARVÆ

**Myasis**—By this term (spelled also myiasis, and myiosis), is meant parasitism by dipterous larvæ. Such parasitism may be normal, as in the cases already described under the heading parasitic Diptera, or it may be facultative, due to free-living larvæ being accidentally introduced into wounds or the body-cavities of man. Of this latter type, there is a multitude of cases on record, relating to comparatively few species. The literature of the subject, like that relating to facultative parasitism in general, is unsatisfactory, for most of the determinations of species have been very loose.

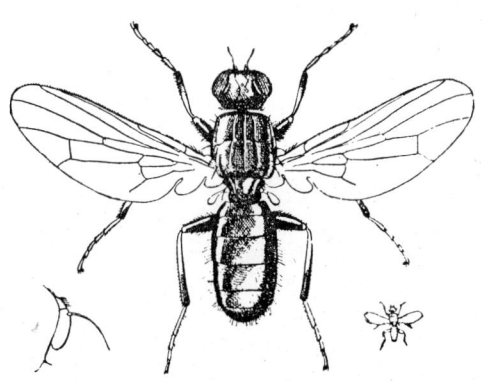

99. Piophila casei. After Graham-Smith.

Indeed, so little has been known regarding the characteristics of the larvæ concerned that in many instances they could not be exactly determined. Fortunately, several workers have undertaken comparative studies along this line. The most comprehensive publication is that of Banks (1912), entitled "The structure of certain dipterous larvæ, with particular reference to those in human food."

Without attempting an exhaustive list, we shall discuss here the more important species of Diptera whose larvæ are known to cause myasis, either external or internal. The following key will serve to determine those most likely to be encountered. The writers would be glad to examine specimens not readily identifiable, if accompanied by exact data relative to occurrence.

*a.* Body more or less flattened, depressed; broadest in the middle, each segment with dorsal, lateral, and ventral fleshy processes, of which the laterals, at least, are more or less spiniferous (fig. 101). *Fannia* (=*Homalomyia*). In *F. canicularis* the dorsal processes are nearly as long as the laterals; in *F. scalaris* the dorsal processes are short spinose tubercles.

*aa.* Body cylindrical, or slender conical tapering toward the head; without fleshy lateral processes (fig. 105).

*b.* With the posterior stigmata at the end of shorter or longer tubercles, or if not placed upon tubercles, then not in pit; usually without a "marginal button" and without a chitinous ring surrounding the three slits; the slits narrowly or broadly oval, not bent (fig. 171 i). *Acalyptrate muscidæ* and some species of *Anthomyiidæ*. To this group belong the cheese skipper (*Piophila casei*, figs. 98, 99), the pomace-fly (*Drosophila ampelophila*), the apple maggot (*Rhagoletis pomonella*), the cherry fruit fly (*Rhagoletis cingulata*), the small dung fly (*Sepsis violacea*, fig. 170), the beet leaf-miner (*Pegomyia vicina*, fig. 171 i), the cabbage, bean and onion maggots (*Phorbia* spp.) et. al.

*bb.* Posterior stigmata of various forms, if the slits are narrowly oval (fig. 171) then they are surrounded by a chitin ring which may be open ventromesally.

*c.* Integument leathery and usually strongly spinulose; larvæ hypodermatic or endoparasitic.....................Bot flies (fig. 171, f, g, k).—*Oestridæ*

*cc.* Integument not leathery and (except in *Protocalliphora*) spinulæ restricted to transverse patches near the incisures of the segments.

*d.* The stigmal plates in a pit; the lip-like margin of the pit with a number of fleshy tubercles; chitin of the stigma not complete; open ventro-mesally, button absent (fig. 171 e).......................Flesh flies.—*Sarcophaga*

*dd.* Stigmata not in a pit.

*e.* The chitin ring open ventra-mesally; button absent (fig. 171 c). Screwworm fly............................................*Chrysomyia*

*ee.* The chitin ring closed.

*f.* Slits of the posterior stigmata straight; marginal "button" present (fig. 171 b); two distinct mouth hooks, fleshy tubercles around the anal area. *Phormia* (fig. 171 f), *Lucilia* and *Calliphora* (fig. 172, a, b), *Protocalliphora* (fig. 171, j), *Cynomyia* (fig. 171, a). Blow flies, bluebottle flies........*Calliphorinæ*

*ff.* Slits of the posterior stigmata sinuous or bent. Subfamily Muscinæ.
*g.* Slits of the posterior stigmata bent; usually two mouth hooks. *Muscina stabulans* (fig. 171, *l*), *Muscina similis, Myiospila meditatunda* (fig. 172, i), and some of the higher *Anthomyiidæ*.
*gg.* Slits of the posterior stigmata sinuous; mouth hooks usually consolidated into one. The house-fly (*Musca domestica* fig. 171, d), the stable fly (*Stomoxys calcitrans*) the horn fly (*Lyperosia irritans*), *Pyrellia, Pseudopyrellia, Morellia, Mesembrina. Polietes,* et. al. (fig. 172 in part).

*Eristalis*—The larvæ of *Eristalis* are the so-called rat-tailed maggots, which develop in foul water. In a few instances these larvæ have been known to pass through the human alimentary canal uninjured. Hall and Muir (1913) report the case of a boy five years of age, who had been ailing for ten weeks and who was under treatment for indigestion and chronic constipation. For some time he had vomited everything he ate. On administration of a vermifuge he voided one of the rat-tailed maggots of *Eristalis*. He admitted having drunk water from a ditch full of all manner of rotting matter. It was doubtless through this that he became infested. It is worth noting that the above described symptoms may have been due to other organisms or substances in the filthy water.

*Piophila casei,* the cheese-fly (fig. 99), deposits its eggs not only in old cheeses, but on ham, bacon, and other fats. The larvæ (fig. 98) are the well-known cheese skippers, which sometimes occur in great abundance on certain kinds of cheese. Indeed, some people have a comfortable theory that such infested cheese is especially good. Such being the case, it is small wonder that this species has been repeatedly reported as causing intestinal myasis. Thebault (1901) describes the case of a girl who, shortly after consuming a large piece of badly infested cheese, became ill and experienced severe pains in the region of the navel. Later these extended through the entire alimentary canal, the excrement was mixed with blood and she suffered from vertigo and severe headaches. During the four following days the girl felt no change, although the excretion of the blood gradually diminished and stopped. On the fourth day she voided two half-digested larvæ and, later, seven or eight, of which two were alive and moving.

That these symptoms may be directly attributed to the larvæ, or "skippers," has been abundantly shown by experimental evidence. Portschinsky cites the case of a dog fed on cheese containing the larvæ. The animal suffered much pain and its excrement contained blood. On *post mortem* it was found that the small intestine throughout almost its entire length was marked by bloody bruises. The papillæ on these places were destroyed, although the walls were not entirely perforated. In the appendix were found two or three dead larvæ. Alessandri (1910) has likewise shown that the larvæ cause intestinal lesions.

According to Graham-Smith, Austen (1912) has recorded a case of myasis of the nose, attended with a profuse watery discharge of several weeks duration and pain, due to the larvæ of *Piophila casei*.

**Anthyomyiidæ**—The characteristic larvæ of two species of *Fannia* (=*Homalomyia* or *Anthomyia*, in part) (fig. 101) are the most commonly reported of dipterous larvæ causing intestinal myasis. Hewitt (1912) has presented a valuable study of the bionomics and of the larvæ of these flies, a type of what is needed for all the species concerned in myasis. We have seen two cases of their having been passed in stools, without having caused any special symptoms. In other instances their presence in the alimentary canal has given rise to symptoms vaguely described as those of tapeworm infestation, or helminthiasis. More specifically, they have been described as causing vertigo, severe headache, nausea and vomiting, severe abdominal pains, and in some instances, bloody diarrhœa.

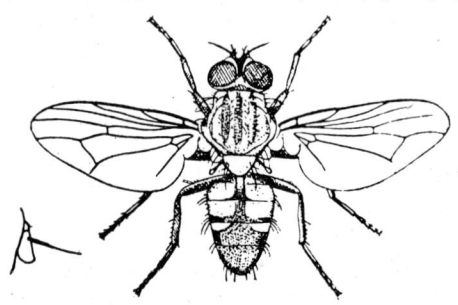

100. Fannia canicularis (x4). After Graham-Smith.

One of the most striking cases is that reported by Blankmeyer (1914), of a woman whose illness began fourteen years previously with nausea and vomiting. After several months of illness she began passing larvæ and was compelled to resort to enemas. Three years previous to the report, she noticed frequent shooting pains in the rectal region and at times abdominal tenderness was marked. There was much mucus in the stools and she "experienced the sensation of larvæ crawling in the intestine." Occipital headaches were marked, with remissions, and constipation became chronic. The appetite was variable, there was a bad taste in the mouth, tongue furred and ridged, and red at the edges. Her complexion was sallow, and general nervousness was marked. As treatment, there were given doses of magnesium sulphate before breakfast and at

4 P. M., with five grain doses of salol four times a day. The customary parasiticides yielded no marked benefit. At the time of the report the patient passed from four to fifty larvæ per day, and was showing some signs of improvement. The nausea had disappeared, her nervousness was less evident, and there was a slight gain in weight.

The case was complicated by various other disorders, but the symptoms given above seem to be in large part attributable to the myasis. There is nothing in the case to justify the assumption that larvæ were continuously present, for years. It seems more reasonable to suppose that something in the habits of the patient favored repeated infestation. Nevertheless, a study of the various cases of intestinal myasis caused by these and other species of dipterous larvæ seems to indicate that the normal life cycle may be considerably prolonged under the unusual conditions.

The best authenticated cases of myasis of the urinary passage have been due to larvæ of *Fannia*. Chevril (1909) collected and described twenty cases, of which seven seemed beyond doubt. One of these was that of a woman of fifty-five who suffered from albuminuria, and urinated with much difficulty, and finally passed thirty to forty larvæ of *Fannia canicularis*.

It is probable that infestation usually occurs through eating partially decayed fruit or vegetables on which the flies have deposited their eggs. Wellman points out that the flies may deposit their eggs in or about the anus of persons using outside privies and Hewitt believes that this latter method of infection is probably the common one in the case of infants belonging to careless mothers. "Such infants are sometimes left about in an exposed and not very clean condition, in consequence of which flies are readily attracted to them and deposit their eggs."

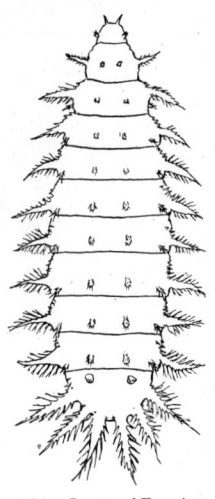

101. Larva of Fannia scalaris.

**Muscinæ**—The larvæ of the common house-fly, *Musca domestica*, are occasionally recorded as having been passed with the feces or vomit of man. While such cases may occur, it is probable that in most instances similar appearing larvæ of other insects have been mistakenly identified.

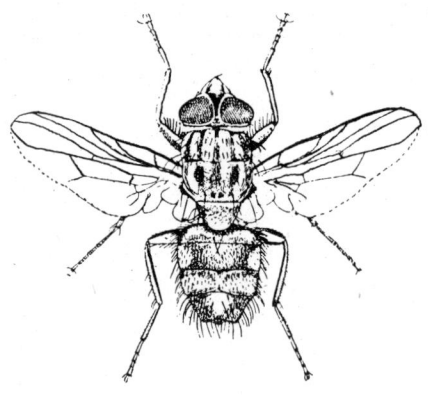

*Muscina stabulans* is regarded by Portschinsky (1913) as responsible for many of the cases of intestinal myasis attributed to other species. He records the case of a peasant who suffered from pains in the lower part of the breast and intestines, and whose stools were mixed with blood. From November until March he had felt particularly ill, being troubled with nausea and vomiting in addition to the pain in his intestines. In March, his physician prescribed injections of a concentrated solution of tannin, which resulted in the expulsion of fifty living larvæ of *Muscina stabulans*. Thereafter the patient felt much better, although he suffered from intestinal catarrh in a less severe form.

102. Muscina stabulans (x4). After Graham Smith.

**Calliphorinæ**—Closely related to the Sarcophagidæ are the *Calliphorinæ*. to which group belong many of the so-called "blue bottle" flies. Their larvæ feed upon dead animals, and upon fresh and cooked meat. Those of *Protocalliphora*, already mentioned, are ectoparasitic on living nestling birds. Larvæ of *Lucilia*, we have taken from tumors on living turtles. To this sub-family belongs also *Aucheromyia luteola*, the Congo floor maggot. Some of these, and at least the last mentioned, are confirmed, rather than facultative parasites. Various species of Calliphorinæ are occassionally met with as facultative parasites of man.

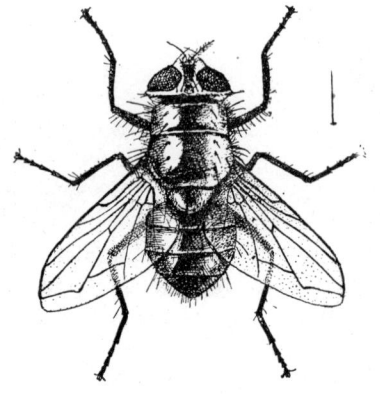

103. Lucilia cæsar, (x3). After Howard.

*Chrysomyia macellaria*, the screw worm fly (fig. 107), is the fly which is responsible for the most serious cases of human myasis in the United States. It is widely distributed in the United States

but is especially abundant in the south. While the larvæ b    n
decaying matter in general, they so commonly breed in the living
flesh of animals that they merit rank as true parasites. The females
are attracted to open wounds of all kinds on cattle and other animals
and quickly deposit large numbers of eggs. Animals which have
been recently castrated, dehorned, or branded, injured by barbed
wire, or even by the attacks of ticks are promptly attacked in the
regions where the fly abounds. Even the navel of young calves or
discharges from the vulva of cows may attract the insect.

Not infrequently the fly attacks man, being attracted by an offensive breath, a chronic catarrh, or a purulent discharge from the
ears. Most common are the cases where the eggs are deposited in

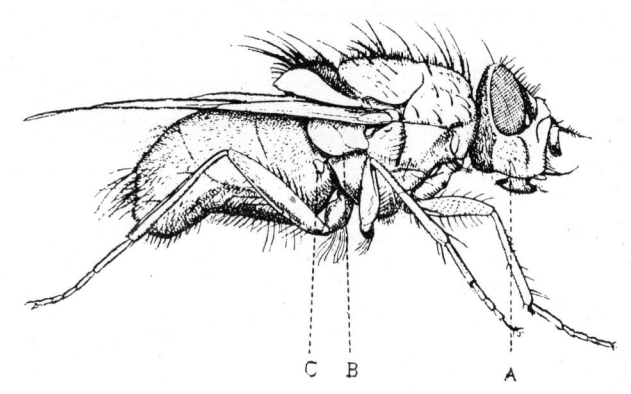

104. Calliphora erythrocephala, (x6). After Graham-Smith.

the nostrils. The larvæ, which are hatched in a day or two, are
provided with strong spines and proceed to bore into the tissues
of the nose, even down into or through the bone, into the frontal
sinus, the pharynx, larynx, and neighboring parts.

Osborn (1896) quotes a number of detailed accounts of the attacks
of the *Chrysomyia* on man. A vivid picture of the symptomology
of rhinal myasis caused by the larvæ of this fly is given by Castellani
and Chalmers: "Some couple of days after a person suffering from
a chronic catarrh, foul breath, or ozæna, has slept in the open or has
been attacked by a fly when riding or driving,—*i.e.*, when the hands
are engaged—signs of severe catarrh appear, accompanied with
inordinate sneezing and severe pain over the root of the nose or the
frontal bone. Quickly the nose becomes swollen, and later the face
also may swell, while examination of the nose may show the presence

of the larvæ. Left untreated, the patient rapidly becomes worse, and pus and blood are discharged from the nose, from which an offensive odor issues. Cough appears as well as fever, and often some delirium. If the patient lives long enough, the septum of the nose may fall in, the soft and hard palates may be pierced, the wall of the pharynx may be destroyed. By this time, however, the course of the disease will have become quite evident by the larvæ dropping out of the nose, and if the patient continues to live all the larvæ may come away naturally."

For treatment of rhinal myasis these writers recommend douching the nose with chloroform water or a solution of chloroform in sweet milk (10–20 per cent), followed by douches of mild antiseptics. Surgical treatment may be necessary.

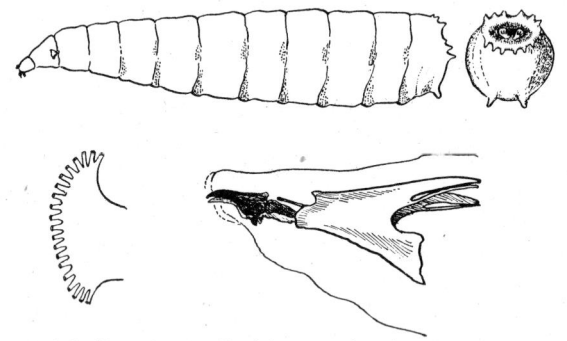

105. Larva of a flesh fly (Sarcophaga). Caudal aspect. Anterior stigmata. Pharyngeal skeleton.

**Sarcophagidæ**—The larvæ (fig. 105) of flies of this family usually feed upon meats, but have been found in cheese, oleomargerine, pickled herring, dead and living insects, cow dung and human feces. Certain species are parasitic in insects. Higgins (1890) reported an instance of "hundreds" of larvæ of *Sarcophaga* being vomited by a child eighteen months of age. There was no doubt as to their origin for they were voided while the physician was in the room. There are many other reports of their occurrence in the alimentary canal. We have recorded elsewhere (Riley, 1906) a case in which some ten or twelve larvæ of *Sarcophaga* were found feeding on the diseased tissues of a malignant tumor. The tumor, a melanotic sarcoma, was about the size of a small walnut, and located in the small of the back of an elderly lady. Although they had irritated and caused a slight hemorrhage, neither the patient nor others of the family knew of their presence. Any discomfort which they had caused had been attributed to the sarcomatous growth. The infestation occurred

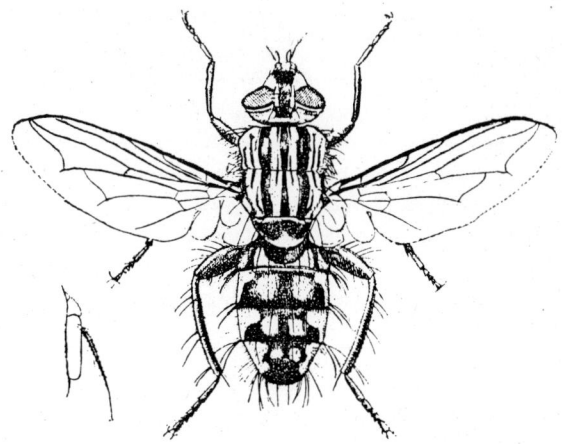

106. A flesh fly (Sarcophaga), (x4). After Graham-Smith.

in mid-summer. It is probable that the adult was attracted by the odor of the discharges and deposited the living maggots upon the diseased tissues.

According to Küchenmeister, *Sarcophaga carnaria* (fig. 106), attracted by the odor, deposits its eggs and larvæ in the vagina of girls and women when they lie naked in hot summer days upon dirty clothes, or when they have a discharge from the vagina. In malignant inflammations of the eyes the larvæ even nestle under the eyelids and in Egypt, for example, produce a very serious addition to the effects of smallpox upon the cornea, as according to Pruner, in such cases perforation of the cornea usually takes place.

*Wohlfartia magnifica* is another Sarcophagid which commonly infests man in the regions where it is abundant. It is found in all Europe but is especially common in Russia, where Portschinsky has devoted much attention to its ravages. It deposits living larvæ in wounds, the nasal fossæ, the ears and the eyes, causing injuries even more revolting than those described for *Chrysomyia*.

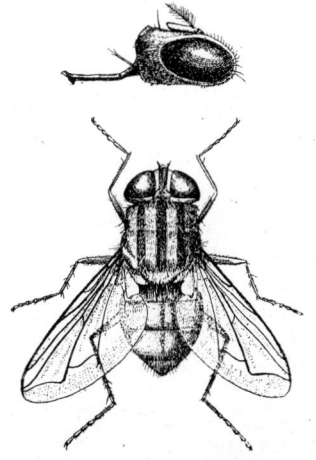

107. Chrysomyia macellaria, (x3)

# CHAPTER V

## ARTHROPODS AS SIMPLE CARRIERS OF DISEASE

The fact that certain arthropods are poisonous, or may affect the health of man as direct parasites has always received attention in the medical literature. We come now to the more modern aspect of our subject,—the consideration of insects and other arthropods as transmitters and disseminators of disease.

The simplest way in which arthropods may function in this capacity is as *simple carriers* of pathogenic organisms. It is conceivable that any insect which has access to, and comes in contact with such organisms and then passes to the food, or drink, or to the body of man, may in a wholly accidental and incidental manner convey infection. That this occurs is abundantly proved by the work of recent years. We shall consider as typical the case against the house-fly, which has attracted so much attention, both popular and scientific. The excellent general treatises of Hewitt (1910), Howard (1911), and Graham-Smith (1913), and the flood of bulletins and popular literature render it unnecessary to consider the topic in any great detail.

### THE HOUSE-FLY AS A CARRIER OF DISEASE

Up to the past decade the house-fly has usually been regarded as a mere pest. Repeatedly, however, it had been suggested that it might disseminate disease. We have seen that as far back as the sixteenth century, Mercurialis suggested that it was the agent in the spread of bubonic plague, and in 1658, Kircher reiterated this view. In 1871, Leidy expressed the opinion that flies were probably a means of communicating contagious diseases to a greater degree than was generally suspected. From what he had observed regarding gangrene in hospitals, he thought flies should be carefully excluded from wounds. In the same year, the editor of the *London Lancet*, referring to the belief that they play a useful rôle in purifying the air said, "Far from looking upon them as dipterous angels dancing attendance on Hygeia, regard them rather in the light of winged sponges spreading hither and thither to carry out the foul behests of Contagion."

These suggestions attracted little attention from medical men, for it is only within very recent years that the charges have been supported by direct evidence. Before considering this evidence, it is necessary that we define what is meant by "house-fly" and that we then consider the life-history of the insect.

There are many flies which are occasionally to be found in houses, but according to various counts, from 95 per cent to 99 per cent of these in warm weather in the Eastern United States belong to the one species *Musca domestica* (fig. 108). This is the dominant house-fly the world over and is the one which merits the name. It has been well characterized by Schiner (1864), whose description has been freely translated by Hewitt, as follows:

"Frons of male occupying a fourth part of the breadth of the head. Frontal stripe of female narrow in front, so broad behind that it entirely fills up the width of the frons. The dorsal region of the thorax dusty grey in color with four equally broad longitudinal stripes. Scutellum gray with black sides. The light regions of the abdomen yellowish, transparent, the darkest parts at least at the base of the ventral side yellow. The last segment and a dorsal line blackish brown. Seen from behind and against the light, the whole abdomen shimmering yellow, and only on each side of the dorsal line on each segment a dull transverse band. The lower part of the face silky yellow, shot with blackish brown. Median stripe velvety black. Antennæ brown. Palpi black. Legs blackish brown. Wings tinged with pale gray with yellowish base. The female has a broad velvety back, often reddishly shimmering frontal stripe, which is not broader at the anterior end than at the bases of the antennæ, but become so very much broader above that the light dustiness of the sides is entirely obliterated. The abdomen gradually becoming darker. The shimmering areas on the separate segments generally brownish. All the other parts are the same as in the male."

The other species of flies found in houses in the Eastern United States which are frequently mistaken for the house or typhoid fly may readily be distinguished by the characters of the following key:

a. Apical cell ($R_s$) of the wide wing open, i.e., the bounding veins parallel or divergent (fig. 100). Their larvæ are flattened, the intermediate body segments each fringed with fleshy, more or less spinose, processes..................................*Fannia*

b. Male with the sides of the second and third abdominal segments translucent yellowish. The larva with three pairs of nearly equal spiniferous appendages on each segment,

arranged in a longitudinal series and in addition two pairs
of series of smaller processes (fig. 100) *F. canicularis*
bb. Male with blackish abdomen, middle tibia with a tubercle
beyond the middle. The larva with spiniferous appendages of which the dorsal and ventral series are short, the
lateral series long and feathered (fig. 101)....*F. scalaris*
aa. Apical cell (R) of the wing more or less narrowed in the
margin; i. e., the bounding veins more or less converging
(fig. 108).
  b. The mouth-parts produced and pointed, fitted for piercing.
    c. Palpi much shorter than the proboscis; a brownish gray
fly, its thorax with three rather broad whitish stripes;
on each border of the middle stripe and on the mesal
borders of the lateral stripes is a blackish brown line.
Abdomen yellowish brown; on the second, third and
fourth segments are three brown spots which may be
faint or even absent. The larvæ live in dung. The
stable-fly (fig. 110).............*Stomoxys calcitrans*
    cc. Palpi nearly as long as the proboscis. Smaller species
than the house-fly. The horn-fly (fig. 167)
*Hæmatobia irritans*
  bb. Mouth-parts blunt, fitted for lapping.
    c. Thorax, particularly on the sides and near the base of the
wings with soft golden yellow hairs among the bristles.
This fly is often found in the house in very early spring
or even in the winter. The cluster-fly, *Pollenia rudis*
    cc. Thorax without golden yellow hairs among the bristles.
      d. The last segment of the vein M with an abrupt
angle. (fig. 108). The larvæ live in manure,
etc...............House-fly, *Musca domestica*
      dd. The last segment of vein M with a broad, gentle
curve (fig. 102).
        e. Eyes microscopically hairy; each abdominal
segment with two spots. Larvæ in dung.
*Myiospila meditabunda*
        ee. Eyes bare; abdomen gray and brown marbled.
*Muscina*
          f. With black legs and palpi. *M. assimilis*

ff. With legs more or less yellowish; palpi yellow. Larvæ in decaying vegetable substances, dung, etc. *M. stabulans*

It is almost universally believed that the adults of *Musca domestica* hibernate, remaining dormant throughout the winter in attics, around chimneys, and in sheltered but cold situations. This belief has been challenged by Skinner (1913), who maintains that all the adult flies die off during the fall and early winter and that the species is carried over in the pupal stage, and in no other way. The cluster-fly, *Pollenia rudis*, undoubtedly does hibernate in attics and similar

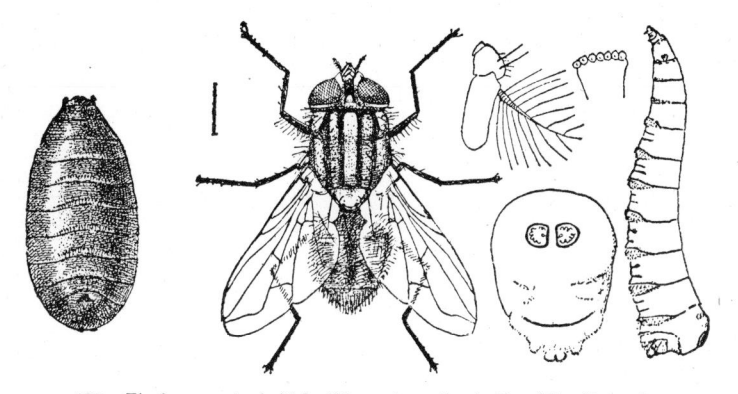

108. The house or typhoid fly (Musca domestica (4x)). After Howard.

situations and is often mistaken for the house-fly. In so far as concerns *Musca domestica*, the important question as to hibernation in the adult stage is an open one. Many observations by one of the writers (Johannsen) tend to confirm Dr. Skinner's conclusion, in so far as it applies to conditions in the latitude of New York State. Opposed, is the fact that various experimentors, notably Hewitt (1910) and Jepson (1909) wholly failed to carry pupæ through the winter.

The house-fly breeds by preference in horse manure. Indeed, Dr. Howard, whose extensive studies of the species especially qualify him for expressing an opinion on the subject, has estimated that under ordinary city and town conditions, more than ninety per cent of the flies present in houses have come from horse stables or their vicinity. They are not limited to such localities, by any means, for it has been found that they would develop in almost any fermenting organic substance. Thus, they have been bred from pig, chicken, and cow manure, dirty waste paper, decaying vegetation, decaying meat, slaughter-house refuse, sawdust-sweepings, and many other sources. A fact which makes them especially dangerous as disease-carriers is that they breed readily in human excrement.

The eggs are pure white, elongate ovoid, somewhat broader at the anterior end. They measure about one millimeter (1-25 inch) in length. They are deposited in small, irregular clusters, one hundred and twenty to one hundred and fifty from a single fly. A female may deposit as many as four batches in her life time. The eggs hatch in from eight to twenty-four hours.

The newly hatched larva, or maggot (fig. 108), measures about two millimeters (1-12 inch) in length. It is pointed at the head end and blunt at the opposite end, where the spiracular openings are borne. It grows rapidly, molts three times and reaches maturity in from six to seven days, under favorable conditions.

The pupal stage, like that of related flies, is passed in the old larval skin which, instead of being molted, becomes contracted and heavily chitinized, forming the so-called *puparium* (fig. 108). The pupal stage may be completed in from three to six days.

Thus during the warm summer months a generation of flies may be produced in ten to twelve days. Hewitt at Manchester, England, found the minimum to be eight days but states that larvæ bred in the open air in horse manure which had an average daily temperature of 22.5 C., occupied fourteen to twenty days in their development, according to the air temperature.

After emergence, a period of time must elapse before the fly is capable of depositing eggs. This period has been termed the *preoviposition period*. Unfortunately we have few exact data regarding this period. Hewitt found that the flies became sexually mature in ten to fourteen days after their emergence from the pupal state and four days after copulation they began to deposit their eggs; in other words the preoviposition stage was fourteen days or longer. Griffith (1908) found this period to be ten days. Dr. Howard believes that the time "must surely be shorter, and perhaps much shorter, under midsummer conditions, and in the freedom of the open air." He emphasizes that the point is of great practical importance, since it is during this period that the trapping and other methods of destroying the adult flies, will prove most useful.

Howard estimates that there may be nine generations of flies a year under outdoor conditions in places comparable in climate to

Washington. The number may be considerably increased in warmer climates.

The rate at which flies may increase under favorable conditions is astounding. Various writers have given estimates of the numbers of flies which may develop as the progeny of a single individual, providing all the eggs and all the individual flies survived. Thus, Howard estimates that from a single female, depositing one hundred and twenty eggs on April 15th, there may be by September 10th, 5,598,720,000,000 adults. Fortunately, living forms do not produce in any such mathematical manner and the chief value of the figures is to illustrate the enormous struggle for existence which is constantly taking place in nature.

Flies may travel for a considerable distance to reach food and shelter, though normally they pass to dwellings and other sources of food supply in the immediate neighborhood of their breeding places. Copeman, Howlett and Merriman (1911) marked flies by shaking them in a bag containing colored chalk. Such flies were repeatedly recovered at distances of eight to one thousand yards and even at a distance of seventeen hundred yards, nearly a mile.

Hindle and Merriman (1914) continued these experiments on a large scale at Cambridge, England. They "do not think it likely that, as a rule, flies travel more than a quarter of a mile in thickly-housed areas." In one case a single fly was recovered at a distance of 770 yards but a part of this distance was across open fen-land. The surprising fact was brought out that flies tend to travel either *against* or across the wind. The actual direction followed may be determined either directly by the action of the wind (positive anemotropism), or indirectly owing to the flies being attracted by any odor that it may convey from a source of food. They conclude that it is likely that the chief conditions favoring the disposal of flies are fine weather and a warm temperature. The nature of the locality is another considerable factor. Hodge (1913) has shown that when aided by the wind they may fly to much greater distances over the water. He reports that at Cleveland, Ohio, the cribs of the water works, situated a mile and a quarter, five miles, and six miles out in Lake Erie are invaded by a regular plague of flies when the wind blows from the city. Investigation showed that there was absolutely nothing of any kind in which flies could breed on the crib.

The omnivorous habits of the house-fly are matters of everyday observation. From our view point, it is sufficient to emphasize that from feeding on excrement, on sputum, on open sores, or on putrifying matter, the flies may pass to the food or milk upon the table or to healthy mucous membranes, or uncontaminated wounds. There is nothing in its appearance to tell whether the fly that comes blithely to sup with you is merely unclean, or whether it has just finished feeding upon dejecta teeming with typhoid bacilli.

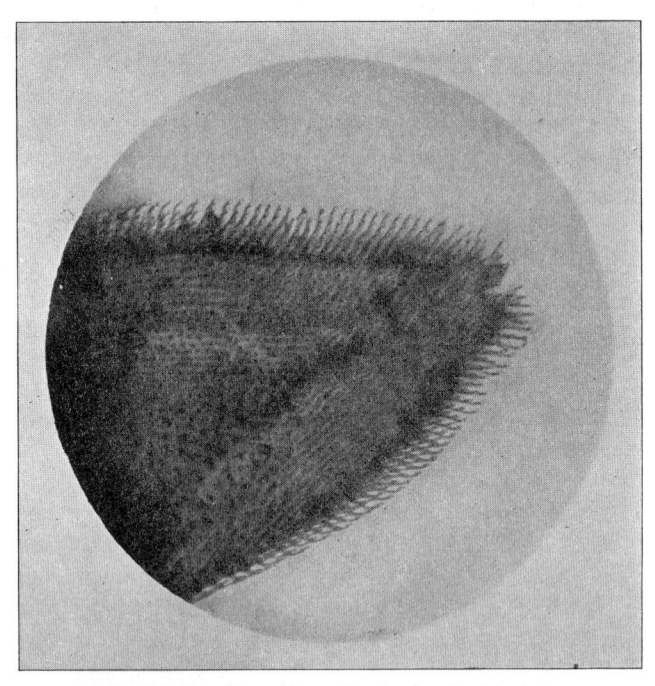

109. Pulvillus of foot of house-fly, showing glandular hairs.

The method of feeding of the house-fly has an important bearing on the question of its ability to transmit pathogenic organisms. Graham-Smith (1910) has shown that when feeding, flies frequently moisten soluble substances with "vomit" which is regurgitated from the crop. This is, of course, loaded with bacteria from previous food. When not sucked up again these drops of liquid dry, and produce round marks with an opaque center and rim and an intervening less opaque area. Fly-specks, then, consist of both vomit spots and feces. Graham-Smith shows a photograph of a cupboard window where, on an area six inches square, there were counted eleven hundred and two vomit marks and nine fecal deposits.

## The House-fly as a Carrier of Disease

From a bacteriologist's viewpoint a discussion of the possibility of a fly's carrying bacteria would seem superfluous. Any exposed object, animate or inanimate, is contaminated by bacteria and will transfer them if brought into contact with suitable culture media, whether such substance be food, or drink, open wounds, or the sterile culture media of the laboratory. A needle point may convey enough germs to produce disease. Much more readily may the house-fly with its covering of hairs and its sponge-like pulvilli (fig. 109) pick up and transfer bits of filth and other contaminated material.

For popular instruction this inevitable transfer of germs by the house-fly is strikingly demonstrated by the oft copied illustration of the tracks of a fly on a sterile culture plate. Two plates of gelatine or, better, agar medium are prepared. Over one of these a fly (with wings clipped) is allowed to walk, the other is kept as a check. Both are put aside at room temperature, to be examined after twenty-four to forty-eight hours. At the end of that time, the check plate is as clear as ever, the one which the fly has walked is dotted with colonies of bacteria and fungi. The value in the experiment consists in emphasizing that by this method we merely render visible what is constantly occurring in nature.

A comparable experiment which we use in our elementary laboratory work is to take three samples of *clean* (preferably, sterile) fresh milk in sterile bottles. One of them is plugged with a pledget of cotton, into the second is dropped a fly from the laboratory and into the third is dropped a fly which has been caught feeding upon garbage or other filth. After a minute or two the flies are removed and the vials plugged as was number one. The three are then set aside at room temperature. When examined after twenty-four hours the milk in the first vial is either still sweet or has a "clean" sour odor; that of the remaining two is very different, for it has a putrid odor, which is usually more pronounced in the case of sample number three.

Several workers have carried out experiments to determine the number of bacteria carried by flies under natural conditions. One of the most extended and best known of these is the series by Esten and Mason (1908). These workers caught flies from various sources in a sterilized net, placed them in a sterile bottle and poured over them a known quantity of sterilized water, in which they were shaken so as to wash the bacteria from their bodies. They found the number of bacteria on a single fly to range from 550 to 6,600,000. Early in the fly season the numbers of bacteria on flies are comparatively small, while later the numbers are comparatively very large. The place where flies live also determines largely the numbers that they carry. The lowest number, 550, was from a fly caught in the bacteriological laboratory, the highest number, 6,600,000 was the average from eighteen swill-barrel flies. Torrey (1912) made examination of "wild" flies from a tenement house district of New York City. He found "that the surface contamination of these 'wild' flies may vary from 570 to 4,400,000 bacteria per insect, and the intestinal bacterial content from 16,000 to 28,000,000."

Less well known in this country is the work of Cox, Lewis, and Glynn (1912). They examined over four hundred and fifty naturally infected house-flies in Liverpool during September and early October. Instead of washing the flies they were allowed to swim on the surface of sterile water for five, fifteen, or thirty minutes, thus giving natural conditions, where infection occurs from vomit and dejecta of the flies, as well as from their bodies. They found, as might be expected, that flies from either insanitary or congested areas of the city contain far more bacteria than those from the more sanitary, less congested, or suburban areas. The number of aerobic bacteria from the former varied from 800,000 to 500,000,000 per fly and from the latter from 21,000 to 100,000. The number of intestinal forms conveyed by flies from insanitary or congested areas was from 10,000 to 333,000,000 as compared with from 100 to 10,000 carried by flies from the more sanitary areas.

Pathogenic bacteria and those allied to the food poisoning group were only obtained from the congested or moderately congested areas and not from the suburban areas, where the chances of infestation were less.

The interesting fact was brought out that flies caught in milk shops apparently carry and obtain more bacteria than those from other shops with exposed food in a similar neighborhood. The writers explained this as probably due to the fact that milk when accessible, especially during the summer months, is suitable culture medium for bacteria, and the flies first inoculate the milk and later reinoculate themselves, and then more of the milk, so establishing a vicious circle.

They conclude that in cities where food is plentiful flies rarely migrate from the locality in which they are bred, and consequently the number of bacteria which they carry depends upon the general standard of cleanliness in that locality. Flies caught in a street of modern, fairly high class, workmen's dwellings forming a sanitary oasis in the midst of a slum area, carried far less bacteria than those caught in the adjacent neighborhood.

Thus, as the amount of dirt carried by flies in any particular locality, measured in the terms of bacteria, bears a definite relation to the habits of the people and to the state of the streets, it demonstrates the necessity of efficient municipal and domestic cleanliness, if the food of the inhabitants is to escape pollution, not only with harmless but also with occasional pathogenic bacteria.

The above cited work is of a general nature, but, especially in recent years, many attempts have been made to determine more specifically the ability of flies to transmit pathogenic organisms. The critical reviews of Nuttall and Jepson (1909), Howard (1911), and Graham-Smith (1913) should be consulted by the student of the subject. We can only cite here a few of the more striking experiments.

Celli (1888) fed flies on pure cultures of *Bacillus typhosus* and declared that he was able to recover these organisms from the intestinal contents and excrement.

Firth and Horrocks (1902), cited by Nuttall and Jepson, "kept *Musca domestica* (also bluebottles) in a large box measuring 4 x 3 x 3 feet, with one side made of glass. They were fed on material contaminated with cultures of *B. typhosus*. Agar plates, litmus, glucose broth and a sheet of clean paper were at the same time exposed in the box. After a few days the plates and broth were removed and incubated with a positive result." Graham-Smith (1910) "carried out experiments with large numbers of flies kept in gauze cages and fed for eight hours on emulsions of *B. typhosus* in syrup. After that time the infested syrup was removed and the flies were fed on plain syrup. *B. typhosus* was isolated up to 48 hours (but not later) from emulsions of their feces and from plates over which they walked."

Several other workers, notably Hamilton (1903), Ficker (1903), Bertarelli (1910) Faichnie (1909), and Cochrane (1912), have isolated *B. typhosus* from "wild" flies, naturally infected. The papers of Faichnie and of Cochrane we have not seen, but they are quoted in *extenso* by Graham-Smith (1913).

On the whole, the evidence is conclusive that typhoid germs not only may be accidentally carried on the bodies of house-flies but may pass through their bodies and be scattered in a viable condition in the feces of the fly for at least two days after feeding. Similar, results have been reached in experiments with cholera, tuberculosis and yaws, the last-mentioned being a spirochæte disease. Darling (1913) has shown that murrina, a trypanosome disease of horses and mules in the Canal zone is transmitted by house-flies which feed upon excoriated patches of diseased animals and then pass to cuts and galls of healthy animals.

Since it is clear that flies are abundantly able to disseminate viable pathogenic bacteria, it is important to consider whether they have access to such organisms in nature. A consideration of the method of spread of typhoid will serve to illustrate the way in which flies may play an important rôle.

Typhoid fever is a specific disease caused by *Bacillus typhosus*, and by it alone. The causative organism is to be found in the excrement and urine of patients suffering from the disease. More than that, it is often present in the dejecta for days, weeks, or even months and years, after the individual has recovered from the disease. Individuals so infested are known as "typhoid carriers" and they, together with those suffering from mild cases, or "walking typhoid," are a constant menace to the health of the community in which they are found.

Human excrement is greedily visited by flies, both for feeding and for ovipositing. The discharges of typhoid patients, or of chronic "carriers," when passed in the open, in box privies, or camp latrines, or the like, serve to contaminate myriads of the insects which may then spread the germ to human food and drink. Other intestinal diseases may be similarly spread. There is abundant epidæmiological evidence that infantile diarrhœa, dysentery, and cholera may be so spread.

Stiles and Keister (1913) have shown that spores of *Lamblia intestinalis*, a flagellate protozoan living in the human intestine, may be carried by house-flies. Though this species is not normally pathogenic, one or more species of *Entamœba* are the cause of a type of a highly fatal tropical dysentery. Concerning it, and another protozoan parasite of man, they say, "If flies can carry *Lamblia* spores measuring 10 to 7$\mu$, and bacteria that are much smaller, and particles of lime that are much larger, there is no ground to assume that flies may not carry *Entamœba* and *Trichomonas* spores.

Tuberculosis is one of the diseases which it is quite conceivable may be carried occasionally. The sputum of tubercular patients is very attractive to flies, and various workers, notably Graham-Smith, have found that *Musca domestica* may distribute the bacillus for several days after feeding on infected material.

A type of purulent opthalmia which is very prevalent in Egypt is often said to be carried by flies. Nuttall and Jepson (1909) consider that the evidence regarding the spread of this disease by flies is conclusive and that the possibility of gonorrhœal secretions being likewise conveyed cannot be denied.

Many studies have been published, showing a marked agreement between the occurrence of typhoid and other intestinal diseases and the prevalence of house-flies. The most clear-cut of these are the studies of the Army Commission appointed to investigate the cause of epidemics of enteric fever in the volunteer camps in the Southern United States during the Spanish-American War. Though their findings as presented by Vaughan (1909), have been quoted very many times, they are so germane to our discussion that they will bear repetition:

"Flies swarmed over infected fecal matter in the pits and fed upon the food prepared for the soldiers in the mess tents. In some instances where lime had recently been sprinkled over the contents of the pits, flies with their feet whitened with lime were seen walking over the food." Under such conditions it is no wonder that "These pests had inflicted greater loss upon American soldiers than the arms of Spain."

Similar conditions prevailed in South Africa during the Boer War. Seamon believes that very much of the success of the Japanese in their fight against Russia was due to the rigid precautions taken to prevent the spread of disease by these insects and other means.

Veeder has pointed out that the characteristics of a typical fly-borne epidemic of typhoid are that it occurs in little neighborhood epidemics, extending by short leaps from house to house, without regard to water supply or anything else in common. It tends to follow the direction of prevailing winds (cf. the conclusions of Hindle and Merriman). It occurs during warm weather. Of course, when the epidemic is once well under way, other factors enter into its spread.

In general, flies may be said to be the chief agency in the spread of typhoid in villages and camps. In cities with modern sewer systems they are less important, though even under the best of such conditions, they are important factors. Howard has emphasized that in such cities there are still many uncared-for box privies and that, in addition, the deposition of feces overnight in uncared-for waste lots and alleys is common.

Not only unicellular organisms, such as bacteria and protozoa, but also the eggs, embryos and larvæ of parasitic worms have been found to be transported by house-flies. Ransom (1911) has found that *Habronema muscæ*, a nematode worm often found in adult flies, is the immature stage of a parasite occurring in the stomach of the horse. The eggs or embryos passing out with the feces of the horse, are taken up by fly larvæ and carried over to the imago stage.

Grassi (1883), Stiles (1889), Calandruccio (1906), and especially Nicoll (1911), have been the chief investigators of the ability of house-flies to carry the ova and embryos of human intestinal parasites. Graham-Smith (1913) summarizes the work along this line as follows:

"It is evident from the investigations that have been quoted that house-flies and other species are greatly attracted to the ova of parasitic worms contained in feces and other materials, and make great efforts to ingest them. Unless the ova are too large they often succeed, and the eggs are deposited uninjured in their feces, in some cases up to the third day at least. The eggs may also be carried on their legs or bodies. Under suitable conditions, food and fluids may be contaminated with the eggs of various parasitic worms by flies, and in one case infection of the human subject has been observed. Feces containing tape-worm segments may continue to be a source of infection for as long as a fortnight. Up to the present, however, there is no evidence to show what part flies play in the dissemination of parasitic worms under natural conditions."

Enough has been said to show that the house-fly must be dealt with as a direct menace to public health. Control measures are not merely matters of convenience but are of vital importance.

Under present conditions the speedy elimination of the house-fly is impossible and the first thing to be considered is methods of protecting food and drink from contamination. The first of these methods is the thorough screening of doors and windows to prevent the entrance of flies. In the case of kitchen doors, the flies, attracted by odors, are likely to swarm onto the screen and improve the first opportunity for gaining an entrance. This difficulty can be largely avoided by screening-in the back porch and placing the screen door at one end rather than directly before the door.

The use of sticky fly paper to catch the pests that gain entrance to the house is preferable to the various poisons often used. Of the latter, formalin (40 per cent formaldehyde) in the proportion of two tablespoonfuls to a pint of water is very efficient, if all other liquids are removed or covered, so that the flies must depend on the formalin for drink. The mixture is said to be made more attractive by the addition of sugar or milk, though we have found the plain solution wholly satisfactory, under proper conditions. It should be emphasized that this formalin mixture is not perfectly harmless, as so often stated. There are on record cases of severe and even fatal poisoning from the accidental drinking of solutions.

When flies are very abundant in a room they can be most readily gotten rid of by fumigation with sulphur, or by the use of pure pyrethrum powder either burned or puffed into the air. Herrick (1913) recommends the following method: "At night all the doors and windows of the kitchen should be closed; fresh powder should be sprinkled over the stove, on the window ledges, tables, and in the air. In the morning flies will be found lying around dead or stupified. They may then be swept up and burned." This method has proved very efficacious in some of the large dining halls in Ithaca.

The writers have had little success in fumigating with the vapors of carbolic acid, or carbolic acid and gum camphor, although these methods will aid in driving flies from a darkened room.

All of these methods are but makeshifts. As Howard has so well put it, "the truest and simplest way of attacking the fly problem is to prevent them from breeding, by the treatment or abolition of all places in which they can breed. To permit them to breed undisturbed and in countless numbers, and to devote all our energy to the problem of keeping them out of our dwellings, or to destroy them after they have once entered in spite of all obstacles, seems the wrong way to go about it."

We have already seen that *Musca domestica* breeds in almost any fermenting organic material. While it prefers horse manure, it breeds also in human feces, cow dung and that of other animals, and in refuse of many kinds. To efficiently combat the insect, these breeding places must be removed or must be treated in some such way as to render them unsuitable for the development of the larvæ. Under some conditions individual work may prove effective, but to be truly efficient there must be extensive and thorough co-operative efforts.

Manure, garbage, and the like should be stored in tight receptacles and carted away at least once a week. The manure may be carted to the fields and spread. Even in spread manure the larvæ may continue their development. Howard points out that "it often happens that after a lawn has been heavily manured in early summer the occupants of the house will be pestered with flies for a time, but finding no available breeding place these disappear sooner or later. Another generation will not breed in the spread manure."

Hutchinson (1914) has emphasized that the larvæ of houseflies have deeply engrained the habit of migrating in the prepupal stage and has shown that this offers an important point of attack in attempts to control the pest. He has suggested that maggot traps might be developed into an efficient weapon in the warfare against the house-fly. Certain it is that the habit greatly simplifies the problem of treating the manure for the purpose of killing the larvæ.

There have been many attempts to find some cheap chemical which would destroy fly larvæ in horse manure without injuring the bacteria or reducing the fertilizing values of the manure. The literature abounds in recommendations of kerosene, lime, chloride of lime, iron sulphate, and other substances, but none of them have met the situation. The whole question has been gone into thoroughly by Cook, Hutchinson and Scales (1914), who tested practically all of the substances which have been recommended. They find that by far the most effective, economical, and practical of the substances is borax in the commercial form in which it is available throughout the country.

"Borax increases the water-soluble nitrogen, ammonia and alkalinity of manure and apparently does not permanently injure the bacterial flora. The application of manure treated with borax at the rate of 0.62 pound per eight bushels (10 cubic feet) to soil does not injure the plants thus far tested, although its cumulative effect, if any, has not been determined."

As their results clearly show that the substances so often recommended are inferior to borax, we shall quote in detail their directions for treating manure so as to kill fly eggs and maggots.

"Apply 0.62 pound borax or 0.75 pound calcined colemanite to every 10 cubic feet (8 bushels) of manure immediately on its removal from the barn. Apply the borax particularly around the outer edges of the pile with a flour sifter or any fine sieve, and sprinkle two or three gallons of water over the borax-treated manure.

"The reason for applying the borax to the fresh manure immediately after its removal from the stable is that the flies lay their eggs on the fresh manure, and borax, when it comes in contact with the eggs, prevents their hatching. As the maggots congregate at the outer edge of the pile, most of the borax should be applied there. The treatment should be repeated with each addition of fresh manure, but when the manure is kept in closed boxes, less frequent applications will be sufficient. When the calcined colemanite is available, it may be used at the rate of 0.75 pound per 10 cubic feet of manure, and is a cheaper means of killing the maggots. In addition to the application of borax to horse manure to kill fly larvæ, it may be applied in the same proportion to other manures, as well as to refuse and garbage. Borax may also be applied to the floors and crevices in barns, stables, markets, etc., as well as to street sweepings, and water should be added as in the treatment of horse manure. After estimating the amount of material to be treated and weighing the necessary amount of borax, a measure may be used which will hold the proper amount, thus avoiding the subsequent weighings.

"While it can be safely stated that no injurious action will follow the application of manure treated with borax at the rate of 0.62 pound for eight bushels, or even larger amounts in the case of some plants, nevertheless the borax-treated manure has not been studied in connection with the growth of all crops, nor has its cumulative effect been determined. It is therefore recommended that not more than 15 tons per acre of the borax-treated manure should be applied to the field. As truckmen use considerably more than this amount, it is suggested that all cars containing borax-treated manure be so marked, and that public-health officials stipulate in their directions for this treatment that not over 0.62 pound for eight bushels of manure be used, as it has been shown that larger amounts of borax will injure most plants. It is also recommended that all public-health officials and others, in recommending the borax treatment for killing fly eggs and maggots in manure, warn the public against the injurious effects of large amounts of borax on the growth of plants."

"The amount of manure from a horse varies with the straw or other bedding used, but 12 or 15 bushels per week represent the approximate amount obtained. As borax costs from five to six cents per pound in 100-pound lots in Washington, it will make the cost of the borax practically one cent per horse, per day. And if calcined colemanite is purchased in large shipments the cost should be considerably less."

Hodge (1910) has approached the problem of fly extermination from another viewpoint. He believes that it is practical to trap flies out of doors during the preoviposition period, when they are sexually immature, and to destroy such numbers of them that the comparatively few which survive will not be able to lay eggs in sufficent numbers to make the next generation a nuisance. To the end of capturing them in enormous numbers he has devised traps to be fitted over garbage cans, into stable windows, and connected with the kitchen window screens. Under some conditions this method of attack has proved very satisfactory.

One of the most important measures for preventing the spread of disease by flies is the abolition of the common box privy. In villages and rural districts this is today almost the only type to be found. It is the chief factor in the spread of typhoid and other intestinal diseases, as well as intestinal parasites. Open and exposed to myriads of flies which not only breed there but which feed upon the excrement, they furnish ideal conditions for spreading contamination. Even where efforts are made to cover the contents with dust, or ashes, or lime, flies may continue to breed unchecked. Stiles and Gardner have shown that house-flies buried in a screened stand-pipe forty-eight inches under sterile sand came to the surface. Other flies of undetermined species struggled up through seventy-two inches of sand.

So great is the menace of the ordinary box privy that a number of inexpensive and simple sanitary privies have been designed for use where there are not modern sewer systems. Stiles and Lumsden (1911) have given minute directions for the construction of one of the best types, and their bulletin should be obtained by those interested.

Another precaution which is of fundamental importance in preventing the spread of typhoid, is that of disinfecting all discharges from patients suffering with the disease. For this purpose, quicklime is the cheapest and is wholly satisfactory. In chamber vessels it should be used in a quantity equal to that of the discharge to be treated. It should be allowed to act for two hours. Air-slaked lime is of no value whatever. Chloride of lime, carbolic acid, or formalin may be used, but are more expensive. Other intestinal diseases demand similar precautions.

**Stomoxys calcitrans, the stable-fly**—It is a popular belief that house-flies bite more viciously just before a rain. As a matter of fact, the true house-flies never bite, for their mouth-parts are not fitted for piercing. The basis of the misconception is the fact that a true biting fly, *Stomoxys calcitrans* (fig. 110), closely resembling the house-fly, is frequently found in houses and may be driven in in greater numbers by muggy weather. From its usual habitat this fly is known as the "stable-fly" or, sometimes as the "biting house-fly."

*Stomoxys calcitrans* may be separated from the house-fly by the use of the key on p. 145. It may be more fully characterized as follows:

The eyes of the male are separated by a distance equal to one-fourth of the diameter of the head, in the female by one-third. The

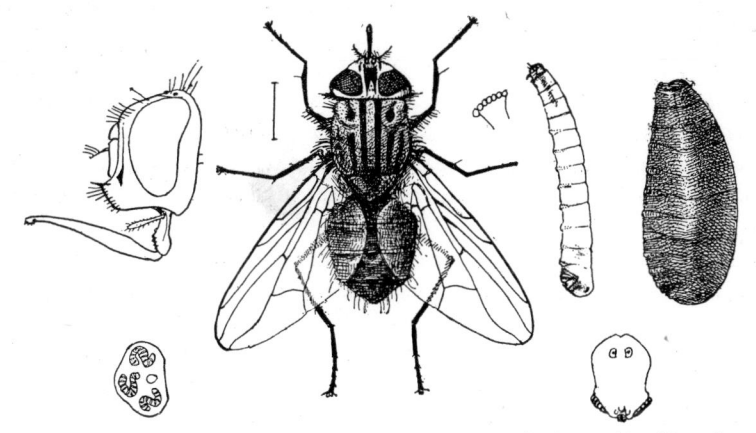

110. Stomoxys calcitrans; adult, larva, puparium and details, (x5). After Howard.

frontal stripe is black, the cheeks and margins of the orbits silvery-white. The antennæ are black, the arista feathered on the upper side only. The proboscis is black, slender, fitted for piercing and projects forward in front of the head. The thorax is grayish, marked by four conspicuous, more or less complete black longitudinal stripes; the scutellum is paler; the macrochætæ are black. The abdomen is gray, dorsally with three brown spots on the second and third segments and a median spot on the fourth. These spots are more pronounced in the female. The legs are black, the pulvilli distinct. The wings are hyaline, the vein $M_{1+2}$ less sharply curved than in the house-fly, the apical cell being thus more widely open (cf. fig. 110). Length 7 mm.

This fly is widely distributed, being found the world over. It was probably introduced into the United States, but has spread to all parts of the country. Bishopp (1913) regards it as of much more importance as a pest of domestic animals in the grain belt than elsewhere in the United States. The life-history and habits of this species have assumed a new significance since it has been suggested that it may transmit the human diseases, infantile paralysis and pellagra. In this country, the most detailed study of the fly is that of Bishopp (1913) whose data regarding the life cycle are as follows:

The eggs like those of the house-fly, are about one mm. in length. Under a magnifying glass they show a distinct furrow along one side. When placed on any moist substance they hatch in from one to three days after being deposited.

The larvæ or maggots (fig. 110) have the typical shape and actions of most maggots of the Muscid group. They can be distinguished from those of the house-fly as the stigma-plates are smaller, much further apart, with the slits less sinuous. Development takes place fairly rapidly when the proper food conditions are available and the growth is completed within eleven to thirty or more days.

The pupa (fig. 110), like that of related flies, undergoes its development within the contracted and hardened last larval skin, or puparium. This is elongate oval, slightly thicker towards the head end, and one-sixth to one-fourth of an inch in length. The pupal stage requires six to twenty days, or in cool weather considerably longer.

The life-cycle of the stable-fly is therefore considerably longer than that of *Musca domestica*. Bishopp found that complete development might be undergone in nineteen days, but that the average period was somewhat longer, ranging from twenty-one to twenty-five days, where conditions are very favorable. The longest period which he observed was forty-three days, though his finding of full grown larvæ and pupæ in straw during the latter part of March, in Northern Texas, showed that development may require about three months, as he considered that these stages almost certainly developed from eggs deposited the previous December.

The favorite breeding place, where available, seems to be straw or manure mixed with straw. It also breeds in great numbers in horse-manure, in company with *Musca domestica*.

Newstead considers that in England the stable-fly hibernates in the pupal stage. Bishopp finds that in the southern part of the United States there is no true hibernation, as the adults have been found to emerge at various times during the winter. He believes that in the northern United States the winter is normally passed in the larval and pupal stages, and that the adults which have been observed in heated stables in the dead of winter were bred out in refuse within the warm barns and were not hibernating adults.

Graham-Smith (1913) states that although the stable-fly frequents stable manure, it is probably not an important agent in distributing the organisms of intestinal diseases. Bishopp makes the important observation that "it has never been found breeding in human excrement and does not frequent malodorous places, which are so attractive to the house-fly. Hence it is much less likely to carry typhoid and other germs which may be found in such places."

Questions of the possible agency of *Stomoxys calcitrans* in the transmission of infantile paralysis and of pellagra, we shall consider later.

**Other arthropods which may serve as simple carriers of pathogenic organisms**—It should be again emphasized that any insect which has access to, and comes in contact with, pathogenic organisms and then passes to the food, or drink, or the body of man, may serve as a simple carrier of disease. In addition to the more obvious illustrations, an interesting one is the previously cited case of the transfer of *Dermatobia cyaniventris* by a mosquito (fig. 81–84). Darling (1913) has shown that in the tropics, the omnipresent ants may be important factors in the spread of disease.

## CHAPTER VI

### ARTHROPODS AS DIRECT INOCULATORS OF DISEASE GERMS

We have seen that any insect which, like the house-fly, has access to disease germs and then comes into contact with the food or drink of man, may serve to disseminate disease. Moreover, it has been clearly established that a contaminated insect, alighting upon wounded or abraded surfaces, may infect them. These are instances of mere accidental, mechanical transfer of pathogenic organisms.

Closely related are the instances of direct inoculation of disease germs by insects and other arthropods. In this type, a blood-sucking species not only takes up the germs but, passing to a healthy individual, it inserts its contaminated mouth-parts and thus directly inoculates its victim. In other words, the disease is transferred just as blood poisoning may be induced by the prick of a contaminated needle, or as the laboratory worker may inoculate an experimental animal.

Formerly, it was supposed that this method of the transfer of disease by arthropods was a very common one and many instances are cited in the earlier literature of the subject. It is, however, difficult to draw a sharp line between such cases and those in which, on the one hand, the arthropod serves as a mere passive carrier or, on the other hand, serves as an essential host of the pathogenic organism. More critical study of the subject has led to the belief that the importance of the rôle of arthropods as direct inoculators has been much overestimated.

The principal reason for regarding this phase of the subject as relatively unimportant, is derived from a study of the habits of the blood-sucking species. It is found that, in general, they are intermittent feeders, visiting their hosts at intervals and then abstaining from feeding for a more or less extended period, while digesting their meal. In the meantime, most species of bacteria or of protozoan parasites with which they might have contaminated their mouth-parts, would have perished, through inability to withstand drying.

In spite of this, it must be recognized that this method of transfer does occur and must be reckoned with in any consideration of the relations of insects to disease. We shall first cite some general illustrations and shall then discuss the rôle of fleas in the spreading of bubonic plague, an illustration which cannot be regarded as typical, since it involves more than mere passive carriage.

## Some Illustrations of Direct Inoculation of Disease Germs by Arthropods

In discussing poisonous arthropods, we have already emphasized that species which are of themselves innocuous to man, may occasionally introduce bacteria by their bite or sting and thus cause more or less severe secondary symptoms. That such cases should occur, is no more than is to be expected. The mouth-parts or the sting of the insect are not sterile and the chances of their carrying pyogenic organisms are always present.

More strictly falling in the category of transmission of disease germs by direct inoculation are the instances where the insect, or related form, feeds upon a diseased animal and passes promptly to a healthy individual which it infects. Of such a nature are the following:

Various species of biting flies are factors in the dissemination of anthrax, an infectious and usually fatal disease of animals and, occasionally, of man. That the bacteria with which the blood of diseased animals teem shortly before death might be transmitted by such insects has long been contended, but the evidence in support of the view has been unsatisfactory. Recently, Mitzmain (1914) has reported a series of experiments which show conclusively that the disease may be so conveyed by a horse-fly, *Tabanus striatus*, and by the stable-fly, *Stomoxys calcitrans*.

Mitzmain's experiments were tried with an artificially infected guinea pig, which died of the disease upon the third day. The flies were applied two and one-half hours, to a few minutes, before the death of the animal. With both species the infection was successfully transferred to healthy guinea pigs by the direct method, in which the flies were interrupted while feeding on the sick animal. The evidence at hand does not warrant the conclusion that insect transmission is the rule in the case of this disease.

The nagana, or tsetse-fly disease of cattle is the most virulent disease of domestic animals in certain parts of Africa. It is caused by a protozoan blood parasite, *Trypanosoma brucei*, which is conveyed to healthy animals by the bite of *Glossina morsitans* and possibly other species of tsetse-flies. The flies remain infective for forty-eight hours after feeding on a diseased animal. The insect also serves as an essential host of the parasite.

Surra, a similar trypanosomiasis affecting especially horses and mules, occurs in southern Asia, Malaysia, and the Philippines where the tsetse-flies are not to be found. It is thought to be spread by various species of blood-sucking flies belonging to the genera *Stomoxys*, *Hæmatobia*, and *Tabanus*. Mitzmain (1913) demonstrated that in the Philippines it is conveyed mechanically by *Tabanus striatus*.

The sleeping sickness of man, in Africa, has also been supposed to be directly inoculated by one, or several, species of tsetse-flies. It is now known that the fly may convey the disease for a short time after feeding, but that there is then a latent period of from fourteen to twenty-one days, after which it again becomes infectious. This indicates that in the meantime the parasite has been undergoing some phase of its life-cycle and that the fly serves as an intermediate host. We shall therefore consider it more fully under that grouping.

These are a few of the cases of direct inoculation which may be cited as of the simpler type. We shall next consider the rôle of the flea in the dissemination of the bubonic plague, an illustration complicated by the fact that the bacillus multiples within the insect and may be indirectly inoculated.

### The Rôle of Fleas in the Transmission of the Plague

The plague is a specific infectious disease caused by *Bacillus pestis*. It occurs in several forms, of which the bubonic and the pneumonic are the most common. According to Wyman, 80 per cent of the human cases are of the bubonic type. It is a disease which, under the name of oriental plague, the pest, or the black death, has ravaged almost from time immemorial the countries of Africa, Asia, and Europe. The record of its ravages are almost beyond belief. In 542 A. D. it caused in one day ten thousand deaths in Constantinople. In the 14th century it was introduced from the East and prevailed throughout Armenia, Asia Minor, Egypt and Northern Africa and Europe. Hecker estimates that one-fourth of the population of Europe, or twenty-five million persons, died in the epidemic of that century. From then until the 17th century it was almost constantly present in Europe, the great plague of London, in 1665 killing 68,596 out of a population of 460,000. Such an epidemic would mean for New York City a proportionate loss of over 600,000 in a single year. It is little wonder that in the face of such an appalling disaster suspicion and credulity were rife and the wildest demoralization ensued.

During the 14th century the Jews were regarded as responsible for the disease, through poisoning wells, and were subjected to the

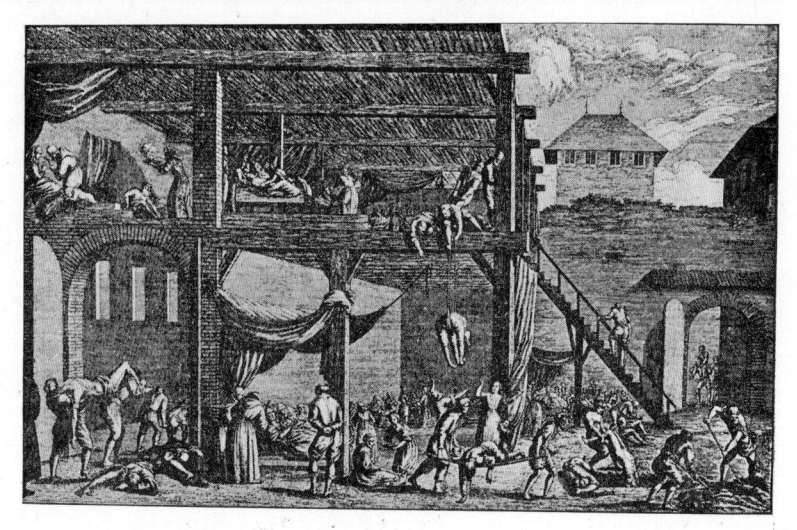

111. A contemporaneous engraving of the pest hospital in Vienna in 1679. After Peters.

most incredible persecution and torture. In Milan the visitation of 1630 was credited to the so-called anointers,—men who were supposed to spread the plague by anointing the walls with magic ointment—and the most horrible tortures that human ingenuity could devise were imposed on scores of victims, regardless of rank or of public service (fig. 112, a). Manzoni's great historical novel, "The Betrothed" has well pictured conditions in Italy during this period.

In modern times the plague is confined primarily to warm climates, a condition which has been brought about largely through general improvement in sanitary conditions.

At present, the hotbed of the disease is India, where there were 1,040,429 deaths in 1904 and where in a period of fifteen years, ending with January 1912, there were over 15,000,000 deaths. The reported deaths in that country for 1913 totaled 198,875.

During the winter of 1910–11 there occurred in Manchuria and North China a virulent epidemic of the pneumonic plague which caused the death of nearly 50,000 people. The question as to its origin and means of spread will be especially referred to later.

Until recent years, the plague had not been known to occur in the New World but there were outbreaks in Brazil and Hawaii in 1899, and in 1900 there occurred the first cases in San Francisco.

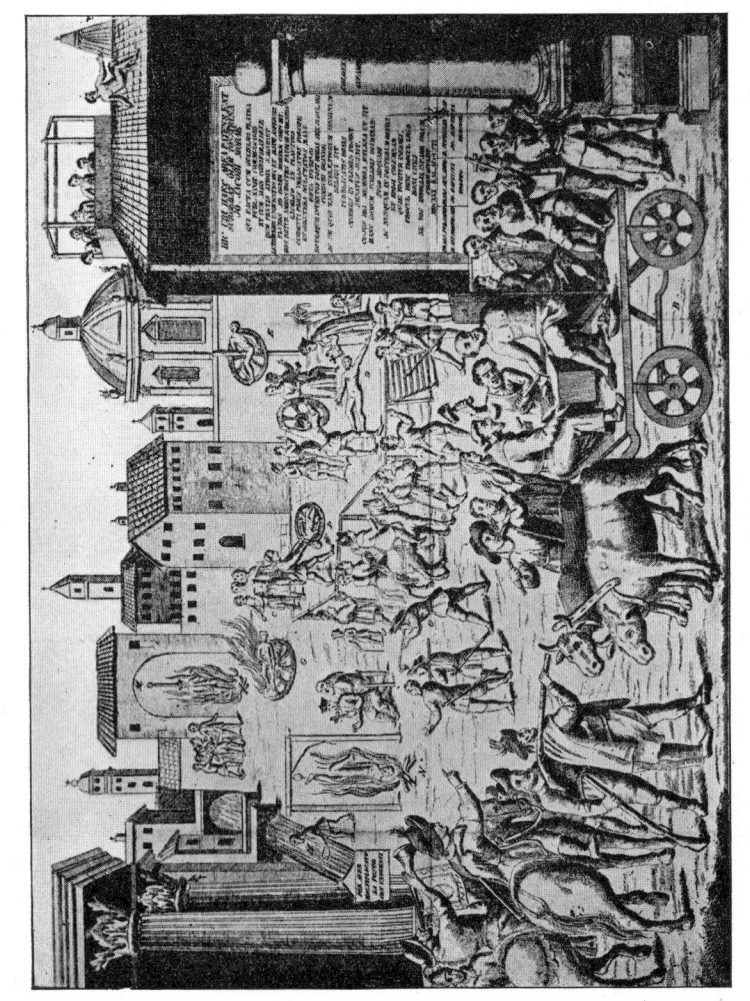

168  *Arthropods as Direct Inoculators of Disease Germs*

112 a. A medieval method of combating the plague. The persecution of the anointers in Milan in 1630. From a copy of "Il processi originale degli untori" in the library of Cornell University.

In California there were 125 cases in the period 1900–04; three cases in the next three years and then from May 1907 to March 1908, during the height of the outbreak, 170 cases. Since that time there have been only sporadic cases, the last case reported being in May 1914. Still more recent were the outbreaks in the Philippine Islands, Porto Rico, and Cuba.

On June 24, 1914, there was recognized a case of human plague in New Orleans. The Federal Health Service immediately took charge, and measures for the eradication of the disease were vigorously enforced. Up to Otcober 10, 1914 there had been reported 30 cases of the disease in man, and 181 cases of plague in rats.

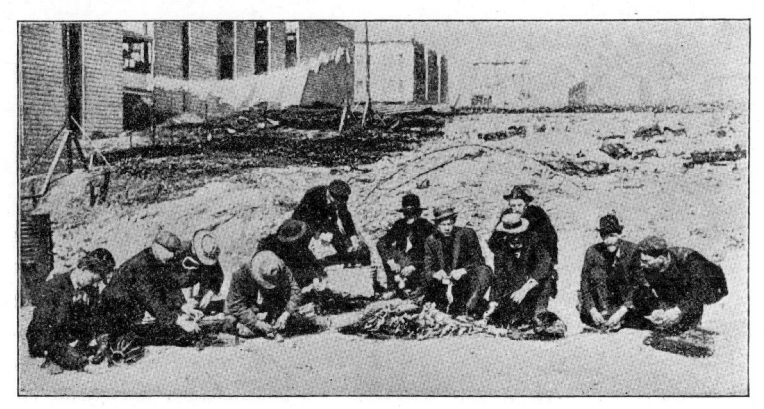

112 b. The modern method of combating the plague. A day's catch of rats in the fight against plague in San Francisco. Courtesy of Review of Reviews.

The present-day methods of combating bubonic plague are well illustrated by the fight in San Francisco. Had it not been for the strenuous and radical anti-plague campaign directed by the United States Marine Hospital Service we might have had in our own country an illustration of what the disease can accomplish. On what newly acquired knowledge was this fight based?

The basis was laid in 1894, when the plague bacillus was first discovered. All through the centuries, before and during the Christian era, down to 1894, the subject was enveloped in darkness and there had been a helpless, almost hopeless struggle in ignorance on the part of physicians, sanitarians, and public health officials against the ravages of this dread disease, Now its cause, method of propagation and means to prevent its spread are matters of scientific certainty.

After the discovery of the causative organism, one of the first advances was the establishment of the identity of human plague and that of rodents. It had often been noted that epidemics of the human disease were preceded by great epizootics among rats and mice. So well established was this fact that with the Chinese, unusual mortality among these rodents was regarded as foretelling a visitation of the human disease. That there was more than an accidental connection between the two was obvious when Yersin, the discoverer of *Bacillus pestis*, announced that during an epidemic the rats found dead in the houses and in the streets almost always contain the bacillus in great abundance in their organs, and that many of them exhibit veritable buboes.

Once it was established that the diseases were identical, the attention of the investigators was directed to a study of the relations between that of rats and of humans, and evidence accumulated to show that the bubonic plague was primarily a disease of rodents and that in some manner it was conveyed from them to man.

There yet remained unexplained the method of transfer from rat to man. As long ago as the 16th century, Mercuralis suggested that house-flies were guilty of disseminating the plague but modern investigation, while blaming the fly for much in the way of spreading disease, show that it is an insignificant factor in this case.

Search for blood-sucking insects which would feed on both rodents and man, and which might therefore be implicated, indicated that the fleas most nearly met the conditions. At first it was urged that rat fleas would not feed upon man and that the fleas ordinarily attacking man would not feed upon rats. More critical study of the habits of fleas soon showed that these objections were not well-founded. Especially important was the evidence that soon after the death of their host, rat fleas deserted its body and might then become a pest in houses where they had not been noticed before.

Attention was directed to the fact that while feeding, fleas are in the habit of squirting blood from the anus and that in the case of those which had fed upon rats and mice dying of the plague, virulent plague bacilli were to be found in such blood. Liston (1905) even found, and subsequent investigations confirmed, that the plague bacilli multiply in the stomach of the insect and that thus the blood ejected was richer in the organisms than was that of the diseased animal. It was found that a film of this infected blood spread out under the body of the flea and that thus the bacilli might be inoculated by the bite of the insect and by scratching.

Very recently, Bacot and Martin (1914) have paid especial attention to the question of the mechanism of the transmission of the plague bacilli by fleas. They believe that plague infested fleas regurgitate blood through the mouth, and that under conditions precluding the possibility of infection by dejecta, the disease may be thus transmitted. The evidence does not seem sufficient to establish that this is the chief method of transmission.

Conclusive experimental proof that fleas transmit the disease is further available from a number of sources. The most extensive series of experiments is that of the English Plague Commission in India, which reported in 1906 that:

On thirty occasions a healthy rat contracted plague in sequence of living in the neighborhood of a plague infected rat under circumstances which prevented the healthy rat coming in contact with either the body or excreta of the diseased animal.

In twenty-one experiments out of thirty-eight, healthy rats living in flea-proof cages contracted plague when exposed to rat fleas (*Xenopsylla cheopis*), collected from rats dead or dying of septicæmic plague.

Close contact of plague-infected with healthy animals, if fleas are excluded, does not give rise to an epizootic among the latter. As the huts were never cleaned out, close contact included contact with feces and urine of infected animals, and contact with, and eating of food contaminated with feces and urine of infected animals, as well as pus from open plague ulcers. Close contact of young, even when suckled by plague-infected mothers, did not give the disease to the former.

If fleas are present, then the epizootic, once started, spreads from animal to animal, the rate of progress being in direct proportion to the number of fleas.

Aerial infection was excluded. Thus guinea-pigs suspended in a cage two feet above the ground did not contract the disease, while in the same hut those animals allowed to run about and those placed two inches above the floor became infected. It had previously been found that a rat flea could not hop farther than about five inches.

Guinea pigs and monkeys were placed in plague houses in pairs, both protected from soil contact infection and both equally exposed to aerial infection, but one surrounded with a layer of tangle-foot paper and the other surrounded with a layer of sand. The following observations were made:

(a) Many fleas were caught in the tangle-foot, a certain proportion of which were found on dissection to contain in their stomachs abundant bacilli microscopically identical with plague bacilli. Out of eighty-five human fleas dissected only one contained these bacilli, while out of seventy-seven rat fleas twenty-three were found thus infected.

(b) The animals surrounded with tangle-foot in no instance developed plague, while several (24 per cent) of the non-protected animals died of the disease.

Thus, the experimental evidence that fleas transmit the plague from rat to rat, from rats to guinea pigs, and from rats to monkeys is indisputable. There is lacking direct experimental proof of its transfer from rodents to man but the whole chain of indirect evidence is so complete that there can be no doubt that such a transfer does occur so commonly that in the case of bubonic plague it must be regarded as the normal method.

Rats are not the only animals naturally attacked by the plague but as already suggested, it occurs in various other rodents. In California the disease has spread from rats to ground squirrels (*Otospermophilus beecheyi*), a condition readily arising from the frequency of association of rats with the squirrels in the neighborhood of towns, and from the fact that the two species of fleas found on them are also found on rats. While the danger of the disease being conveyed from squirrels to man is comparatively slight, the menace in the situation is that the squirrels may become a more or less permanent reservoir of the disease and infect rats, which may come into more frequent contact with man.

The tarbagan (*Arctomys bobac*), is a rodent found in North Manchuria, which is much prized for its fur. It is claimed that this animal is extremely susceptible to the plague and there is evidence to indicate that it was the primary source of the great outbreak of pneumonic plague which occurred in Manchuria and North China during the winter of 1910-11.

Of fleas, any species which attacks both rodents and man may be an agent in the transmission of the plague. We have seen that in India the species most commonly implicated is the rat flea, *Xenopsylla cheopis*, ( = *Lœmopsylla* or *Pulex cheopis*) (fig. 89). This species has also been found commonly on rats in San Francisco. The cat flea, *Ctenocephalus felis*, the dog flea, *Ctenocephalus canis*, the human flea, *Pulex irritans*, the rat fleas, *Ceratophyllus fasciatus* and *Ctenopsyllus musculi* have all been shown to meet the conditions.

But, however clear the evidence that fleas are the most important agent in the transfer of plague, it is a mistake fraught with danger to assume that they are the only factor in the spread of the disease. The causative organism is a bacillus and is not dependent upon any insect for the completion of its development.

Therefore, any blood-sucking insect which feeds upon a plague infected man or animal and then passes to a healthy individual, conceivably might transfer the bacilli. Verjbitski (1908) has shown experimentally that bed-bugs may thus convey the disease. Hertzog found the bacilli in a head-louse, *Pediculus humanus*, taken from a child which had died from the plague, and McCoy found them in a louse taken from a plague-infected squirrel. On account of their stationary habits, the latter insects could be of little significance in spreading the disease.

Contaminated food may also be a source of danger. While this source, formerly supposed to be the principal one, is now regarded as unimportant, there is abundant experimental evidence to show that it cannot be disregarded. It is believed that infection in this way can occur only when there is some lesion in the alimentary canal.

Still more important is the proof that in pneumonic plague the patient is directly infective and that the disease is spread from man to man without any intermediary. Especially conclusive is the evidence obtained by Drs. Strong and Teague during the Manchurian epidemic of 1910-11. They found that during coughing, in pneumonic plague cases, even when sputum visible to the naked eye is not expelled, plague bacilli in large numbers may become widely disseminated into the surrounding air. By exposing sterile plates before patients who coughed a single time, very numerous colonies of the baccilus were obtained.

But the great advance which has been made rests on the discovery that bubonic plague is in the vast majority of cases transmitted by the flea. The pneumonic type forms a very small percentage of the human cases and even with it, the evidence indicates that the original infection is derived from a rodent through the intermediary of the insect.

So modern prophylactic measures are directed primarily against the rat and fleas. Ships coming from infected ports are no longer disinfected for the purpose of killing the plague germs, but are fumigated to destroy the rats and the fleas which they might harbor. When anchored at infected ports, ships must observe strenuous precautions to prevent the ingress of rats. Cargo must be inspected just before being brought on board, in order to insure its freedom from rats. Even lines and hawsers must be protected by large metal discs or funnels, for rats readily run along a rope to reach the ship. Once infested, the ship must be thoroughly fumigated, not only to avoid carrying the disease to other ports but to obviate an outbreak on board.

When an epidemic begins, rats must be destroyed by trapping and poisoning. Various so-called biological poisons have not proved practicable. Sources of food supply should be cut off by thorough cleaning up, by use of rat-proof garbage cans and similar measures. Hand in hand with these, must go the destruction of breeding places, and the rat-proofing of dwellings, stables, markets, warehouses, docks and sewers. All these measures are expensive, and a few years ago would have been thought wholly impossible to put into practice but now they are being enforced on a large scale in every fight against the disease.

Rats and other rodents are regularly caught in the danger zone and examined for evidence of infection, for the sequence of the epizootic and of the human disease is now understood. In London, rats are regularly trapped and poisoned in the vicinity of the principal docks, to guard against the introduction of infected animals in shipping. During the past six years infected rats have been found yearly, thirteen having been found in 1912. In Seattle, Washington, seven infected rats were found along the water front in October, 1913, and infected ground squirrels are still being found in connection with the anti-plague measures in California.

The procedure during an outbreak of the human plague was well illustrated by the fight in San Francisco. The city was districted, and captured rats, after being dipped in some fluid to destroy the fleas, were carefully tagged to indicate their source, and were sent to the laboratory for examination. If an infected rat was found, the officers in charge of the work in the district involved were immediately notified by telephone, and the infected building was subjected to a thorough fumigation. In addition, special attention was given to all the territory in the four contiguous blocks.

By measures such as these, this dread scourge of the human race is being brought under control. Incidentally, the enormous losses due to the direct ravages of rats are being obviated and this alone would justify the expenditure many times over of the money and labor involved in the anti-rat measures.

## CHAPTER VII

### ARTHROPODS AS ESSENTIAL HOSTS OF PATHOGENIC ORGANISMS

We now have to consider the cases in which the arthropod acts as the essential host of a pathogenic organism. In other words, cases in which the organism, instead of being passively carried or merely accidentally inoculated by the bite of its carrier, or *vector*, is taken up and undergoes an essential part of its development within the arthropod.

In some cases, the sexual cycle of the parasite is undergone in the arthropod, which then serves as the *definitive* or *primary host*. In other cases, it is the asexual stage of the parasite which is undergone, and the arthropod then acts as the *intermediate host*. This distinction is often overlooked and all the cases incorrectly referred to as those in which the insect or other arthropod acts as intermediate host.

We have already emphasized that this is the most important way in which insects may transmit disease, for without them the particular organisms concerned could never complete their development. Exterminate the arthropod host and the life cycle of the parasite is broken, the disease is exterminated.

As the phenomenon of alternation of generations, as exhibited by many of the parasitic protozoa, is a complicated one and usually new to the student, we shall first take up some of the grosser cases illustrated by certain parasitic worms. There is the additional reason that these were the first cases known of arthropod transmission of pathogenic organisms.

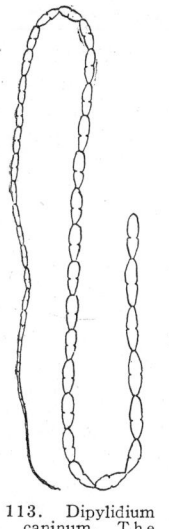

113. Dipylidium caninum. The double pored tapeworm of the dog.

### INSECTS AS INTERMEDIATE HOSTS OF TAPEWORMS

A number of tapeworms are known to undergo their sexual stage in an insect or other arthropod. Of these at least two are occasional parasites of man.

*Dipylidium caninum* (figs. 113 and 114), more generally known as *Taenia cucumerina* or *T. elliptica*, is the commonest intestinal parasite of pet dogs and cats. It is occasionally found as a human parasite, 70 per cent of the cases reported being in young children.

176  *Arthropods as Essential Hosts of Pathogenic Organisms*

In 1869, Melnikoff found in a dog louse, *Trichodectes canis*, some peculiar bodies which Leuckart identified as the larval form of this tapeworm. The worm is, however, much more common in dogs and cats than is the skin parasite, and hence it appears that the *Trichodectes* could not be the only intermediate host. In 1888, Grassi found that it could also develop in the cat and dog fleas, *Ctenocephalus felis* and *C. canis*, and in the human flea, *Pulex irritans*.

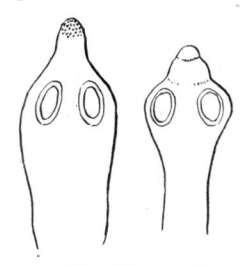

114. Dipylidium caninum. Rostrum evaginated and invaginated. After Blanchard.

The eggs, scattered among the hairs of the dog or cat, are ingested by the insect host and in its body cavity they develop into pyriform bodies, about 300μ in length, almost entirely destitute of a bladder, but in the immature stage provided with a caudal appendage (fig. 115). Within the pear-shaped body (fig. 116) are the invaginated head and suckers of the future tapeworm. This larval form is known as a cysticercoid, in contradistinction to the bladder-like cysticercus of many other cestodes. It is often referred to in literature as *Cryptocystis trichodectis* Villot.

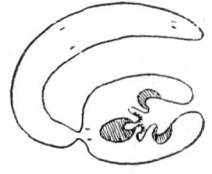

As many as fifty of the cysticercoids have been found in the body cavity of a single flea. When the dog takes up an infested flea or louse, by biting itself, or when the cat licks them up, the larvæ quickly develop into tapeworms, reaching sexual maturity in about twenty days in the intestine of their host. Puppies and kittens are quickly infested when suckling a flea-infested mother, the developing worms having been found in the intestines of puppies not more than five or six days old.

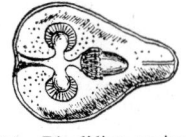

115. Dipylidium caninum. Immature cysticercoid. After Grassi and Rovelli.

Infestation of human beings occurs only through accidental ingestion of an infested flea. It is natural that such cases should occur largely in children, where they may come about in some such way as illustrated in the accompanying figures 117 and 118.

116. Dipylidium caninum. Cysticercoid. After Villot.

*Hymenolepis diminuta*, very commonly living in the intestine of mice and rats, is also known to occur in man. Its cysticercoid develops in the body cavity of a surprising range of meal-infesting insects. Grassi and Rovelli (abstract in Ransom, 1904) found it in the

## Insects as Intermediate Hosts of Tapeworms 177

larvæ and adult of a moth, *Asopia farinalis*, in the earwig, *Anisolabis annulipes*, the Tenebrionid beetles *Akis spinosa* and *Scaurus striatus*. Grassi considers that the lepidopter is the normal intermediate host. The insect takes up the eggs scattered by rats and mice. It has been experimentally demonstrated that man may develop the tapeworm by swallowing infested insects. Natural infection probably occurs by ingesting such insects with cereals, or imperfectly cooked foods.

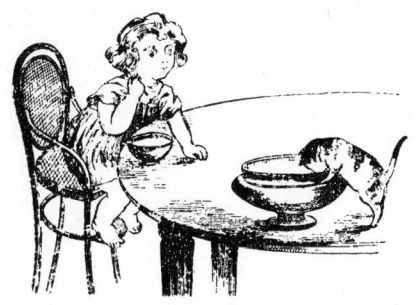

117. One way in which Dipylidium infection in children may occur. After Blanchard.

*Hymenolepis lanceolata*, a parasite of geese and ducks, has been reported once for man. The supposed cysticercoid occurs in various small crustaceans of the family Cyclopidæ.

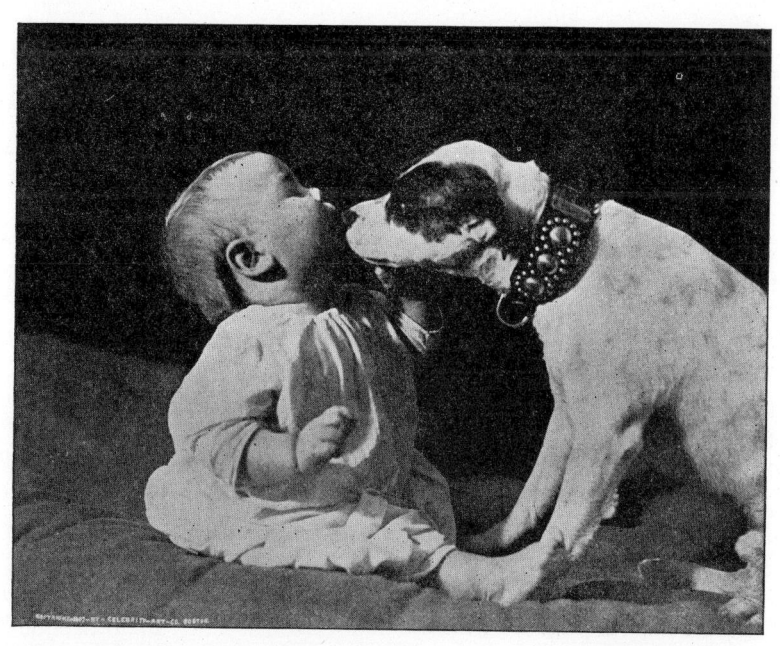

118. The probable method by which Dipylidium infection usually occurs.

Several other cestode parasites of domestic animals are believed to develop their intermediate stage in certain arthropods. Among these may be mentioned:

*Choanotænia infundibulformis*, of chickens, developing in the housefly (Grassi and Rovelli);

*Davainea cesticillus*, of chickens, in some lepidopter or coleopter (Grassi and Rovelli);

*Hymenolepis anatina*, *H. gracilis*, *H. sinuosa*, *H. coronula* and *Fimbriaria fasciolaris*, all occurring in ducks, have been reported as developing in small aquatic crustaceans. In these cases, cysticercoids have been found which, on account of superficial characters, have been regarded as belonging to the several species, but direct experimental evidence is scant.

## Arthropods as Intermediate Hosts of Nematode Worms

**Filariasis and Mosquitoes**—A number of species of Nematode worms belonging to the genus *Filaria*, infest man and other vertebrates and in the larval condition are to be found in the blood. Such infestation is known as *filariasis*. The sexually mature worms are to be found in the blood, the lymphatics, the mesentery and subcutaneous connective tissue. In the cases best studied it has been found that the larval forms are taken up by mosquitoes and undergo a transformation before they can attain maturity in man.

The larvæ circulating in the blood are conveniently designated as microfilariæ. In this stage they are harmless and only one species, *Filaria bancrofti*, appears to be of any great pathological significance at any stage.

*Filaria bancrofti* in its adult state, lives in the lymphatics of man. Though often causing no injury it has been clearly established that they and their eggs may cause various disorders due to stoppage of the lymphatic trunks (fig. 119). Manson lists among other effects, abscess, varicose groin glands, lymph scrotum, chyluria, and elephantiasis.

The geographical distribution of this parasite is usually given as coextensive with that of elephantiasis, but it is by no means certain that it is the only cause of this disease and so actual findings of the parasites are necessary. Manson reports that it is "an indigenous parasite in almost every country throughout the tropical and subtropical world, as far north as Spain in Europe and Charlestown in the United States, and as far south as Brisbane in Australia." In some sections, fully 50 per cent of the natives are infested. Labredo (1910) found 17.82 per cent infestation in Havana.

The larval forms of *Filaria bancrofti* were first discovered in 1863, by Demarquay, in a case of chylous dropsy. They were subsequently noted under similar conditions, by several workers, and by Wücherer in the urine of twenty-eight cases of tropical chyluria, but in 1872 Lewis found that the blood of man was the normal habitat, and gave them the name *Filaria sanguinis hominis*. The adult worm was found in 1876 by Bancroft, and in 1877, Cobbold gave it the name *Filaria bancrofti*. It has since been found repeatedly in various parts of the lymphatic system, and its life-history has been the subject of detailed studies by Manson (1884), Bancroft (1899), Low (1900), Grassi and Noé (1900), Noé (1901) and Fülleborn (1910).

The larvæ, as they exist in the circulating blood, exhibit a very active wriggling movement, without material progression. They may exist in enormous numbers, as many as five or six hundred swarming in a single drop of blood. This is the more surprising when we consider that they measure about $300\mu \times 8\mu$, that is, their width is equal to the diameter of the red blood corpuscle of their host and their length over thirty-seven times as great.

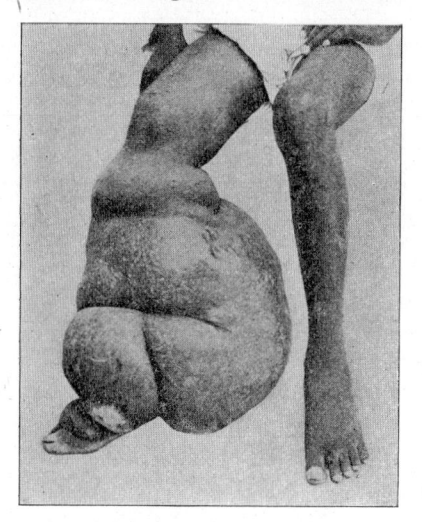

119. Elephantiasis in Man. From "New Sydenham Society's Atlas."

Their organs are very immature and the structure obscure. When they have quieted down somewhat in a preparation it may be seen that at the head end there is a six-lipped and very delicate prepuce, enclosing a short "fang" which may be suddenly exserted and retracted. Completely enclosing the larva is a delicate sheath, which is considerably longer than the worm itself. To enter into further details of anatomy is beyond the scope of this discussion and readers interested are referred to the work of Manson and of Fülleborn.

One of the most surprising features of the habits of these larvæ is the periodicity which they exhibit in their occurrence in the peripheral blood. If a preparation be made during the day time there may be no evidence whatever of filarial infestation, whereas a preparation from the same patient taken late in the evening or during the night may be literally swarming with the parasites. Manson quotes Mackenzie as having brought out the further interesting fact that should a "filarial subject be made to sleep during the day and remain awake at night, the periodicity is reversed; that is to say, the parasites come into the blood during the day and disappear from it during the night." There have been numerous attempts to explain this peculiar phenomenon of periodicity but in spite of objections which have been raised, the most plausible remains that of Manson, who believes that it is an adaptation correlated with the life-habits of the liberating agent of the parasite, the mosquito.

The next stages in the development of *Filaria nocturna* occur in mosquitoes, a fact suggested almost simultaneously by Bancroft and Manson in 1877, and first demonstrated by the latter very soon thereafter. The experiments were first carried out with *Culex quinquefasciatus* (= *fatigans*) as a host, but it is now known that a number of species of mosquitoes, both anopheline and culicine, may serve equally well.

When the blood of an infested individual is sucked up and reaches the stomach of such a mosquito, the larvæ, by very active movements, escape from their sheaths and within a very few hours actively migrate to the body cavity of their new host and settle down primarily in the thoracic muscles. There in the course of sixteen to twenty days they undergo a metamorphosis of which the more conspicuous features are the formation of a mouth, an alimentary canal and a trilobed tail. At the same time there is an enormous increase in size, the larvæ which measured .3 mm. in the blood becoming 1.5 mm. in length. This developmental period may be somewhat shortened in some cases and on the other hand may be considerably extended. The controlling factor seems to be the one of temperature.

The transformed larvæ then reenter the body cavity and finally the majority of them reach the interior of the labium (fig. 120). A few enter the legs and antennæ, and the abdomen, but these are wanderers which, it is possible, may likewise ultimately reach the labium, where they await the opportunity to enter their human host.

It was formerly supposed that when the infested mosquito punctured the skin of man, the mature larvæ were injected into the circulation. The manner in which this occurred was not obvious, for when the insect feeds it inserts only the stylets, the labium itself remaining on the surface of the skin. Fülleborn has cleared up the question by showing that at this time the filariæ escape and, like the hookworm, actively bore into the skin of their new host.

Once entered, they migrate to the lymphatics and there quickly become sexually mature. The full grown females measure 85–90 mm. in length by .24–.28 mm. in diameter, while the males are less than

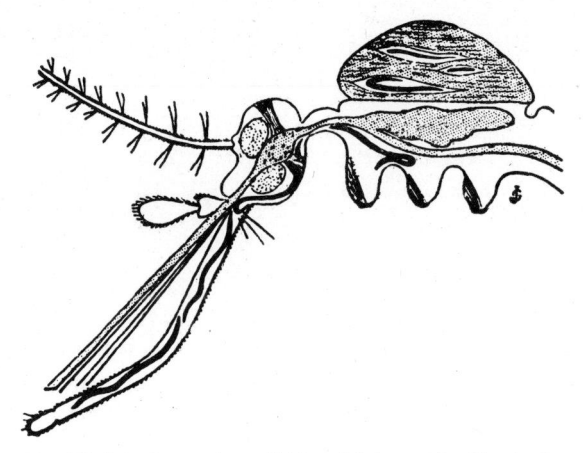

120. Filaria in the muscles and labium of Culex. After Blanchard.

half this size, being about 40 mm. by .1 mm. Fecundation occurs and the females will be found filled with eggs in various stages of development, for they are normally viviparous.

*Filaria philippinensis* is reported by Ashburn and Craig (1907) as a common blood filaria in the Philippine Islands. As they describe it, it differs from *Filaria bancrofti* primarily in that it does not exhibit periodicity. Its development has been found to occur in *Culex quinquefasciatus*, where it undergoes metamorphosis in about fourteen or fifteen days. There is doubt as to the species being distinct from *bancrofti*.

Several other species occur in man and are thought to be transferred by various insects, among which have been mentioned Tabanidæ and tsetse-flies, but there is no experimental proof in support of such conjectures.

*Filaria immitis* is a dangerous parasite of the dog, the adult worm living in the heart and veins of this animal. It is one of the species which has been clearly shown to undergo its development in the mosquito, particularly in *Anopheles maculipennis* and *Aedes calopus* (= Stegomyia). The larval form occurs in the peripheral blood, especially at night. When taken up by mosquitoes they differ from *Filaria bancrofti* in that they undergo their development in the Malpighian tubules rather than in the thoracic muscles. In about twelve days they have completed their growth in the tubules, pierce the distal end, and pass to the labium. This species occurs primarily in China and Japan, but is also found in Europe and in the United States. It is an especially favorable species for studying the transformations in the mosquito.

*Filariæ* are also commonly found in birds, and in this country this is the most available source of laboratory material. We have found them locally (Ithaca, N. Y.) in the blood of over sixty per cent of all the crows examined, at any season of the year, and have also found them in English sparrows.

In the crows, they often occur in enormous numbers, as many as two thousand having been found in a single drop of the blood of the most heavily infested specimen examined. For study, a small drop of blood should be mounted on a clean slide and the coverglass rung with vaseline or oil to prevent evaporation. In this way they can be kept for hours.

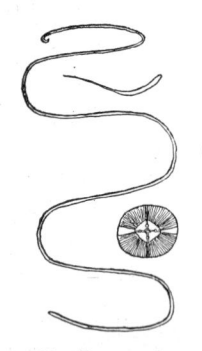

121. Dracunculus medinensis; female; mouth; embryo. After Bastian and Leuckart.

Permanent preparations may be made by spreading out the blood in a film on a perfectly clean slide and staining. This is easiest done by touching the fresh drop of blood with the end of a second slide which is then held at an angle of about 45° to the first slide and drawn over it without pressure. Allow the smear to dry in the air and stain in the usual way with hæmatoxylin.

## Other Nematode Parasites of Man and Animals Developing in Arthropods

*Dracunculus medinensis* (fig. 121), the so-called guinea-worm, is a nematode parasite of man which is widely distributed in tropical Africa, Asia, certain parts of Brazil and is occasionally imported into North America.

The female worm is excessively long and slender, measuring nearly three feet in length and not more than one-fifteenth of an inch in diameter. It is found in the subcutaneous connective tissue and when mature usually migrates to some part of the leg. Here it pierces the skin and there is formed a small superficial ulcer through which the larvæ reach the exterior after bursting the body of the mother.

Fedtschenko (1879) found that when these larvæ reach the water they penetrate the carapace of the little crustacean, *Cyclops* (fig. 122). Here they molt several times and undergo a metamorphosis. Fedtschenko, in Turkestan, found that these stages required about five weeks, while Manson who confirmed these general results, found that eight or nine weeks were required in the cooler climate of Engand.

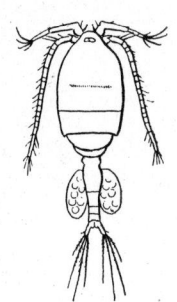

122. Cyclops. the intermediate host of Dracunculus.

Infection of the vertebrate host probably occurs through swallowing infested cyclops in drinking water. Fedtschenko was unable to demonstrate this experimentally and objection has been raised against the theory, but Leiper (1907), and Strassen (1907) succeeded in infesting monkeys by feeding them on cyclops containing the larvæ.

*Habronema muscæ* is a worm which has long been known in its larval stage, as a parasite of the house-fly. Carter found them in 33 per cent of the house-flies examined in Bombay during July, 1860, and since that time they have been shown to be very widely distributed. Italian workers reported them in 12 per cent to 30 per cent of the flies examined. Hewitt reported finding it rarely in England. In this country it was first reported by Leidy who found it in about 20 per cent of the flies examined at Philadelphia, Pa. Since then it has been reported by several American workers. We have found it at Ithaca, N. Y., but have not made sufficient examinations to justify stating percentage. Ransom (1913) reports it in thirty-nine out of one hundred and thirty-seven flies, or 28 per cent.

Until very recently the life-history of this parasite was unknown but the thorough work of Ransom (1911, 1913) has shown clearly that the adult stage occurs in the stomach of horses. The embryos, produced by the parent worms in the stomach of the horse, pass out with the feces and enter the bodies of fly larvæ which are developing in the manure. In these they reach their final stage of larval development at about the time the adult flies emerge from the pupal stage. In the adult fly they are commonly found in the head.

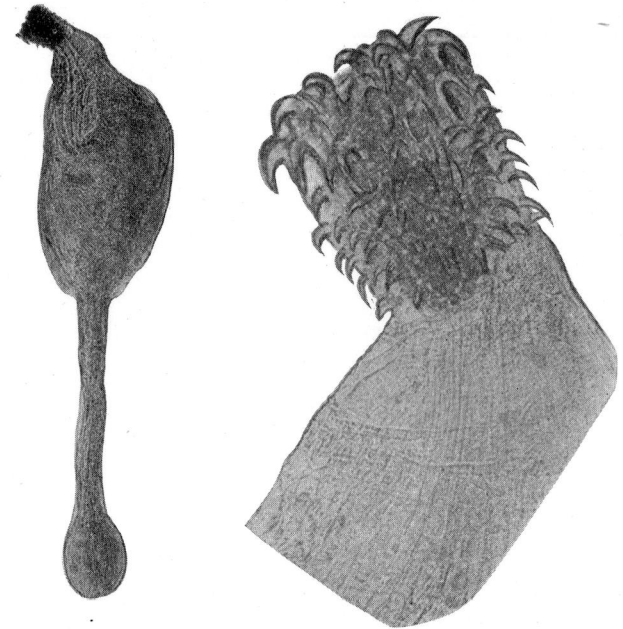

184  *Arthropods as Essential Hosts of Pathogenic Organisms*

123. An Echinorhynchid, showing the spinose retractile proboscis.

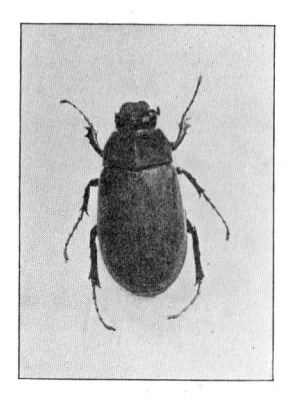

124. June beetle (Lachnosterna).                    Larva

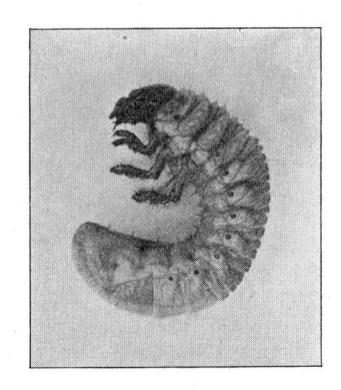

frequently in the proboscis, but they occur also in the thorax and abdomen. Infested flies are accidentally swallowed by horses and the parasite completes its development to maturity in the stomach of its definitive host.

*Gigantorhynchus hirudinaceus* (=*Echinorhynchus gigas*) is a common parasite of the pig and has been reported as occurring in man. The adult female is 20–35 cm. long and 4–9 mm. in diameter. It lacks an alimentary canal and is provided with a strongly spined protractile rostrum, by means of which it attaches to the intestinal mucosa of its host.

The eggs are scattered with the feces of the host and are taken up by certain beetle larvæ. In Europe the usual intermediate hosts are the larvæ of the cockchafer, *Melolontha vulgaris*, or of the flower beetle, *Cetonia aurata*. Stiles has shown that in the United States the intermediate host is the larva of the June bug, *Lachnosterna* (fig. 124). It is probable that several of the native species serve in this capacity.

A number of other nematode parasites of birds and mammals have been reported as developing in arthropods but here, as in the case of the cestodes, experimental proof is scant. The cases above cited are the better established and will serve as illustrations.

## CHAPTER VIII

### ARTHROPODS AS ESSENTIAL HOSTS OF PATHOGENIC PROTOZOA

#### Mosquitoes and Malaria

Under the name of malaria is included a group of morbid symptoms formerly supposed to be due to a miasm or bad air, but now known to be caused by protozoan parasites of the genus *Plasmodium*, which attack the red blood corpuscles. It occurs in paroxysms, each marked by a chill, followed by high fever and sweating. The fever is either intermittent or remittent.

There are three principal types of the disease, due to different species of the parasite. They are:

1. The benign-tertian, caused by *Plasmodium vivax*, which undergoes its schizogony or asexual cycle in the blood in forty-eight hours or even less. This type of the disease,—characterized by fever every two days, is the most wide-spread and common.

2. The quartan fever is due to the presence of *Plasmodium malariæ*, which has an asexual cycle of seventy-two hours, and therefore the fever recurs every three days. This type is more prevalent in temperate and sub-tropical regions, but appears to be rare everywhere.

3. The sub-tertian "æstivo-autumnal," or "pernicious" fever is caused by *Plasmodium falciparum*. Schizogony usually occurs in the internal organs, particularly in the spleen, instead of in the peripheral circulation, as is the case of the tertian and quartan forms. The fever produced is of an irregular type and the period of schizogony has not been definitely determined. It is claimed by some that the variations are due to different species of malignant parasites.

It is one of the most wide-spread of human diseases, occurring in almost all parts of the world, except in the polar regions and in waterless deserts. It is most prevalent in marshy regions.

So commonplace is malaria that it causes little of the dread inspired by most of the epidemic diseases, and yet, as Ross says, it is perhaps the most important of human diseases. Figures regarding its ravages are astounding. Celli estimated that in Italy it caused an average annual mortality of fifteen thousand, representing about two million cases. In India alone, according to Ross (1910) "it has been officially estimated to cause a mean annual death-rate of five per thousand; that is, to kill every year, on the average, one million one hundred and thirty thousand." In the United States it is widespread and though being restricted as the country develops, it still causes enormous losses. During the year 1911, "in Alabama alone there were seventy thousand cases and seven hundred and seventy deaths." The weakening effects of the disease, the invasion of other diseases due to the attacks of malaria, are among the very serious results, but they cannot be estimated.

Not only is there direct effect on man, but the disease has been one of the greatest factors in retarding the development of certain regions. Everywhere pioneers have had to face it, and the most fertile regions have, in many instances been those most fully dominated by it. Herrick (1903) has presented an interesting study of its effects on the development of the southern United States and has shown that some parts, which are among the most fertile in the world, are rendered practically uninhabitable by the ravages of malaria. Howard (1909) estimates that the annual money loss from the disease in the United States is not less than $100,000,000.

It was formerly supposed that the disease was due to a miasm, to a noxious effluvia, or infectious matter rising in the air from swamps. In other words its cause was, as the name indicated "mal aria," and the deep seated fear of night air is based largely on the belief that this miasm was given off at night. Its production was thought to be favored by stirring of the soil, dredging operations and the like.

The idea of some intimate connection between malaria and mosquitoes is not a new one. According to Manson, Lancisi noted that in some parts of Italy the peasants for centuries have believed that malaria is produced by the bite of mosquitoes. Celli states that one not rarely hears from such peasants the statement that "In such a place, there is much fever, because it is full of mosquitoes." Koch points out that in German East Africa the natives call malaria and the mosquito by the same name, *Mbù*. The opinion was not lacking support from medical men. Celli quotes passages from the writings of the Italian physician, Lancisi, which indicate that he favored the view in 1717.

Dr. Josiah Nott is almost universally credited with having supported the theory, in 1848, but as we have already pointed out his work has been misinterpreted. The statements of Beauperthuy, (1853) were more explicit.

The clearest early presentation of the circumstantial evidence in favor of the theory of mosquito transmission was that of A. F. A. King, an American physician, in 1883. He presented a series of epidemiological data and showed "how they may be explicable by the supposition that the mosquito is the real source of the disease, rather than the inhalation or cutaneous absorption of a marsh vapor." We may well give the space to summarizing his argument here for it has been so remarkably substantiated by subsequent work:

1. Malaria, like mosquitoes, affects by preference low and moist localities, such as swamps, fens, jungles, marshes, etc.

2. Malaria is hardly ever developed at a lower temperature than 60° Fahr., and such a temperature is necessary for the development of the mosquito.

3. Mosquitoes, like malaria, may both accumulate in and be obstructed by forests lying in the course of winds blowing from malarious localities.

4. By atmospheric currents malaria and mosquitoes are alike capable of being transported for considerable distances.

5. Malaria may be developed in previously healthy places by turning up the soil, as in making excavations for the foundation of houses, tracks for railroads, and beds for canals, because these operations afford breeding places for mosquitoes.

6. In proportion as countries, previously malarious, are cleared up and thickly settled, periodical fevers disappear, because swamps and pools are drained so that the mosquito cannot readily find a place suitable to deposit her eggs.

7. Malaria is most dangerous when the sun is down and the danger of exposure after sunset is greatly increased by the person exposed sleeping in the night air. Both facts are readily explicable by the mosquito malaria theory.

8. In malarial districts the use of fire, both indoors and to those who sleep out, affords a comparative security against malaria, because of the destruction of mosquitoes.

9. It is claimed that the air of cities in some way renders the poison innocuous, for, though a malarial disease may be raging outside, it does not penetrate far into the interior. We may easily conceive that mosquitoes, while invading cities during their nocturnal pilgrimages will be so far arrested by walls and houses, as well as attracted by lights in the suburbs, that many of them will in this way be prevented from penetrating "far into the interior."

10. Malarial diseases and likewise mosquitoes are most prevalent toward the latter part of summer and in the autumn.

11. Various writers have maintained that malaria is arrested by canvas curtains, gauze veils and mosquito nets and have recommended the use of mosquito curtains, "through which malaria can seldom or never pass." It can hardly be conceived that these intercept marsh-air but they certainly do protect from mosquitoes.

12. Malaria spares no age, but it affects infants much less frequently than adults, because young infants are usually carefully housed and protected from mosquito inoculation.

Correlated with the miasmatic theory was the belief that some animal or vegetable organism which lived in marshes, produced malaria, and frequent searches were made for it. Salisbury (1862) thought this causative organism to be an alga, of the genus *Palmella;* others attributed it to certain fungi or bacteria.

In 1880, the French physician, Laveran, working in Algeria, discovered an amœboid organism in the blood of malarial patients and definitely established the parasitic nature of this disease. Pigmented granules had been noted by Meckel as long ago as 1847, in the spleen and blood of a patient who had died of malaria, and his observations had been repeatedly verified, but the granules had been regarded as degeneration products, and the fact that they occurred in the body of a foreign organism had been overlooked.

Soon after the discovery of the parasites in the blood, Gerhardt (1884) succeeded in transferring the disease to healthy individuals by inoculation of malarious blood, and thus proved that it is a true infection. This was verified by numerous experimenters and it was found that inoculation with a very minute quantity of the diseased blood would not only produce malaria but the particular type of disease.

Laveran traced out the life cycle of the malarial parasite as it occurs in man. The details as we now know them and as they are illustrated by the accompanying figure 125, are as follows:

The infecting organism or *sporozoite*, is introduced into the circulation, penetrates a red blood corpuscle, and forms the amœboid *schizont*. This lives at the expense of the corpuscle and as it develops there are deposited in its body scattered black or reddish black particles. These are generally called melanin granules, but are much better referred to as hæmozoin, as they are not related to

190        *Arthropods as Hosts of Pathogenic Protozoa*

melanin. The hæmozoin is the most conspicuous part of the parasite, a feature of advantage in diagnosing from unstained preparations.

As the schizont matures, its nucleus breaks up into a number of daughter nuclei, each with a rounded mass of protoplasm about it, and finally the corpuscles are broken down and these rounded bodies

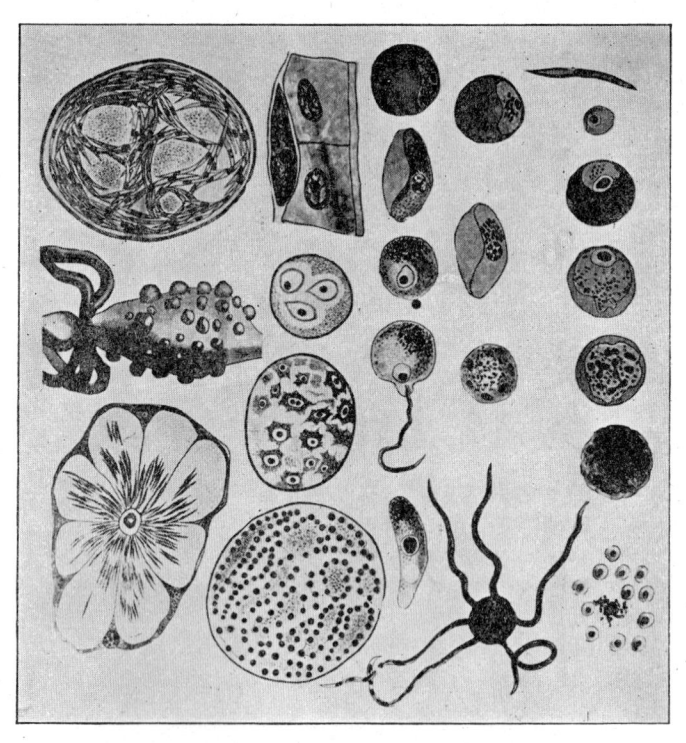

125. Life cycle of the malaria parasite. Adapted from Leuckart's chart, by Miss Anna Stryke.

are liberated in the plasma as *merozoites*. These merozoites infect new corpuscles and thus the asexual cycle is continued. The malarial paroxysm is coincident with sporulation.

As early as Laveran's time it was known that under conditions not yet determined there are to be found in the blood of malarious patients another phase of the parasite, differing in form according to the type of the disease. In the pernicious type these appear as large, crescent-shaped organisms which have commonly been called "crescents." We now know that these are sexual forms.

When the parasite became known there immediately arose speculations as to the way in which it was transferred from man to man. It was thought by some that in nature it occurred as a free-living amœba, and that it gained access to man through being taken up with impure water. However, numerous attempts to infect healthy persons by having them drink or inhale marsh water, or by injecting it into their circulation resulted in failure, and influenced by Leuckart's and Melnikoff's work on *Dipylidium*, that of Fedtschenko on *Dracunculus*, and more especially by that of Manson on *Filaria*, search was made for some insect which might transfer the parasite.

Laveran had early suggested that the rôle of carrier might be played by the mosquito, but Manson first clearly formulated the hyopthesis, and it was largely due to his suggestions that Ross in India, undertook to solve the problem. With no knowledge of the form or of the appearance in this stage, or of the species of mosquito concerned, Ross spent almost two and a half years of the most arduous work in the search and finally in August, 1897, seventeen years after the discovery of the parasite in man, he obtained his first definite clue. In dissecting a "dappled-winged mosquito," "every cell was searched and to my intense disappointment nothing whatever was found, until I came to the insect's stomach. Here, however, just as I was about to abandon the examination, I saw a very delicate circular cell, apparently lying amongst the ordinary cells of the organ and scarcely distinguishable from them. On looking further, another and another similar object presented itself. I now focused the lens carefully on one of these, and found that it contained a few minute granules of some black substance, exactly like the pigment of the parasite of malaria. I counted altogether twelve of these cells in the insect."

Further search showed that "the contents of the mature pigment cells did not consist of clear fluid but of a multitude of delicate, thread-like bodies which on the rupture of the parent cell, were poured into the body cavity of the insect. They were evidently spores."

With these facts established, confirmation and extension of Ross's results quickly followed, from many different sources. We cannot trace this work in detail but will only point out that much of the credit is due to the Italian workers, Grassi, Bignami, and Bastianelli, and to Koch and Daniels.

It had already been found that when fresh blood was mounted and properly protected against evaporation, a peculiar change occurred in these crescents after about half an hour's time. From certain of them there were pushed out long whip-like processes which moved with a very active, lashing movement. The parasite at this stage is known as the "flagellated body." Others, differing somewhat in details of structure, become rounded but do not give off "flagella." The American worker, MacCallum (1897), in studying bird malaria as found in crows, first recognized the true nature of these bodies. He regarded them as sexual forms and believed that the so-called flagella played the part of spermatozoa. Thus, the "flagellated body" is in reality a *microgametoblast*, producing *microgametes*, or the male sexual element, while the others constitute the *macrogametes*, or female elements.

It was found that when blood containing these sexual forms was sucked up by an Anopheline mosquito and taken into its stomach, a microgamete penetrated and fertilized a macrogamete in a way analogous to what takes place in the fertilization of the egg in higher forms. The resultant, mobile organism is known as the *migratory ookinete*. In this stage the parasite bores through the epithelial lining of the "stomach" (mid-intestine) of the mosquito and becomes encysted under the muscle layers. Here the *oocyst*, as it is now known, matures and breaks up into the body cavity and finally its products come to lie in the salivary glands of the mosquito. Ten to twelve days are required for these changes, after which the mosquito is infective, capable of introducing the parasite with its saliva, when feeding upon a healthy person.

Thus the malarial parasite is known to have a double cycle, an alternation of generations, of which the asexual stage is undergone in man, the sexual in certain species of mosquitoes. The mosquito is therefore the definitive host rather than the *intermediate*, as usually stated.

The complicated cycle may be made clearer by the diagram of Miss Stryke (1912) which, by means of a double-headed mosquito (fig. 126) endeavors to show how infection takes place through the biting of the human victim, (at A), in whom asexual multiplication then takes place, and how the sexual stages, taken up at B in the diagram, are passed in the body of the mosquito.

The experimental proof that mosquitoes of the Anopheline group are necessary agents in the transmission of malaria was afforded in 1900 when two English physicians, Drs. Sambon and Low lived for the three most malarial months in the midst of the Roman Campagna,

## Mosquitoes and Malaria 193

a region famous for centuries as a hot-bed of malaria. The two experimenters moved about freely throughout the day, exposed

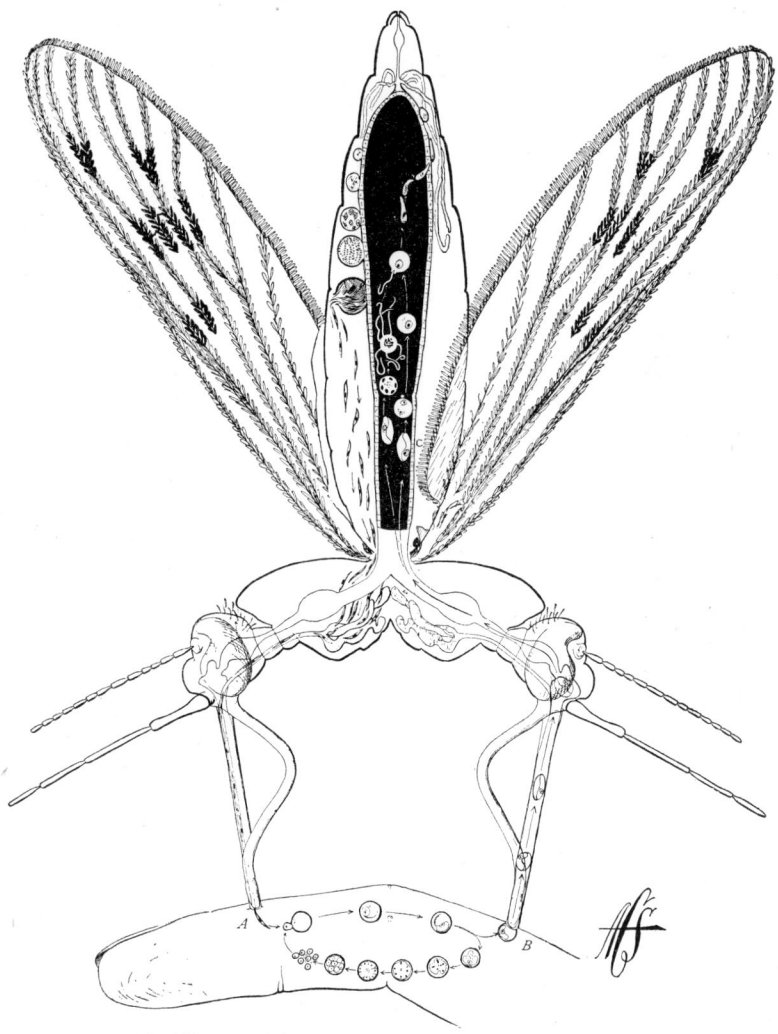

126. Life cycle of the malarial parasite. After Miss Anna Stryke.

themselves to rains and all kinds of weather, drank marsh water, slept exposed to the marsh air, and, in short, did everything which was supposed to cause malaria, except that they protected themselves thoroughly from mosquito bites, retiring at sunset to a mosquito-proof hut. Though they took no quinine and all of their neighbors suffered from malaria, they were absolutely free from the disease.

To complete the proof, mosquitoes which had fed in Rome on malarious patients were sent to England and allowed to bite two volunteers, one of them Dr. Manson's own son, who had not been otherwise exposed to the disease. Both of these gentlemen contracted typical cases of malaria and the parasites were to be found in abundance in their blood.

Since that time there have been many practical demonstrations of the fact that malaria is transmitted exclusively by the bite of mosquitoes and that the destruction of the mosquitoes means the elimination of the disease.

We have said that the malarial parasite is able to undergo its development only in certain species of mosquitoes belonging to the Anopheline group. It is by no means certain that all of this group even, are capable of acting as the definitive host of the parasites, and much careful experiment work is still needed along this line. In the United States, several species have been found to be implicated, *Anopheles quadrimaculatus* and *Anopheles crucians* being the most common. The characteristics of these species and the distinctions between them and other mosquitoes will be discussed in Chapter XII.

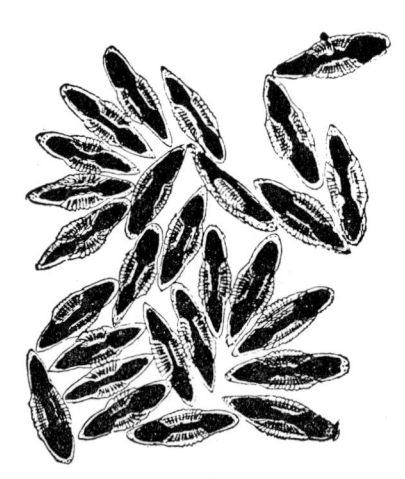

127. Eggs of Anopheles. After Howard.

In antimalarial work it is desirable to distinguish the anopheline mosquitoes from the culicine species in all stages. The following tabulation presents the more striking distinctions between the groups as represented in the United States.

| *Anopheles* | *Culex, Aedes, etc.* |
| --- | --- |
| *Eggs:* Laid singly in small numbers upon the surface of the water. Eggs lie upon their sides and float by means of lateral expansions (fig. 127). | Deposited in clumps in the form of a raft (Culex group) or deposited singly in the water or on the ground in places which may later be submerged. |

*Larva:* When at rest floats in a horizontal position beneath the surface film. No respiratory tube but instead a flattened area on the eighth abdominal segment into which the two spiracles open (fig. 128).

*Adults:* Palpi in both sexes nearly or quite as long as the proboscis. Proboscis projecting forward nearly on line with the axis of the body. When at rest on a vertical wall the body is usually held at an angle with the vertical (fig. 128). Wings frequently spotted (fig. 130).

When at rest (with few exceptions) floats suspended in an oblique or vertical position, or more rarely nearly horizontal, with the respiratory tube in contact with the surface film (fig. 128).

Palpi short in the female, in the male usually elongate. Proboscis projects forward at an angle with the axis of the body. When at rest on a vertical wall the body is usually held parallel or the tip of the abdomen inclined towards the wall (fig. 128). Wings usually not spotted.

These malarial-bearing species are essentially domesticated mosquitoes. They develop in any accumulation of water which stands for a week or more. Ponds, puddles, rain barrels, horse troughs, cess-pools, cans, even the foot-prints of animals in marshy ground may afford them breeding places.

128. (*a*) Normal position of the larvae of Culex and Anopheles in the water. Culex, left; Anopheles, middle; Culex pupa, right hand figure.

It is clear from what has been said regarding the life cycle of the malarial parasite that the mosquito is harmless if not itself diseased. Hence malarial-bearing species may abound in the neighborhood where there is no malaria, the disease being absent simply because the mosquitoes are uninfected. Such a locality is potentially malarious and needs only the introduction of a malarial patient who is exposed to the mosquitoes. It is found that such patients may harbor the parasites in their blood long after they are apparently well and thus may serve as a menace, just as do the so-called typhoid carriers. In some malarious regions as high as 80–90 per cent of the natives are such malaria-carriers and must be reckoned with in antimalaria measures.

Based upon our present day knowledge of the life cycle of the malarial parasite the fight against the disease

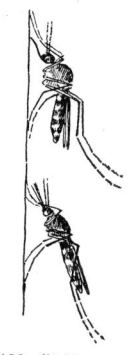

128. (*b*) Norma position of Culex and Anopheles on the wall.

becomes primarily a problem in economic entomology,—it is a question of insect control, in its broadest interpretation.

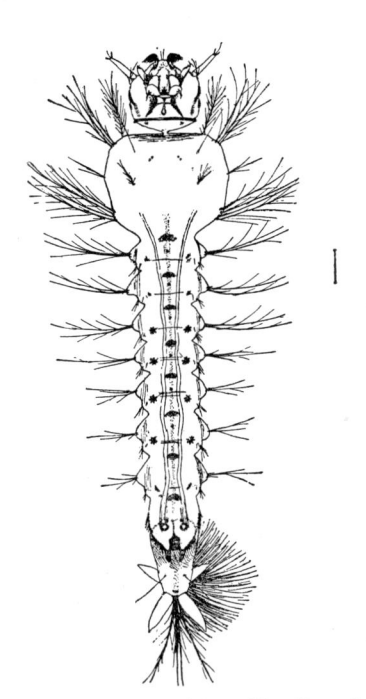

The lines of defence and offence against the disease as outlined by Boyce (1909) are:

1. Measures to avoid the reservoir (man):
   Segregation.
   Screening of patients.
2. Measures to avoid Anopheles:
   Choice of suitable locality, when possible.
   Screening of houses and porches.
   Sleeping under mosquito nets.
3. Measures to exterminate the Anopheles:
   Use of natural enemies.
   Use of culicides, oiling ponds, etc.
   Drainage and scavenging to destroy breeding places.
   Enforcement of penalties for harboring larvæ or keeping stagnant water.
   Educational methods.
4. Systematic treatment with quinine to exterminate the parasites.

129. Larva of Anopheles. After Howard.

## Mosquitoes and Yellow Fever

Yellow fever was until recently one of the most dreaded of epidemic diseases. It is an acute, specific and infectious disease, non-contagious in character but occurring in epidemics, or endemics, within a peculiarly limited geographical area. It is highly fatal, but those who recover are generally immune from subsequent attacks.

It is generally regarded as an American disease, having been found by Cortez, in Mexico, and being confined principally to the American continents and islands. It also occurs in Africa and attempts have been made to show that it was originally an African disease but there is not sufficient evidence to establish this view.

There have been many noted outbreaks in the United States. Boston suffered from it in 1691 and again in 1693; New York in 1668 and as late as 1856; Baltimore in 1819. In 1793 occurred the great epidemic in Philadelphia, with a death rate of one in ten of the population. In the past century it was present almost every year in some locality of our Southern States, New Orleans being the greatest sufferer. In the latter city there were 7848 deaths from the disease in 1853, 4854 in 1858, and 4046 in 1878. The last notable outbreak

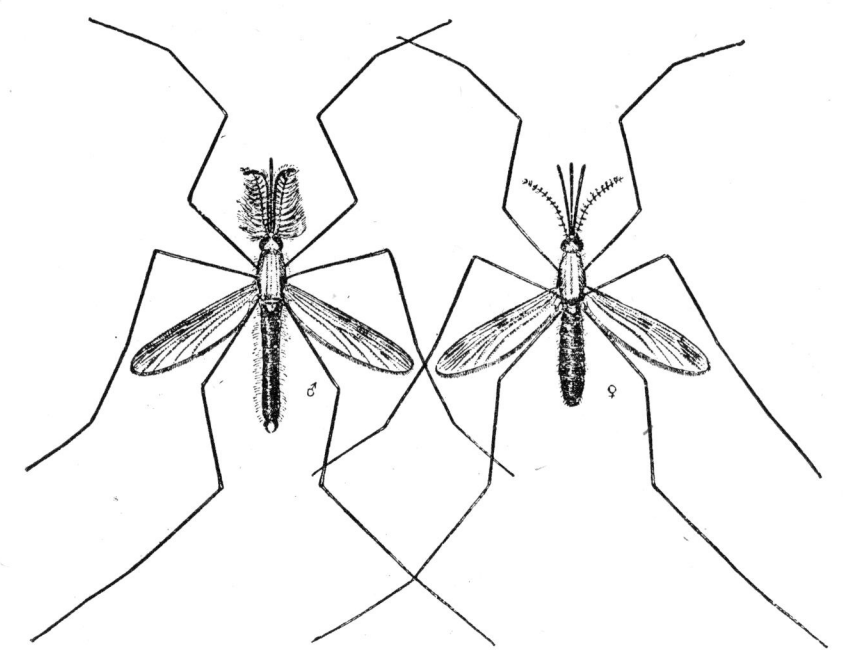

130. Anopheles quadrimaculatus, male and female, (x3½). After Howard.

was in 1905. Reed and Carroll (1901) estimated that during the period from 1793 to 1900 there had not been less than 500,000 cases in the United States.

As in the case of the plague, the most stringent methods of control proved ineffective and helplessness, almost hopelessness marked the great epidemics. A vivid picture of conditions is that given by Mathew Cary, 1793 (quoted by Kelly, 1906) in "A Short Account of the Malignant Fever Lately Prevalent in Philadelphia."

"The consternation of the people of Philadelphia at this period was carried beyond all bounds. Dismay and affright were visible in the countenance of almost every person. Of those who remained, many shut themselves in their houses and were afraid to walk the streets. * * * The corpses of the most respectable citizens, even those who did not die of the epidemic, were carried to the grave on the shafts of a chair (chaise), the horse driven by a negro, unattended by friends or relative, and without any sort of ceremony.

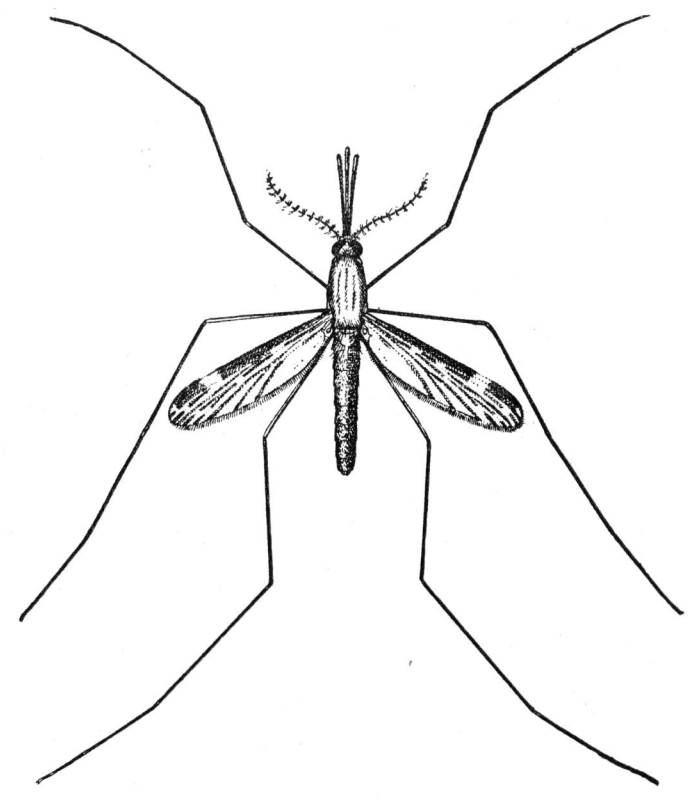

131. Anopheles punctipennis. Female, (x4). After Howard.

People hastily shifted their course at the sight of a hearse coming toward them. Many never walked on the footpath, but went into the middle of the streets to avoid being infected by passing by houses wherein people had died. Acquaintances and friends avoided each other in the streets and only signified their regard by a cold nod. The old custom of shaking hands fell into such disuse that many shrunk back with affright at even the offer of the hand. A person with a crape, or any appearance of mourning was shunned l ke a viper. And many valued themselves highly on the skill and address with which they got to the windward of every person they met. Indeed, it is not probable that London, at the last stage of the plague, exhibited stronger marks of terror than were to be seen in Phila-

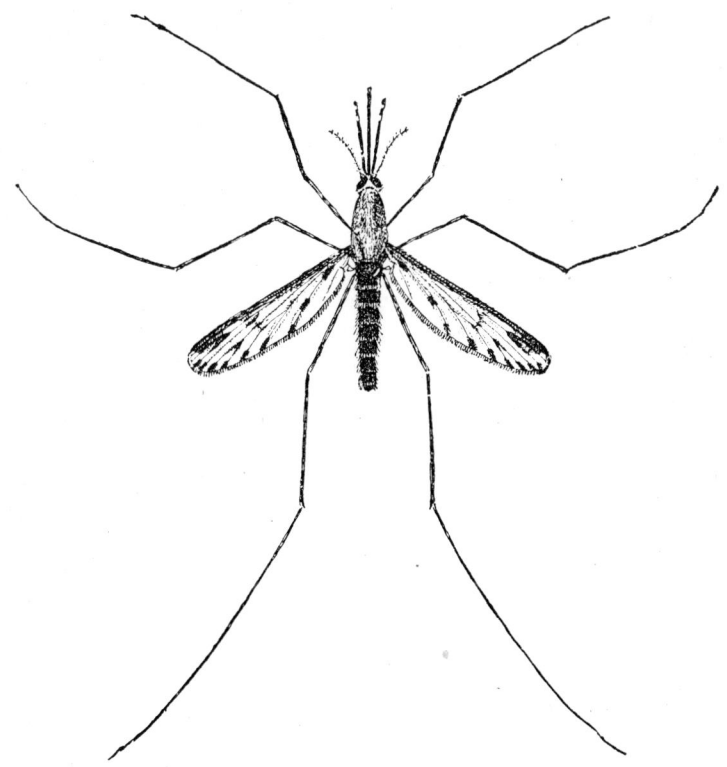

132. Anopheles crucians. Female (x4). After Howard.

delphia from the 24th or 25th of August until pretty late in September."

Such was the condition in Philadelphia in 1793 and, as far as methods of control of the disease were concerned, there was practically no advance during the last century. The dominant theory was that yellow fever was spread by *fomites*, that is, exposed bedding, clothing, baggage, and the like. As late as 1898 a bulletin of the United States Marine Hospital Service stated:

"While yellow fever is a communicable disease, it is not contagious in the ordinary acceptance of the term, but is spread by the infection of places and articles of bedding, clothing, and furniture."

Based upon this theory, houses, baggage, freight, even mail, were disinfected, and the most rigid quarantine regulations were enforced. The hardships to which people of the stricken regions were subjected and the financial losses are incalculable. And withal, the only efficient check upon the disease seemed to be the heavy frosts.

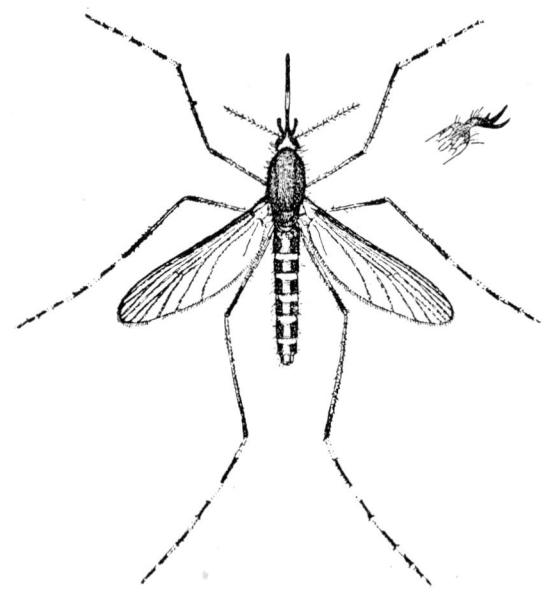

133. Culex sollicitans. Female (x4). After Howard.

It was found that for some reason, the epidemic abated with cold weather,—a measure beyond human control.

It is not strange that among the multitude of theories advanced to explain the cause and method of dissemination of the disease there should be suggestions that yellow fever was transmitted by the mosquito. We have seen that Beauperthuy (1855) clearly urged this theory.

More detailed, and of the greatest influence in the final solution of the problem were the arguments of Dr. Cárlos Finlay, of Havana. In 1881, in a paper presented before the "Rea Academia de Ciencias Médicas, Fisicis y Naturales de la Habana," he said:

"I feel convinced that any theory which attributes the origin and the propagation of yellow fever to atmospheric influences, to miasmatic or meteorological conditions, to filth, or to the neglect of general hygienic precautions, must be considered as utterly indefensible."

He postulated the existence of a material transportable substance causing yellow fever,—"something tangible which requires to be conveyed from the sick to the healthy before the disease can be propagated" and after discussing the peculiarities of the spread of the disease and the influence of meteorological conditions, he decides that the carriers of the disease must be sought among insects. He continues:

"On the other hand, the fact of yellow fever being characterized both clinically and (according to recent findings) histologically, by lesions of the blood vessels and by alterations of the physical and chemical conditions of the blood, suggested that the insect which should convey the infectious particles from the patient to the healthy should be looked for among those which drive their sting into blood vessels in order to suck human blood. Finally, by reason of other considerations which need not be stated here, I came to think that the mosquito might be the transmitter of yellow fever."

"Assimilating the disease to small-pox and to vaccination, it occurred to me that in order to inoculate yellow fever it would be necessary to pick out the inoculable material from within the blood vessels of a yellow fever patient and to carry it likewise into the interior of a blood vessel of a person who was to be inoculated. All of which conditions the mosquito satisfies most admirably through its bite."

In the course of his study of the problem, Finlay made detailed studies of the life history and habits of the common mosquitoes at Havana, and arrived at the conclusion that the carrier of the yellow fever was the *Culex mosquito* or *Aëdes calopus*, as it is now known. With this species he undertook direct experimental tests, and believed that he succeeded in transmitting the disease by the bite of infected mosquitoes in three cases. Unfortunately, possibility of other exposure was not absolutely excluded, and the experiments attracted little attention.

Throughout the next twenty years Finlay continued his work on yellow fever, modifying his original theory somewhat as time went on. Among his later suggestions was that in the light of Smith's work on Texas fever, his theory must be "somewhat modified so as to include the important circumstance that the faculty of transmitting the yellow fever germ need not be limited to the parent insect, directly contaminated by stinging a yellow fever patient (or perhaps by contact with or feeding from his discharges), but may be likewise inherited by the next generation of mosquitoes issued from the contaminated parent." He believed that the bite of a single mosquito produced a light attack of the disease and was thus effective in immunizing the patient. Throughout the period, many apparently successful attempts to transmit the disease by mosquitoes were made. In the light of present day knowledge we must regard these as defective not only because possibility of other infection was not absolutely excluded but because no account was taken of the incubation period within the body of the mosquito.

In 1900, while the American army was stationed in Cuba there occurred an epidemic of yellow fever and an army medical board was appointed for "the purpose of pursuing scientific investigations with reference to the acute infectious diseases prevalent on the island." This was headed by Walter Reed and associated with him were James Carroll, Jesse W. Lazear and Aristides Agramonte, the latter a Cuban immune. For a detailed summary of this work the lay reader cannot do better than read Dr. Kelly's fascinating biography "Walter Reed and Yellow Fever."

Arriving at the army barracks near Havana the Commission first took up the study of *Bacillus icteroides*, the organism which Sanarelli, an Italian physician, had declared the causative agent in yellow fever. They were unable to isolate this bacillus either from the blood during life or from the blood and organs of cadavers and therefore turned their attention to Finlay's theory of the propagation of yellow fever by means of the mosquito. In this work they had the unselfish and enthusiastic support of Dr. Finlay himself, who not only consulted with them and placed his publications at their disposal, but furnished eggs from which their experimental mosquitoes were obtained. Inoculations of eleven non-immunes through the bite of infected mosquitoes were made, and of these, two gave positive results. The first of the two was Dr. Carroll who allowed himself to be bitten by a mosquito which had been caused to feed upon four cases of yellow fever, two of them severe and two mild. The first patient had been bitten twelve days before.

Three days after being bitten, Dr. Carroll came down with a typical case of yellow fever. So severe was the attack that for three days his life hung in the balance. During his convalescence an incident occurred which showed how the theory of mosquito transmission of the disease was generally regarded. We quote from Dr. Kelly: "One of his nurses who came from Tennessee had had considerable experience with yellow fever, having indeed, lost her husband and several children from it. One day early in his illness Dr. Carroll mentioned to her that he had contracted the disease through the bite of a mosquito, and noticed that she looked surprised. Some time later, when well enough to look over the daily records of his condition, he found this entry: 'Says he got his illness through the bite of a mosquito,—delirious'."

The second case was that of an American who was bitten by four mosquitoes, two of which had bitten severe (fatal) cases of yellow fever twelve days previously, one of which had bitten a severe case (second day) sixteen days before and one which had bitten a severe case eight days before. Five days later, the subject developed a well pronounced but mild case of the disease.

In the meantime, another member of the Commission, Dr. Lazear, was accidentally bitten by a mosquito while collecting blood from yellow fever patients. Five days later he contracted a typical case which resulted fatally.

So clear was the evidence from these preliminary experiments that the commission felt warranted in announcing, October 27, 1900, that, "The mosquito serves as the intermediate host for the parasite of yellow fever, and it is highly probable that the disease is only propagated through the bite of this insect."

In order to extend the experimental evidence under conditions which could leave no possibility of infection from other sources, a special experimental sanitary station, named in honor of the deceased member of the Commission, was established in an open field near the town of Quemados, Cuba. Here there were constructed two small buildings known respectively as the "infected clothing building" and the "infected mosquito building."

The infected clothing building, 14 x 20 feet in size, was purposely so constructed as to exclude anything like efficient ventilation, but was thoroughly screened to prevent the entrance of mosquitoes. Into this building were brought sheets, pillow-slips, blankets, etc., contaminated by contact with cases of yellow fever and their discharges,—many of them purposely soiled with a liberal quantity of black vomit, urine, and fecal matter from patients sick with yellow fever. Nothing could better serve as the fomites which were supposed to convey the dread disease.

Three non-immunes unpacked these articles, giving each a thorough handling and shaking in order to disseminate through the air of the room the specific agent of the disease. They were then used in making up the beds which the volunteers occupied each night for a period of twenty days. The experiment was repeated three times, volunteers even sleeping in the soiled garments of yellow fever victims but in not a single case was there the slightest symptom of disease. The theory of the spread of yellow fever by fomites was completely demolished.

The infected mosquito building, equal in size to its companion, was the antithesis as far as other features were concerned. It was so constructed as to give the best possible ventilation, and bedding which was brought into it was thoroughly sterilized. Like the infected clothing building it was carefully screened, but in this case it was in order to keep mosquitoes in it as well as to prevent entrance of others. Through the middle of the room ran a mosquito-proof screen.

On December 5, 1900, a non-immune volunteer who had been in the quarantine camp for fifteen days and had had no other possible exposure, allowed himself to be bitten by five mosquitoes which had fed on yellow fever patients fifteen or more days previously. The results were fully confirmatory of the earlier experiments of the Commission—at the end of three days, nine and a half hours, the subject came down with a well marked case of yellow fever.

In all, ten cases of experimental yellow fever, caused by the bite of infected mosquitoes were developed in Camp Lazear. Throughout the period of the disease, other non-immunes slept in the little building, separated from the patient only by the mosquito-proof screen, but in no circumstances did they suffer any ill effects.

It was found that a yellow fever patient was capable of infecting mosquitoes only during the first three or four days after coming down with the disease. Moreover, after the mosquito has bitten such a patient, a period of at least twelve days must elapse before the insect is capable of transmitting the disease.

Once the organism has undergone its twelve day development, the mosquito may remain infective for weeks. In experiments of the Commission, two of the mosquitoes transmitted the disease to a volunteer fifty-seven days after their contamination. No other volunteers presenting themselves, one of these mosquitoes died the sixty-ninth and one the seventy-first day after their original contamination, without it being determined whether they were still capable of transmitting the disease.

So carefully carried out was this work and so conclusive were the results that Dr. Reed was justified in writing:

"Six months ago, when we landed on this island, absolutely nothing was known concerning the propagation and spread of yellow fever—it was all an unfathomable mystery—but today the curtain has been drawn—its mode of propagation is established and we know that a case minus mosquitoes is no more dangerous than one of chills and fever."

The conclusions of the Commission were fully substantiated by numerous workers, notably Dr. Guiteras of the Havana Board of Health, who had taken a lively interest in the work and whose results were made known in 1901, and by the Brazilian and French Commission at Sao Paulo, Brazil, in 1903.

Throughout the work of the Army Commission and down to the present time many fruitless efforts have been made to discover the specific organism of yellow fever. It was clearly established that the claims of Sanarelli for *Bacillus icteroides* were without foundation. It was found, too, that whatever the infective agent might be it was capable of passing through a Berkefeld filter and thus belongs to the puzzling group of "filterable viruses." It was further found that the virus was destroyed by heating up to 55° C for ten minutes. It is generally believed that the organism is a Protozoan.

The question of the hereditary transmission of the yellow fever organism within the mosquito was left unsettled by the Army Commission, though, as we have seen, it was raised by Finlay. Marchoux and Simond, of the French Commission devoted much attention to this phase of the problem and basing their conclusions on one apparently positive case, they decided that the disease could be transmitted through the egg of an infected *Aëdes calopus* to the second generation and thence to man. The conclusion, which is of very great importance in the control of yellow fever, has not been verified by other workers.

Once clearly established that yellow fever was transmitted solely by mosquitoes, the question of the characteristics, habits, and geographical distribution of the insect carrier became of vital importance.

*Aëdes calopus*, more commonly known as *Stegomyia fasciata* or *Stegomyia calopus* (fig. 134) is a moderate sized, rather strikingly marked mosquito. The general color is dark-brown or reddish-brown, but the thorax has a conspicuous broad, silvery-white curved line on each side, with two parallel median silvery lines. Between the latter there is a slender, broken line. The whole gives a lyre-shaped pattern to the thorax. The abdomen is dark with silvery-white basal bands and silvery white spots on each side of the abdominal segments. Legs black with rings of pure white at the base of the segments.

Size of the female 3.3 to 5 mm.; male 3 to 4.5 mm.

It is pre-eminently a domesticated species, being found almost exclusively about the habitation of man. "Its long association with man is shown by many of its habits. It approaches stealthily from behind. It retreats upon the slightest alarm. The ankles and, when one is sitting at a table or desk, the underside of the hands and wrists are favorable points of attack. It attacks silently, whereas other mosquitoes have a piping or humming note. The warning sound has doubtless been suppressed in the evolutionary process of its adaptation to man. It is extremely wary. It hides whenever it can, concealing itself in garments, working into the pockets, and under the lapels of coats, and crawling up under the clothes to bite the legs. In houses, it will hide

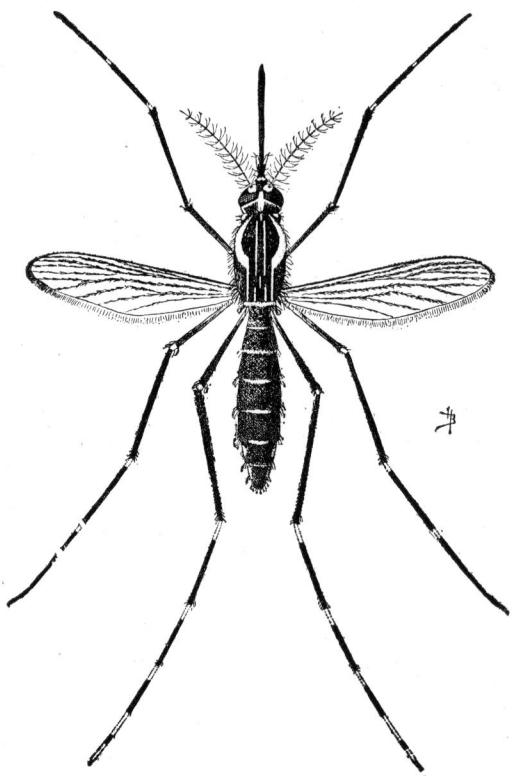

134. The yellow fever mosquito (Aëdes calopus), (x7). After Howard.

in dark corners, under picture moldings and behind the heads of old-fashioned bedsteads. It will enter closets and hide in the folds of garments."—Howard.

It was claimed by the French Commission, and subsequently often stated in discussions of the relation of the mosquito to yellow fever that the mature *Aëdes calopus* will bite only at night. If this were true it would be of the greatest importance in measures to avoid the disease. Unfortunately, the claim was illy founded and numerous workers have clearly established that the exact converse is more nearly true, this mosquito being pre-eminently a day species, feeding most actively in early morning, about sunrise, and late in the afternoon. On cloudy days it attacks at any time during the day. Thus there is peril in the doctrine that infected regions may be visited with perfect safety during the daytime and that measures to avoid the mosquito attack need be taken only at night.

Dr. Finlay maintained that the adult, even when starved, would not bite when the temperature was below 23° C, but subsequent studies have shown that this statement needs modification. The French Commission, working at Rio de Janeiro, found that *Aëdes calopus* would bite regularly at temperatures between 22° and 25° and that the optimum temperature was between 27° and 30° C, but their experiments led them to believe that it would bite in nature at a temperature as low as 17° C.

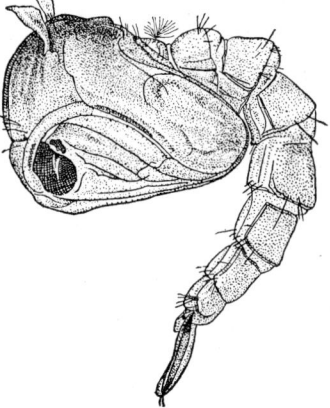

135a. Aëdes calopus. Pupa. After Howard.

The yellow fever mosquito breeds in cisterns, water barrels, pitchers and in the various water receptacles about the house. In our own Southern States it very commonly breeds in the above-ground cisterns which are in general use. Often the larvæ (fig. 135b) are found in flower vases, or even in the little cups of water which are placed under the legs of tables to prevent their being overrun by ants. They have been repeatedly found breeding in the holy water font in churches. In short, they breed in any collection of water in close proximity to the dwellings or gathering places of man.

The life cycle under favorable conditions is completed in from twelve to fifteen days. These figures are of course very dependent upon the temperature. The Army Commission in Cuba found that the cycle might be completed in as brief a period as nine and a half days. Under less favorable conditions it may be greatly lengthened.

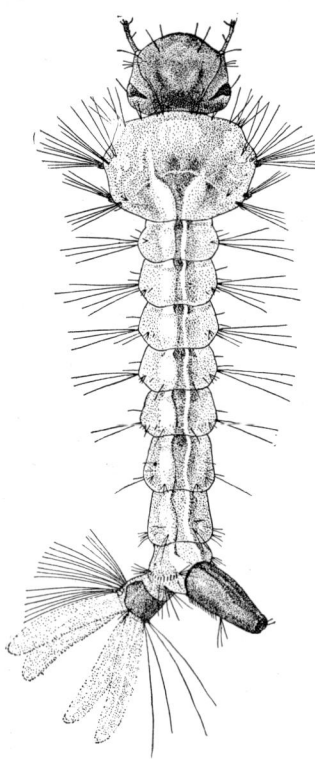

The adults are long lived. We have seen that during the experimental work in Cuba specimens were kept in captivity for sixty-nine and seventy-one days, respectively, and that they were proved to retain their infectivity for at least fifty-seven days. Dr. Guiteras subsequently kept an infected adult for one hundred and fifty-four days.

Low temperatures have a very great effect not only on development, but on the activity and even life of the adults. Long before the method of transmission of yellow fever was discovered it was well known that the epidemics were brought to a close by heavy frosts, and it is now known that this is due to the killing of the mosquitoes which alone could spread the disease.

*Aëdes calopus* has a very wide distribution since, as Howard says, being a domestic mosquito, having a fairly long life in the adult stage, and having the custom of hiding itself in the most ingenious ways, it is particularly subject to carriage for long distances on board vessels, in railway trains, even packed in baggage. In general, its permanent distribution is from 40 degrees north latitude to 40 degrees south latitude (Brumpt), in a belt extending around the world. In the United States it breeds in most of our Southern States.

135*b*. Aëdes calopus; larva. (x7). After Howard.

Thus, as in the case of malaria, there are many places where the insect carrier is abundant but where yellow fever does not occur. Such, for instance, are Hawaii, Australia and Asia. An outbreak may occur at any time that a patient suffering from the disease is allowed to enter and become a source of infection for the mosquitoes. In this connection various writers have called attention to the menace from the Panama Canal. When it is completed, it will allow of direct passage from regions where yellow fever is endemic and this will greatly increase the possibility of its introduction into these places where it is now unknown. The result, with a wholly non-immune population, would be appalling.

On the other hand, there are places wholly outside of the normal range of *Aëdes calopus* where the disease has raged. Such are New York, Boston, and even Philadelphia, which have suffered notable epidemics. These outbreaks have been due to the introduction of infected mosquitoes during the heat of summer, when they have not only conveyed the disease but have found conditions favorable for their multiplication. Or, uninfected mosquitoes have been thus accidentally brought in and developed in large numbers, needing then only the accidental introduction of cases of the disease to start an epidemic.

Methods of control of various diseases have been revolutionized by the discovery that they were insect-borne, but in no other case has the change been as radical or the results as spectacular as in the case of yellow fever. The "shot-gun quarantine," the sufferings and horrors, the hopelessness of fighting absolutely blindly have given way to an efficient, clear-cut method of control, based upon the knowledge that the disease is carried from man to man solely by the mosquito, *Aëdes calopus*. The lines of defense and offense are essentially as follows:

In the first place, when a case of yellow fever occurs, stringent precautions must be adopted to prevent the infection of mosquitoes and the escape of any already infected. This means that the patient must be removed to a mosquito-proof room, or ward beyond reach of the insects, and that the infected room must be thoroughly fumigated at once, to kill the mosquitoes hiding within it. All cracks and openings should be closed with strips of paper and fumigation with burning sulphur or pyrethrum carefully carried out.

It should be remembered that if the first case noted is that of a resident rather than imported, it means that the mosquito carriers became infected more than two weeks before the case was diagnosed, for as we have seen, the germ must undergo a twelve-day period of development within its insect host. Therefore a careful search must be made for mild cases which, though unrecognized, may serve as foci for the spread of the disease.

In face of a threatened epidemic one of the most essential measures is to educate the citizens and to gain their complete coöperation in the fight along modern lines. This may be done through the schools, the pulpit, places of amusement, newspapers and even bulletin boards.

Emphasis should be placed on the necessity of both non-immunes and immunes using mosquito curtains, and in all possible ways avoiding exposure to the mosquitoes.

Then the backbone of the fight must be the anti-mosquito measures. In general, these involve screening and fumigating against adults, and control of water supply, oiling, and drainage against the larvæ. The region involved must be districted and a thorough survey undertaken to locate breeding places, which must, if possible, be eradicated. If they are necessary for water supplies, such as casks, or cisterns, they should be carefully screened to prevent access of egg-laying adults.

The practical results of anti-mosquito measures in the fight against yellow fever are well illustrated by the classic examples of the work in Havana, immediately following the discoveries of the Army Commission and by the stamping out of the New Orleans epidemic in 1905.

The opportunities for an immediate practical application of the theories of the Army Commission in Havana were ideal. The city had always been a hotbed of yellow fever and was the principal source from which the disease was introduced year after year into our Southern States. It was under martial law and with a military governor who was himself a physician and thoroughly in sympathy with the views of the Commission, the rigid enforcement of the necessary regulations was possible. The story of the first campaign has been often told, but nowhere more clearly than in Dr. Reed's own account, published in the *Journal of Hygiene* for 1902.

Closer home was the demonstration of the efficacy of these measures in controlling the yellow fever outbreak in New Orleans in 1905. During the spring and early summer of the year the disease had, unperceived, gained a firm foothold in that city and when, in early July the local Board of Health took cognizance of its existence, it was estimated that there had been in the neighborhood of one hundred cases.

Conditions were not as favorable as they had been under martial law in Havana for carrying on a rigid fight along anti-mosquito lines.

The densely populated city was unprepared, the public had to be educated, and an efficient organization built up. The local authorities actively began a general fight against the mosquito but in spite of their best efforts the disease continued to spread. It was recognized that more rigid organization was needed and on August 12th the United States Public Health and Marine Hospital Service was put in absolute charge of the fight. Up to this time there had been one hundred and forty-two deaths from a total of nine hundred and thirteen cases and all of the conditions seemed to threaten an outbreak to exceed the memorable one of 1878 when, as we have seen there were four thousand and forty-six deaths.

With the hearty coöperation of the citizens,—physicians and laymen alike,—the fight was waged and long before frost or any near approach thereto the disease was stamped out,—a thing unheard of in previous epidemics. The total loss of life was four hundred and sixty—about 11 per cent as great as that from the comparable epidemic of 1878. If the disease had been promptly recognized and combated with the energy which marked the fight later in the summer, the outbreak would have made little headway and the great proportion of these lives would have been saved.

## CHAPTER IX

**ARTHROPODS AS ESSENTIAL HOSTS OF PATHOGENIC PROTOZOA**

### Insects and Trypanosomiases

By trypanosomiasis is meant a condition of animal parasitism, common to man and the lower animals, in which trypanosomes, peculiar flagellate protozoa, infest the blood. Depending upon the species, they may be harmless, producing no appreciable ill-effect, or pathogenic, giving rise to conditions of disease. A number of these are known to be transferred by insects.

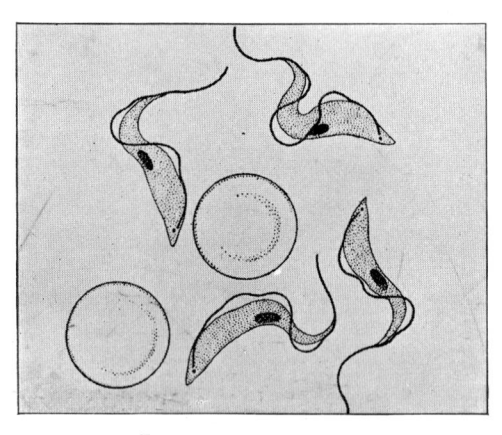

In order that we may consider more fully the developmental stage of these parasites within their insect host, it is necessary that we describe briefly the structure of the blood-inhabiting stage.

The trypanosomes are elongated, usually pointed, flagellated protozoa (fig. 136) in which the single flagellum, bent under the body, forms the outer limit of a delicate undulating membrane. It arises near one end of the organism from a minute centrosome-like body which is known as the blepheroplast, and at the opposite end extends for a greater or less distance as a free flagellum. Enclosing, or close beside the blepheroplast is the small kinetonucleus. The principal nucleus, round or oval in form, is situated near the center of the body. Asexual reproductions occurs in this stage, by longitudinal fission, the nucleus and the blepheroplast dividing independently of one another. From the blepheroplast of one of the daughter cells a new flagellum is formed.

Among the pathogenic species are to be found the causative organisms of some of the most serious diseases of domestic animals and even of man. It is probable that these pathogenic species secrete

136. Trypanosome brucei. After Bruce.

a specific poison. The majority of them are tropical in distribution.

Though we are concerned especially with the species which infest man, we shall first consider two of the trypanosomes of lower animals, known long before any of those of man had been found.

**Fleas and Lice as Carriers of Trypanosoma lewisi.**—*Trypanosoma lewisi*, the first mammalian trypanosome known, is to be found in the blood of wild rats. Like its host, it appears to be cosmopolitan in distribution, having been reported from several localities in the United States, Brazil, Argentine, England, Germany, France, Italy, Russia, Asia and Africa.

This species is usually regarded as non-pathogenic, but in experimental work, especially with white rats, heavy infestations often result fatally, and naturally infested specimens sometimes show evidence of injury. Rats which have been infested exhibit at least temporary immunity against new infection.

*Trypanosoma lewisi* is transmitted from rat to rat by fleas and by lice. Rabinowitsch and Kempner (1899) first found that healthy rats which were kept with infested rats, showed trypanosomes in their blood after about two weeks. They found the trypanosomes in the alimentary canal of fleas which had fed on the diseased rats. On teasing such fleas in physiological salt solution and inoculating them into fresh rats they were able to produce the infection. Finally, they showed that the fleas which had fed upon infested rats were able to carry the parasites to healthy rats. Corresponding experiments with lice were not successful. Prowazek (1905) found in the rat louse (*Hæmatopinus spinulosus*) organisms which he regarded as developmental stages of the *Trypanosoma lewisi*. He believed that the sexual cycle was undergone in this insect.

Nuttall (1908) readily transmitted the trypanosomes through the agency of fleas, (*Ceratophyllus fasciatus* and *Ctenopthalmus agyrtes*). He believes that these insects are probably the chief transmitters of the parasite. He was also able to transmit it from diseased to healthy rats through the agency of the rat louse. He was unable to trace any developmental stages in the louse and inclined to the opinion that Prowazek was deceived by the presence of extraneous flagellates such as are known to exist in a number of blood-sucking arthropods.

Nuttall concludes that since three distinct kinds of blood-sucking insects are capable of transmitting *Trypanosoma lewisi* it appears doubtful that this flagellate is a parasite of the invertebrate "host" in the sense claimed by Prowazek and other investigators.

**Tsetse-flies and Nagana**—One of the greatest factors in retarding the development of certain regions of Africa has been the presence of a small fly, little larger than the common house-fly. This is the tsetse-fly, *Glossina morsitans* (fig. 165) renowned on account of the supposed virulence of its bite for cattle, horses and other domestic mammals.

The technical characteristics of the tsetse-flies, or Glossinas, and their several species, will be found in a later chapter. We need emphasize only that they are blood-sucking Muscidæ and that, unlike the mosquitoes, the sexes resemble each other closely in structure of the mouth-parts, and in feeding habits.

In 1894, Colonel David Bruce discovered that the fly was not in itself poisonous but that the deadly effect of its bite was due to the fact that it transmitted a highly pathogenic blood parasite, *Trypanosoma brucei*. This trypanosome Bruce had discovered in the blood of South African cattle suffering from a highly fatal disease known as "nagana". On inoculating the blood of infected cattle into horses and dogs he produced the disease and found the blood teeming with the causative organism. In the course of his work he established beyond question that the "nagana" and the tsetse-fly disease were identical.

Tsetse-flies of the species *Glossina morsitans*, which fed upon diseased animals, were found capable of giving rise to the disease in healthy animals up to forty-eight hours after feeding. Wild tsetse-flies taken from an infected region to a region where they did not normally occur were able to transmit the disease to healthy animals. It was found that many of the wild animals in the tsetse-fly regions harbored *Trypanosoma brucei* in their blood, though they showed no evidence of disease. As in the case of natives of malarial districts, these animals acted as reservoirs of the parasite. Non-immune animals subjected to the attacks of the insect carrier, quickly succumbed to the disease.

A question of prime importance is as to whether the insect serves as an essential host of the pathogenic protozoan or whether it is a mere mechanical carrier. Bruce inclined to the latter view. He was unable to find living trypanosomes in the intestines or excrements of the fly or to produce the disease on the many occasions when he injected the excrement into healthy animals. Moreover, he had found that the experimental flies were infective only during the first forty-eight hours and that if wild flies were taken from the infected region, "kept without food for three days and then fed on a healthy dog, they never gave rise to the disease."

Koch had early described what he regarded as sexual forms from the intestine of the fly but it remained for Kleine (1909) to experimentally demonstrate that a part of the life cycle of the parasite was undergone in the fly. Working with *Glossina palpalis*, he found that for a period of ten days or longer after feeding on an animal suffering from nagana it was non-infective, but that then it became infective and was able to transmit the disease for weeks thereafter. He discovered and described developmental stages of the parasite within the intestine of the insect. In other words, the tsetse-fly (in nature, *Glossina morsitans*), serves as an essential host, within which an important part of the life cycle of the parasite is undergone. These conclusions were quickly verified by Bruce and numerous other workers and are no longer open to question. Klein and Taute are even inclined to think that mechanical transmission plays practically no rôle in nature, unless the fly is interrupted while feeding and passes immediately to a new animal.

**Tsetse-flies and Sleeping Sickness of Man**—About the beginning of the present century a hitherto little known disease of man began to attract great attention on account of its ravages in Uganda and the region of Victoria Nyanza in South Africa. It was slow, insiduous and absolutely fatal, characterized in its later stages by dullness, apathy, and finally absolute lethargy all day long, symptoms which gave it the name of "sleeping sickness."

It was soon found that the disease was not a new one but that it had been known for over a hundred years on the west coast of Africa. Its introduction into Central and East Africa and its rapid spread have been attributed primarily to the development of the country, the formation of new trade routes and the free mingling of native tribes formerly isolated. It is estimated that in the first ten years of the present century there were approximately two hundred thousand deaths from the disease in the Uganda protectorate. In the British province Bugosa, on the Victoria Nyanza there were thirty thousand deaths in the period from 1902–1905.

While the disease is peculiarly African there are a number of instances of its accidental introduction into temperate regions. Slaves suffering from it were occasionally brought to America in the early part of the last century and cases have sometimes been imported into England. In none of the cases did the disease gain a foothold or spread at all to other individuals.

In 1902 Dutton described a trypanosome, *T. gambiense*, which he and Forde had found the year before in the blood of a patient suffering from a peculair type of fever in Gambia. In 1902–1903 Castellani found the same parasite in the cerebro-spinal fluid of sleeping-sickness patients and definitely reported it as the causative organism of the disease. His work soon found abundant confirmation, and it was discovered that the sleeping sickness was but the ultimate phase of the fever discovered by Dutton and Forde.

When Castellani made known his discovery of the trypanosome of sleeping sickness, Brumpt, in France, and Sambon, in England, independently advanced the theory that the disease was transmitted by the tsetse-fly, *Glossina palpalis*. This theory was based upon the geographical distribution and epidemiology of the disease. Since then it has been abundantly verified by experimental evidence.

Fortunately for the elucidation of problems relating to the methods of transfer of sleeping sickness, *Trypanosoma gambiense* is pathogenic for many species of animals. In monkeys it produces symptoms very similar to those caused in man. Bruce early showed that *Glossina palpalis* "fed on healthy monkeys eight, twelve, twenty-four and forty-eight hours after having fed on a native suffering from trypanosomiasis, invariably transmitted the disease. After three days the flies failed to transmit it." In his summary in Osler's Modern Medicine, he continues "But this is not the only proof that these flies can carry the infective agent. On the lake shore there was a large native population among whom we had found about one-third to be harboring trypanosomes in their blood. The tsetse-flies caught on this lake shore, brought to the laboratory in cages, and placed straightway on healthy monkeys, gave them the disease in every instance, and furnished a startling proof of the danger of loitering along the lake shore among those infected flies."

As in the case of nagana, Bruce and most of the earlier investigators supposed the transmission of the sleeping sickness trypanosome by *Glossina palpalis* to be purely mechanical. The work of Kleine (1909) clearly showed that for *Trypanosoma gambiense* as well as for *Trypanosoma brucei* the fly served as an essential host. Indeed, Kleine and many subsequent investigators are inclined to think that there is practically no mechanical transmission of trypanosomes from animal to animal by *Glossina* in nature, and that the many successful experiments of the earlier investigators were due to the fact that they used wild flies which already harbored the transformed parasite rather than directly inoculated it from the blood of the diseased experimental animals. While the criticism is applicable to some of the work, this extreme view is not fully justified by the evidence at hand.

Kleine states (1912) that *Glossina palpalis* can no longer be regarded as the sole transmitter of sleeping sickness. Taute (1911) had shown that under experimental conditions *Glossina morsitans* was capable of transferring the disease and Kleine calls attention to the fact that in German East Africa, in the district of the Rovuma River, at least a dozen cases of the disease have occurred recently, though only *Glossina morsitans* exists in the district. It appears, however, that these cases are due to a different parasite, *Trypanosoma rhodesiense*. This species, found especially in north-east Rhodesia and in Nyassaland, is transferred by *Glossina morsitans*.

Other workers maintain that the disease may be transmitted by various blood-sucking flies, or even bugs and lice which attack man. Fülleborn and Mayer (1907) have shown by conclusive experiments that *Aedes* (*Stegomyia*) *calopus* may transmit it from one animal to another if the two bites immediately succeed each other.

It is not possible that insects other than the tsetse-flies (and only certain species of these), play an important rôle in the transmission of the disease, else it would be much more wide-spread. Sambon (1908) pointed out that the hypothesis that is spread by *Aedes calopus* is opposed by the fact that the disease never spread in the Antilles, though frequently imported there by West African slaves. The same observation would apply also to conditions in our own Southern States in the early part of the past century.

Since *Glossina palpalis* acts as an essential host of the parasite and the chief, if not the only, transmitter, the fight against sleeping sickness, like that against malaria and yellow fever, becomes primarily a problem in economic entomology. The minutest detail of the life-history, biology, and habits of the fly, and of its parasites and other natural enemies becomes of importance in attempts to eradicate the disease. Here we can consider only the general features of the subject.

218     *Arthropods as Essential Hosts of Pathogenic Protozoa*

*Glossina palpalis* lives in limited areas, where the forest and undergrowth is dense, along the lake shore or river banks. According to Hodges, the natural range from shore is under thirty yards, though the distance to which the flies may follow man greatly exceed this.

It is a day feeder, a fact which may be taken advantage of in avoiding exposure to its attacks. The young are brought forth alive and full-grown, one every nine or ten days. Without feeding, they enter the ground and under favorable conditions, complete their development in a month or more.

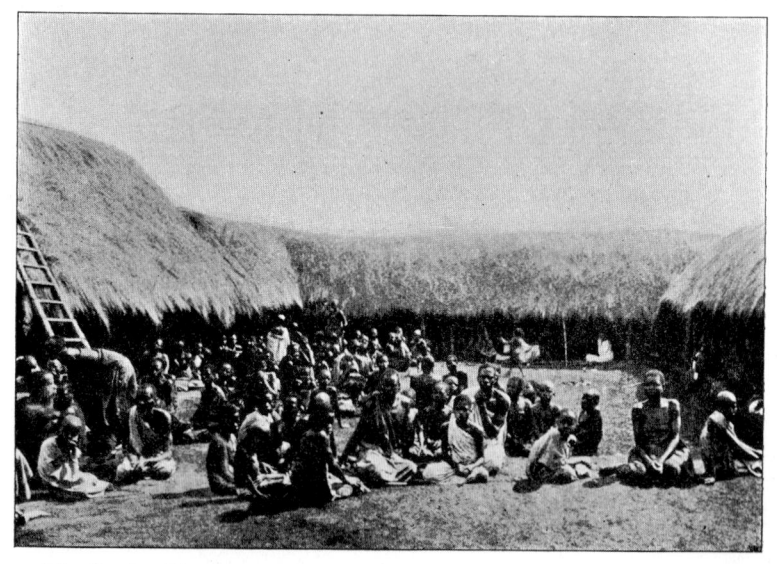

137.  Sleeping sickness concentration camp in German East Africa.  Report of German Commission.

Methods of control of the disease must look to the prevention of infection of the flies, and to their avoidance and destruction. Along the first line, much was hoped from temporary segregation of the sick in regions where the fly was not found. On the assumption that the flies acted as carriers only during the first two or three days, it was supposed that even the "fly belts" would become safe within a few days after the sick were removed. The problem was found to be a much more difficult one when it was learned that after a given brief period the fly again became infective and remained so for an indeterminate period. Nevertheless, isolation of the sick is one of the most important measures in preventing the spread of the disease into new districts. Much, too, is being accomplished by moving native villages from the fly belts. (c.f. fig. 137.)

All measures to avoid the flies should be adopted. This means locating and avoiding the fly belts as far as possible, careful screening of houses, and protection of the body against bites.

Clearing the jungle along the water courses for some yards beyond the natural range of the fly has proved a very important measure. Castellani recommends that the area be one hundred yards and around a village three hundred yards at least.

Detailed studies of the parasites and the natural enemies of the tsetse-fly are being undertaken and may ultimately yield valuable results.

**South American Trypanosomiasis**—The tsetse-flies are distinctively African in distribution and until recently there were no tryanosomes known to infest man in America. In 1909 Dr. Chagas, of Rio de Janeiro described a new species, *Trypanosoma cruzi*, pathogenic to man.

*Trypanosoma cruzi* is the causative organism of a disease common in some regions of Brazil, where it is known as "opilacao." It is especially to be met with in children and is characterized by extreme anemia, wasting, and stunted development associated with fever, and enlargenemt of the thyroid glands. The disease is transmitted by the bites of several species of assassin-bugs, or Reduviidæ, notably by *Conorhinus megistus*. The evolution of the parasite within the bug has been studied especially by Chagas and by Brumpt. From the latter's text we take the following summary.

The adult tryanosomes, ingested by a *Conorhinus megistus*, of any stage, first change into Crithidia-like forms and then those which remain in the stomach become ovoid and non-motile. Brumpt found these forms in immense numbers, in a *Cornohinus* which had been infested fourteen months before. The forms which pass into the intestine quickly assume the *Crithidia* form and continue to develop rapidly under this form. Some weeks later they evolve into the trypanosome forms, pathogenic for man. They then pass out with the excrement of the bug and infect the vertebrate host as soon as they come in contact with any mucous layer (buccal, ocular or rectal). More rarely they enter through the epidermis.

Brumpt showed that the development could take place in three species; bed-bugs (*Cimex lectularius, C. hemipterus*) and in the tick

*Ornithodoros moubata.* The evolution proceeds in the first two species of bed-bugs as rapidly as in Conorhinus, or even more rapidly, but they remain infective for a much shorter time and hence Brumpt considers that they play a much less important rôle in the spread of the disease.

*Conorhinus megistus*, like related forms in our Southern States, very commonly frequents houses and attacks man with avidity. Chagas states that the bites are painless and do not leave any traces. They are usually inflicted on the lips, or the cheeks and thus the buccal mucosa of a sleeper may be soiled by the dejections of the insect and the bite serving as a port of entry of the virus, remain unnoticed.

The possibility of some of our North American Reduviidæ playing a similar rôle in the transmission of disease should not be overlooked.

**Leishmanioses and Insects**—Closely related to the trypanosomes is a group of intracellular parasites which have recently been grouped by Ross under the genus *Leishmania*. Five species are known to affect man. Three of these produce local skin infestations, but two of them, *Leishmania donovani* and *L. infantum*, produce serious and often fatal systemic diseases.

The first of these, that produced by *L. donovani*, is an exceedingly virulent disease common in certain regions of India and China. It is commonly known as "Kala-azar," or "dum-dum" fever, and more technically as tropical leishmaniasis. Patton (1907) believes that the parasite is transmitted by the bed-bug *Cimex hemipterus*, and has described a developmental cycle similar to that which can be found in artificial cultures. On the other hand, Donovan was unable to confirm Patton's work and believes that the true intermediate host is a Reduviid bug, *Conorhinus rubrofasciatus*.

*Leishmania infantum* is the cause of the so-called infantile splenic leishmaniasis, occurring in northern Africa, Spain, Portugal, Italy, and possibly other parts of Europe. The parasite occurs habitually in the dog and is only accidentally transferred to children, Alvares and da Silva, in Portugal (according to Brumpt, 1913) have found that the excrement of a flea from a diseased dog contains flagellates, and they suggest that the infection may be transmitted by the accidental inoculation of this excrement by means of the proboscis of the flea, as has been thought to occur in the case of the plague. To this

Brumpt objects that they and other workers who thought to trace the development of *Leishmania infantum* were apparently misled by the presence of a harmless *Herpetomonas* which infests dog fleas in all countries, even where the leishmaniasis is unknown.

Basile (1910 and 1911) however, carried on numerous experiments indicating that the disease was transferred from children to dogs and from dog to dog by the dog flea, and was able to find in the tissues of the insects forms perfectly identical with those found in children and in dogs suffering from leishmaniasis. He also found that *Pulex irritans* was capable of acting as the carrier.

Of the cutaneous type of leishmaniasis, the best known is the so-called "Oriental sore," an ulcerative disease of the skin which is epidemic in many tropical and subtropical regions. The causative organism is *Leishmania tropica*, which occurs in the diseased tissues as bodies very similar to those found in the spleen in cases of kala-azar. The disease is readily inoculable and there is no doubt that it may be transferred from the open sores to abraded surfaces of a healthy individual by house-flies. It is also believed by a number of investigators that it may be transferred and directly inoculated by various blood-sucking insects.

## Ticks and Diseases of Man and Animals

We have seen that the way to the discoveries of the relations of arthropods to disease was pointed out by the work of Leuckart and Melnikoff on the life cycle of *Dipylidium*, and of Fedtschenko and Manson on that of *Filaria*. They dealt with grosser forms, belonging to well-recognized parasitic groups.

This was long before the rôle of any insect as a carrier of pathogenic micro-organisms had been established, and before the Protozoa were generally regarded as of importance in the causation of disease. The next important step was taken in 1889 when Smith and Kilbourne conclusively showed that the so-called Texas fever of cattle, in the United States, is due to an intracorpuscular blood parasite transmitted exclusively by a tick. This discovery, antedating by eight years the work on the relation of the mosquito to malaria, had a very great influence on subsequent studies along these lines.

While much of the recent work has dealt with the true insects, or hexapods, it is now known that several of the most serious diseases of animals, and at least two important diseases of man are tick borne. These belong to the types known collectively as *babesioses* (or "*piroplasmoses*"), and *spirochætoses*.

## 222   Arthropods as Essential Hosts of Pathogenic Protozoa

The term *babesiosis* is applied to a disease of man or animals which is caused by minute protozoan parasites of the genus *Babesia*, living in the red blood corpuscles. These parasites have usually been given the generic name *Piroplasma* and hence the type of disease which they cause is often referred to as "*piroplasmosis*." The best known illustration is the disease known in this country as Texas fever of cattle.

**Cattle Ticks and Texas Fever**—The cattle disease, which in the United States is known as Texas fever, is a widely distributed, exceedingly acute disease. In Australia it is known as *redwater fever* and in Europe as hæmoglobinuria, due to the fact that the urine of the diseased animals is discolored by the breaking down of the red blood corpuscles infested by the parasite.

In their historical discussion, Smith and Kilbourne, point out that as far back as 1796 it was noted that Southern cattle, in a state of apparent health, might spread a fatal disease among Northern herds. As observations accumulated, it was learned that this infection was carried only during the warm season of the year and in the depth of winter Southern cattle were harmless. Moreover, Southern cattle after remaining for a short time in the North lost their power to transmit the disease, and the same was true of cattle which had been driven for a considerable distance.

Very significant was the fact that the infection was not communicated directly from the Southern to Northern cattle but that the ground over which the former passed was infected by them, and that the infection was transmitted thence to susceptible cattle *after a period of not less than thirty days had elapsed*.

Of course a disease as striking as this, and which caused such enormous losses of cattle in the region invaded was fruitful in theories concerning its causation. The most widespread was the belief that pastures were infected by the saliva, urine, or manure of Southern cattle. There were not wanting keen observers who suggested that the disease was caused by ticks, but little weight was given to their view.

Various workers had described bacteria which they had isolated from the organs of the diseased animals, but their findings could not be verified. In 1889, Smith and Kilbourne discovered a minute, pear-shaped organism (fig. 138) in the red blood corpuscles of a cow which had succumbed to Texas fever. On account of their shape they were given the generic name *Pyrososma* and because they were usually found two in a corpuscle, the specific name, *bigeminum*. It is now generally accepted that the parasite is the same which Babes had observed the year before in Roumanian cattle suffering from hæmoglobinuria, and should be known as *Babesia bovis* (Babes).

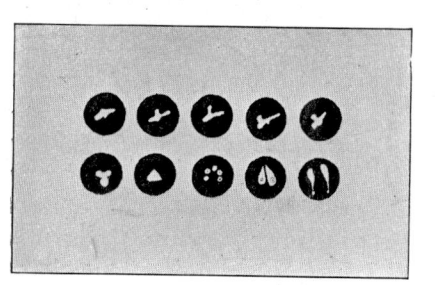

138. Babesia bovis in blood corpuscles. After Calli.

By a series of perfectly conclusive experiments carried on near Washington, D. C., Smith and Kilbourne showed that this organism was carried from Southern cattle to non-immune animals by the so-called Southern cattle tick, *Boophilus annulatus* (= *Margaropus annulatus*) (fig. 139).

Of fourteen head of native cattle placed in a field with tick-infested Northern cattle all but two contracted the disease. This experiment was repeated with similar results. Four head of native cattle kept in a plot with three North Carolina cattle which had been carefully freed from ticks remained healthy. A second experiment the same year gave similar results.

Still more conclusive was the experiment showing that fields which had not been entered by Southern cattle but which had been infected by mature ticks taken from such animals would produce Texas fever in native cattle. On September 13, 1889, several thousand ticks collected from cattle in North Carolina three and four days before, were scattered in a small field near Washington. Three out of four native animals placed in

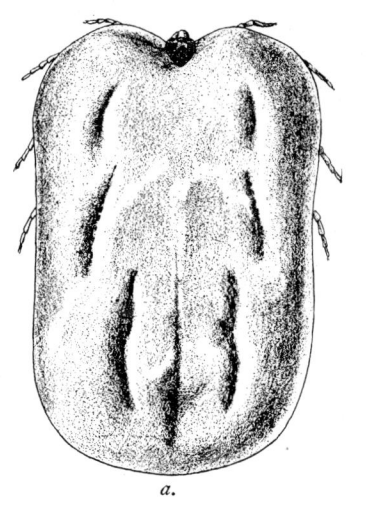

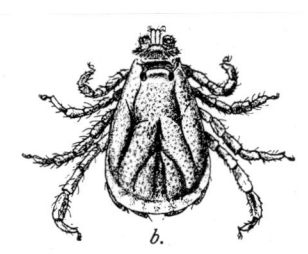

139. The cattle tick (Boophilus annulatus). (*a*) Female; (*b*) male. After Comstock.

this field contracted the disease. The fourth animal was not examined as to its blood but it showed no external symptoms of the disease.

In these earlier experiments it was believed that the cattle tick acted as a carrier of the disease between the Southern cattle and the *soil* of the Northern pastures. "It was believed that the tick obtained the parasite from the blood of its host and in its dissolution on the pasture a certain resistant spore form was set free which produced the disease when taken in with the food." The feeding of one animal for some time with grass from the most abundantly

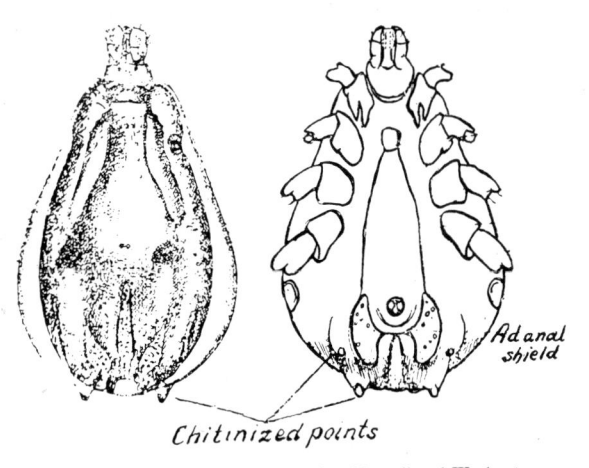

140. Hyalomma aegypticum. After Nuttall and Warburton.

infected field, without any appearance of the disease, made this hypothesis untenable.

In the experimental work in 1890 the astonishing fact was brought out that the disease was conveyed neither by infected ticks disintegrating nor by their directly transferring the parasite, but that it was conveyed by the young hatched from eggs of infected ticks. In other words, the disease was hereditarily transferred to ticks of the second generation and they alone were capable of conveying it.

Thus was explained the fact that Texas fever did not appear immediately along the route of Southern cattle being driven to Northern markets but that after a certain definite period it manifested itself. It was conveyed by the progeny of ticks which had dropped from the Southern cattle and deposited their eggs on the ground.

These results have been fully confirmed by workers in different parts of the world,—notably by Koch, in Africa, and by Pound, in Australia.

The disease is apparently transmitted by *Boophilus annulatus* alone, in the United States, but it, or an almost identical disease, is conveyed by *Ixodes hexagonus* in Norway, *Ixodes ricinus* in Finland and France and by the three species, *Boophilus decoloratus*, *Hyalomma ægypticum* (fig. 140 and 141), and *Hæmaphysalis punctata* in Africa.

In spite of the detailed study which it has received, the life cycle of *Babesia bovis* has not been satisfactorily worked out. The asexual reproduction in the blood of the vertebrate host has been described but the cycle in the tick is practically unknown.

More successful attempts have been made to work out the life cycle of a related species, *Babesia canis*, which causes malignant jaundice in dogs in Africa and parts of Southern Europe. In this instance, also, the disease is transmitted by heredity to the ticks of the second generation. Yet the larval, or "seed ticks," from an infected female are not capable of conveying the disease, but only the nymphs and adults. Still more complicated is the condition in the case of *Babesia ovis* of sheep, which Motas has shown can be conveyed solely by the adult, sexually mature ticks of the second generation.

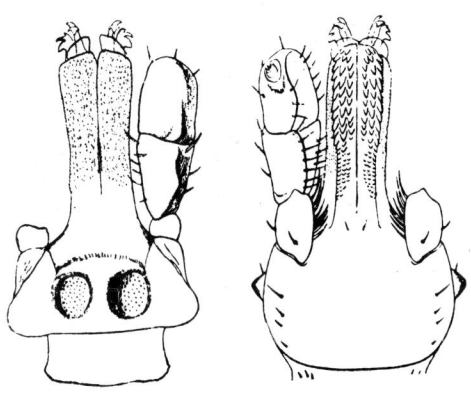

141. Hyalomma aegypticum. Capitulum of female; (*a*) dorsal, (*b*) ventral aspect.

In *Babesis canis*, Christopher (1907) observed developmental stages in the tick. He found in the stomach of adult ticks, large motile club-shaped bodies which he considered as oökinetes. These bodies pass to the ovaries of the tick and enter the eggs where they become globular in form and probably represent an oöcyst. This breaks up into a number of sporoblasts which enter the tissues of the developing tick and give rise to numerous sporozoites, which collect in the salivary glands and thence are transferred to the vertebrate host. A number of other species of *Babesia* are known to infest vertebrates and in all the cases where the method has been worked out it has been found that the conveyal was by ticks. We shall not consider the cases more fully here, as we are concerned especially with the method of transfer of human diseases.

**Ticks and Rocky Mountain Spotted Fever of Man**—Ever since 1873 there has been known in Montana and Idaho a peculiar febrile disease of man, which has gained the name of "Rocky Mountain spotted fever." Its onset is marked by chills and fever which rapidly become acute. In about four to seven days there appears a characteristic eruption on the wrists, ankles or back, which quickly covers the body.

McClintic (1912) states that the disease has now been reported from practically all of the Rocky Mountain States, including Arizona, California, Colorado, Idaho, Montana, Nevada, Oregon, Utah, Washington, and Wyoming. "Although the disease is far more prevalent in Montana and Idaho than in any of the other States, its spread has assumed such proportions in the last decade as to call for the gravest consideration on the part of both the state and national health authorities. In fact, the disease has so spread from state to state that it has undoubtedly become a very serious interstate problem demanding the institution of measures for its control and suppression."

A peculiar feature of the Rocky Mountain spotted fever is a marked variation in its severity in different localities. In Montana, and especially in the famous Bitter Root Valley, from 33 per cent to 75 per cent of the cases result fatally. On the other hand, the fatality does not exceed four per cent in Idaho.

In 1902, Wilson and Chowning reported the causative organism of spotted fever to be a blood parasite akin to the *Babesia* of Texas fever, and made the suggestion that the disease was tick-borne. The careful studies of Stiles (1905) failed to confirm the supposed discovery of the organism, and the disease is now generally classed as due to an invisible virus. On the other hand, the accumulated evidence has fully substantiated the hypothesis that it is tick-borne.

According to Ricketts (1907) the experimental evidence in support of this hypothesis was first afforded by Dr. L. P. McCalla and Dr. H. A. Brereton, in 1905. These investigators transmitted the disease from man to man in two experiments. "The tick was obtained 'from the chest of a man very ill with spotted fever' and 'applied to the arm of a man who had been in the hospital for two months and a half, and had lost both feet from gangrene due to freezing.' On the eighth day the patient became very ill and passed through a mild course of spotted fever, leaving a characteristic eruption. The experiment was repeated by placing the tick on a woman's leg and she likewise was infected with spotted fever."

The most detailed studies were those of the late Dr. H. T. Ricketts, and it was he who clearly established the tick hypothesis. In the summer of 1906 he found that guinea pigs and monkeys are very susceptible to spotted fever and can readily be infected by inoculation of blood from patients suffering from the disease. This opened the way to experimental work on tick transmission. A female tick was fed upon an infected guinea pig for two days, removed and isolated for two days and then placed upon a healthy guinea pig. After an incubation period of three and a half days the experimental animal contracted a well-marked case of the disease.

A similar result was obtained at the same time by King, and later in the season Ricketts proved that the male tick was also capable of transmitting the disease. He found that there was a very intimate relation of the virus to the tick and that the transmission must be regarded as biological throughout. Ticks remained infective as long as they lived and would feed for a period of several months. If they acquired the disease in the larval or nymphal stage they retained it during molting and were infective in the subsequent stages. In a few cases the larvæ from an infected female were infective.

The evidence indicated that the tick suffers from a relatively harmless, generalized infection and the virus proliferates in its body. The disease probably is transferred through the salivary secretion of the tick since inoculation experiments show that the salivary glands of the infected adult contain the virus.

It is probable that in nature the reservoir of the virus of spotted fever is some one or more of the native small animals. Infected ticks have been found in nature, and as various wild animals are susceptible to the disease, it is obvious that it may exist among them unnoticed. Wilson and Chowning suggested that the ground squirrel plays the principal rôle.

Unfortunately, much confusion exists regarding the correct name of the tick which normally conveys the disease. In the medical literature it is usually referred to as *Dermacentor occidentalis*, but students of the group now agree that it is specifically distinct.

Banks has designated it as *Dermacentor venustus* and this name is used in the publications of the Bureau of Entomology. On the other hand, Stiles maintains that the common tick of the Bitter Root Valley, and the form which has been collected by the authors who have worked on Rocky Mountain spotted fever in that region, is separable from *D. venustus*, and he has described it under the name of *Dermacentor andersoni*.

Maver (1911) has shown experimentally that spotted fever may be transmitted by several different species of ticks, notably *Dermacentor marginatus*, *Dermacentor variabilis* and *Amblyomma americanum*. This being the case, the question of the exact systematic status of the species experimented upon in the Bitter Root Valley becomes less important, for since *Dermacentor occidentalis*, *Dermacentor venustus* and *Dermacentor andersoni* all readily attack man, it is probable that either species would readily disseminate the disease if it should spread into their range.

Hunter and Bishop (1911) have emphasized the fact that in the eastern and southern United States there occur several species which attack man, and any one of which might transmit the disease from animal to animal and from animal to man. The following species, they state, would probably be of principal importance in the Southern and Eastern States: the lone star tick (*Amblyomma americanum*); the American dog tick (*Dermacentor variabilis*); and the gulf-coast tick (*Amblyomma maculatum*). In the extreme southern portions of Texas, *Amblyomma cajennense*, is a common pest of man.

Since the evidence all indicates that Rocky Mountain spotted fever is transmitted solely by the tick, and that some of the wild animals serve as reservoirs of the virus, it is obvious that personal prophylaxis consists in avoiding the ticks as fully as possible, and in quickly removing those which do attack. General measures along the line of tick eradication must be carried out if the disease is to be controlled. That such measures are feasible has been shown by the work which has been done in controlling the tick-borne Texas fever of cattle, and by such work as has already been done against the spotted fever tick, which occurs on both wild and domestic animals. Detailed consideration of these measures is to be found in the publications of the Public Health and Marine Hospital Service, and the Bureau of Entomology. Hunter and Bishopp give the following summarized recommendations for control or eradication measures in the Bitter Root Valley.

(1) A campaign of education, whereby all the residents of the valley will be made thoroughly familiar with the feasibility of the plan of eradication, and with what it will mean in the development of the valley.

(2) The obtaining of legislation to make it possible to dip or oil all live stock in the Bitter Root Valley.

(3) The obtaining of an accurate census of the horses, cattle, sheep, mules, and dogs in the valley.

(4) The construction of ten or more dipping vats.

(5) The providing of materials to be used in the dipping mixture.

(6) The organization of a corps of workers to carry on the operations.

(7) The systematic dipping of the horses, cattle, sheep, and dogs of the valley on a definite weekly schedule from approximately March 10 to June 9.

(8) The treatment by hand of the animals in localities remote from vats, on the same schedule.

They estimate that after three seasons' operations a very small annual expenditure would provide against reinfestation of the valley by the incoming of cattle from other places.

Supplementary measures consist in the killing of wild mammals which may harbor the tick; systematic burning of the brush and debris on the mountain side; and in clearing, since the tick is seldom found on land under cultivation.

# CHAPTER X

**ARTHROPODS AS ESSENTIAL HOSTS OF PATHOGENIC PROTOZOA**
[*Continued*]

### Arthropods and Spirochætoses of Man and Animals

The term spirochætoses is applied to diseases of man or animals which are due to protistan parasites belonging to the group of slender, spiral organisms known as spirochætes.

There has been much discussion concerning the relationship of the spirochætes. Formerly, they were regarded as bacteria closely related to the forms grouped in the genus *Spirillum*. The results of the detailed study which the spirochætes have received in recent years, have led most of the workers to consider them as belonging to the protozoa. The merits of the discussion we are not concerned with here, but rather with the fact that a number of diseases caused by spirochætes are arthropod-borne. The better known of these we shall discuss.

**African Relapsing Fever of Man**—It has long been known to the natives of Africa and to travelers in that country, that the bite of a certain tick, *Ornithodoros moubata*, may be followed by severe or even fatal fever of the relapsing type. Until recent years, it was supposed that the effect was due to some special virulence of the tick, just as nagana of cattle was attributed to the direct effect of the bite of the tsetse-fly. The disease is commonly known as "tick-fever" or by the various native names of the tick.

In 1904, Ross and Milne, in Uganda, and Dutton and Todd on the Congo, discovered that the cause of the disease is a spirochæte which is transmitted by the tick. This organism has been designated by Novy and Knapp as *Spirochæta duttoni*.

*Ornithodoros moubata* (fig. 142), the carrier of African relapsing fever, or "tick-fever," is widely distributed in tropical Africa, and occurs in great numbers in the huts of natives, in the dust, cracks and crevices of the dirt floors, or the walls. It feeds voraciously on man as well as upon birds and mammals. Like others of the *Argasidæ*, it resembles the bed-bug in its habit of feeding primarily at night. Dutton and Todd observed that the larval stage is undergone in the egg and that the first free stage is that of the octopod nymph.

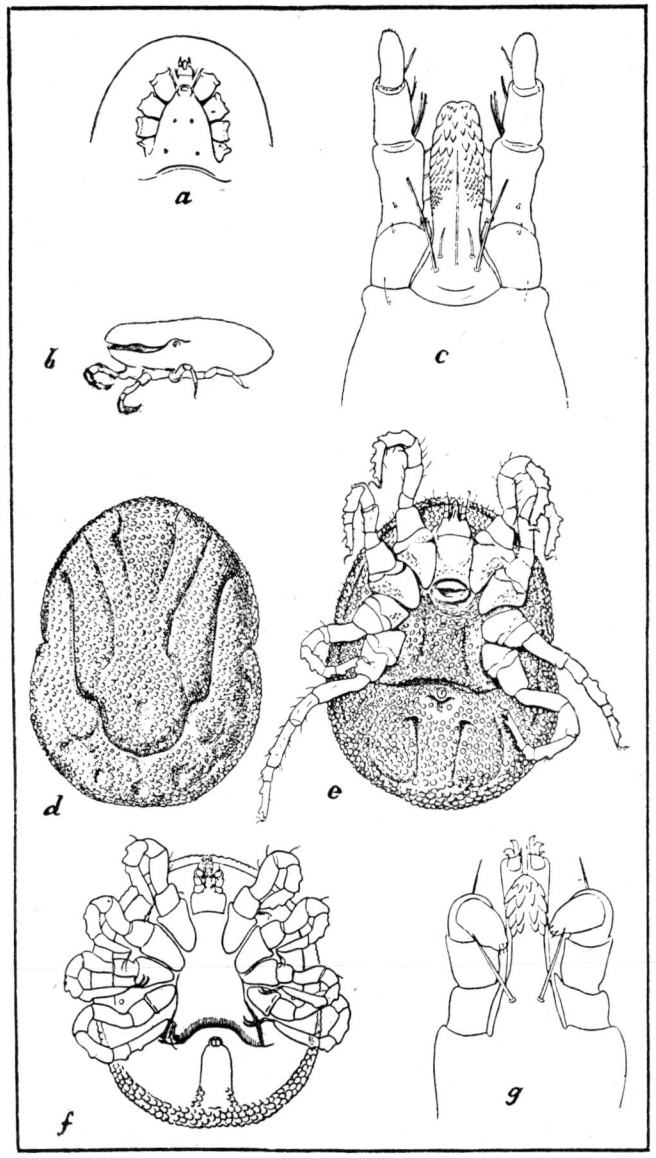

142. Ornithodoros moubata. (a) Anterior part of venter; (b) second stage nymph; (c) capitulum; (d) dorsal and (e) ventral aspect of female; (f) ventral aspect of nymph; (g) capitulum of nymph. After Nuttall and Warburton.

The evidence that the fever is transmitted by this tick is conclusive. Koch found that from five per cent to fifteen per cent, and in some places, fifty per cent of the ticks captured, harbored the spirochæte. The disease is readily transmitted to monkeys, rats, mice and other animals and the earlier experiments along these lines have been confirmed by many workers.

Not only are the ticks which have fed on infected individuals capable of conveying the disease to healthy animals but they transmit the causative organism to their progeny. Thus Möllers (1907), working in Berlin, repeatedly infected monkeys through the bites of nymphs which had been bred in the laboratory from infected ticks. Still more astonishing was his discovery that ticks of the third generation were infective. In other words, if the progeny of infected ticks were fed throughout life on healthy animals, and on maturity deposited eggs, the nymphs which hatched from these eggs would still be capable of carrying the infection.

The developmental cycle of the spirochæte within the tick has not been fully worked out, though the general conclusions of Leishman (1910) have been supported by the recent works of Balfour (1911 and 1912), and Hindle (1912), on the life cycle of spirochætes affecting fowls.

*Spirochæta duttoni* ingested by *Ornithodoros moubata* apparently disappear within a few days, but Leishman believed that in reality they break up into minute granules which are to be found in the alimentary canal, the salivary glands and the Malpighian tubes of the tick. These granules, or "coccoid bodies," as Hindle calls them, are supposed to be the form in which the spirochætes infect the new host. We shall see later that Marchoux and Couvy (1913) dissent wholly from this interpretation.

According to Leishman, and Hindle, the coccoid bodies are not injected into the vertebrate host with the saliva of the tick, as are the sporozoites of malaria with that of the mosquito. Instead, they pass out with the excrement and secondarily gain access to the wound inflicted by the tick.

Nuttall (1912) calls attention to the fact that the geographical distribution of *Ornithodoros moubata* is far wider than our present records show for the distribution of the relapsing fever in man and that there is every reason to fear the extension of the disease. Huts where the ticks occur should be avoided and it should be remembered that in infected localities there is special danger in sleeping on the ground.

**European Relapsing Fever**—There is widely distributed in Europe a type of relapsing fever which is caused by *Spirochæta recurrentis*. It has long been supposed that this disease is spread by the bed-bug and there is some experimental evidence to show that it may be conveyed by these insects.

In 1897, Tictin found that he could infect monkeys by inoculating the contents of bed-bugs which had fed upon a patient within forty-eight hours. Nuttall, in 1907, in one experiment succeeded in transmitting *Spirochæta recurrentis* from mouse to mouse by bites of bed-bugs. The bugs, thirty-five in number, were transferred at short intervals from one mouse to another, not being allowed to take a full meal on the first, or infected mouse.

On the other hand, there is much clinical evidence to show that the European relapsing fever like various other types of the disease is transmitted from man to man by head and body lice (*Pediculus humanus* and *Pediculus corporis*).

Interesting supplementary evidence is that of Bayon's observations (1912), in Moscow. "Having visited the big municipal night hospitals at Moscow I soon noticed that they were kept with such scrupulous cleanliness, disinfected so lavishly, the beds of iron, the floor cemented, that it was not possible for bed-bugs to thrive to any extent on the premises. The people sleeping there were allowed, however, to sleep in their own clothes. The introduction of these model homes had not had any effect on the incidence of relapsing fever, for the places were still hot-beds of the fever during winter. On the other hand, though I changed my rooms several times, I found bugs in every successive lodging, and I was told in Moscow, this can hardly be avoided. Yet no foreigner, or Russian of the better class, ever catches relapsing fever. To this may be added the fact that when I asked for clothes-lice and promised to pay a kopec for two, the attendants from the night hostel brought me next morning a small ounce bottle crammed with *Pediculus capitis* (= *P. humanus*), and *Pediculus vestimentorum* (= *P. corporis*) collected off the sleepers. If relapsing fever were transmitted by bed-bugs, it would be much more disseminated than it is at present in Moscow."

Direct experimental evidence of the agency of lice in transmitting relapsing fever is especially clear in the case of a type of the disease prevalent in parts of North Africa. We shall consider this evidence later.

**Other Types of Relapsing Fever of Man**—In addition to the three types of human relapsing fever already referred to, several others have been distinguished and have been attributed to distinct species of spirochætes. The various spirochætoses of man are:

African, caused by *S. duttoni;* European, caused by *S. recurrentis;* North African, caused by *S. berbera;* East African, caused by *S. rossi;* East Indian, caused by *S. carteri;* North American, caused by *S. novyi;* South American, caused by *S. duttoni*(?).

Nuttall (1912) in his valuable resumé of the subject, has emphasized that "in view of the morphological similarity of the supposedly different species of spirochætes and their individual variations in virulence, we may well doubt if any of the 'species' are valid. As I pointed out four years ago, the various specific names given to the spirochætes causing relapsing fever in man may be used merely for convenience *to distinguish strains or races* of different origin. They cannot be regarded as valid names, in the sense of scientific nomenclature, for virulence and immunity reactions are not adequate tests of specificity."

**North African Relapsing Fever of Man**—The type of human relapsing fever to be met with in Algeria, Tunis, and Tripoli, is due to a *Spirochæta* which does not differ morphologically from *Spirochæta duttoni*, but which has been separated on biological grounds as *Spirochæta berberi*.

Experimenting with this type of disease in Algeria, Sergent and Foly (1910), twice succeeded in transmitting it from man to monkeys by inoculation of crushed body lice and in two cases obtained infection of human subjects who had received infected lice under their clothing and who slept under coverings harboring many of the lice which had fed upon a patient. Their results were negative with *Argas persicus, Cimex lectularius, Musca domestica, Hæmatopinus spinulosus* and *Ceratophyllus fasciatus*. They found body lice associated with every case of relapsing fever which they found in Algeria.

Nicolle, Blaizot, and Conseil (1912) showed that the louse did not transmit the parasite by its bite. Two or three hours after it has fed on a patient, the spirochætes begin to break up and finally they disappear, so that after a day, repeated examinations fail to reveal them. They persist, nevertheless, in some unknown form, for if the observations are continued they reappear in eight to twelve days. These new forms are virulent, for a monkey was infected by inoculating a single crushed louse which had fed on infected blood fifteen days before.

Natural infection is indirect. Those attacked by the insect scratch, and in this act they excoriate the skin, crush the lice and contaminate their fingers. The least abrasion of the skin serves for the entrance of the spirochætes. Even the contact of the soiled fingers on the various mucosa, such as the conjunctive of the eye, is sufficient.

As in the case of *Spirochæta duttoni*, the organism is transmitted hereditarily in the arthropod vector. The progeny of lice which have fed on infected blood may themselves be infective.

**Spirochætosis of Fowls**—One of the best known of the spirochætes transmitted by arthropods is *Spirochæta gallinarum*, the cause of a very fatal disease of domestic fowls in widely separated regions of the world. According to Nuttall, it occurs in Southeastern Europe, Asia, Africa, South America and Australia.

In 1903, Marchoux and Salimbeni, working in Brazil, made the first detailed study of the disease, and showed that the causative organism is transmitted from fowl to fowl by the tick *Argas persicus*. They found that the ticks remained infective for at least five months. Specimens which had fed upon diseased birds in Brazil were sent to Nuttall and he promptly confirmed the experiments. Since that date many investigators, notably Balfour and Hindle, have contributed to the elucidating of the life-cycle of the parasite. Since it has been worked out more fully than has that of any of the human spirochætes, we present Hindle's diagram (fig. 143) and quote the brief summary from his preliminary paper (1911b).

"Commencing with the ordinary parasite in the blood of the fowl, the spirochæte grows until it reaches a certain length (16–19μ) and then divides by transverse division. This process is repeated, and is probably the only method of multiplication of the parasite within the blood. When the spirochætes disappear from the circulation, some of them break up into the coccoid bodies which, however, do not usually develop in the fowl. When the spirochætes are ingested by *Argas persicus*, some of them pass through the gut wall into the cœlomic fluid. From this medium they bore their way into the cells of the various organs of the tick and there break up into a number of coccoid bodies. These intracellular forms multiply by

236   *Arthropods as Essential Hosts of Pathogenic Protozoa*

ordinary fission in the cells of the Malpighian tubules and gonads. Some of the coccoid bodies are formed in the lumen of the gut and Malpighian tubules. The result is that some of the coccoid bodies may be present in the Malpighian secretion and excrement of an infected tick and when mixed with the coxal fluid may gain entry into another fowl by the open wound caused by the tick's bite. They

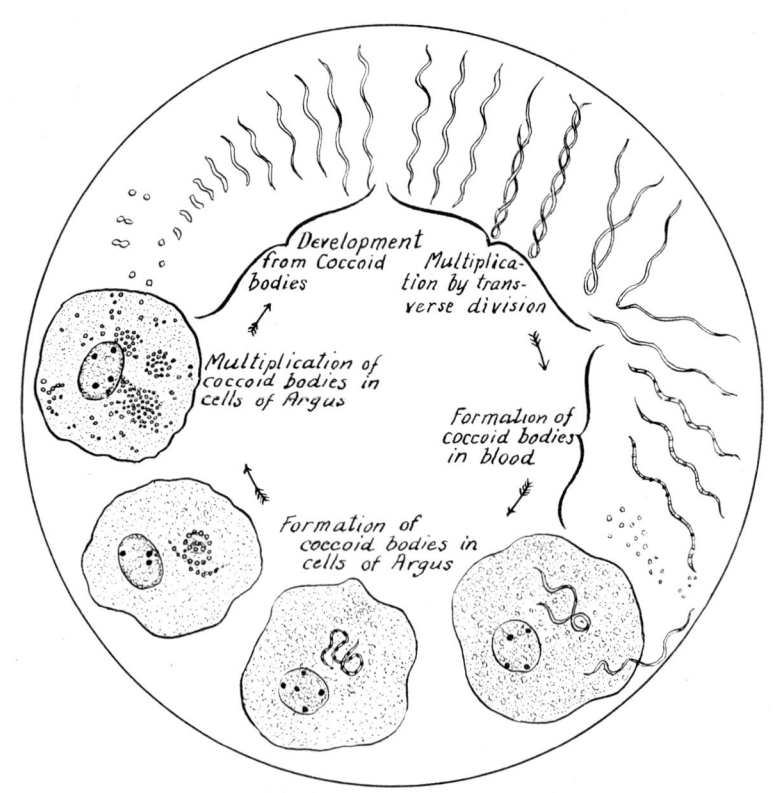

143. Spirochæta gallinarum.   After Hindle.

then elongate and redevelop into ordinary spirochætes in the blood of the fowl, and the cycle may be repeated.

Hindle's account is clear cut and circumstantial, and is quite in line with the work of Balfour, and of Leishman. Radically different is the interpretation of Marchoux and Couvy (1913). These investigators maintain that the granules localized in the Malpighian tubules in the larvæ and, in the adult, also in the ovules and the genital ducts of the male and female, are not derived from spirochætes but that they exist normally in many acariens. They interpret the supposed disassociation of the spirochæte into granules as simply the first phase, not of a process of multiplication, but of a degeneration ending in the death of the parasite. The fragmented chromatin has lost its affinity for stains, remaining always paler than that of the normal spirochætes. On the other hand, the granules of Leishman stain energetically with all the basic stains.

Further, according to Marchoux and Couvy, infection takes place without the emission of the coxal fluid and indeed, soiling of the host by the coxal fluid diluting the excrement is exceptional. All of the organs of the Argasid are invaded by the parasites, but they pass from the cœlom into the acini of the salivary glands and collect in its efferent canal. The saliva serves as the vehicle of infection.

Thus, the question of the life cycle of *Spirochæta gallinarum*, and of spirochætes in general, is an open one.

It should be noted that *Argas persicus*, the carrier of *Spirochæta gallinarum*, is a common pest of poultry in the southwestern United States. Though the disease has not been reported from this country, conditions are such that if accidentally introduced, it might do great damage.

**Other Spirochæte Diseases of Animals**—About a score of other blood inhabiting spirochætes have been reported as occurring in mammals, but little is known concerning their life-histories. One of the most important is *Spirochæta theileri* which produces a spirochætosis of cattle in the Transvaal. Theiler has determined that it is transmitted by an Ixodid tick, *Margaropus decoloratus*.

## TYPHUS FEVER AND PEDICULIDÆ

Typhus is an acute, and continued fever, formerly epidemically prevalent in camps, hospitals, jails, and similar places where persons were crowded together under insanitary conditions. It is accompanied by a characteristic rash, which gives the disease the common name of "spotted" or "lenticular" fever. The causative organism is unknown.

Typhus fever has not generally been supposed to occur in the United States, but there have been a few outbreaks and sporadic cases recognized. According to Anderson and Goldberger (1912a), it has been a subject of speculation among health authorities why, in spite of the arrival of occasional cases in this country and of many persons from endemic foci of the disease, typhus fever apparently does not gain a foothold in the United States. These same workers showed that the so-called Brill's disease, studied especially in New York City, is identical with the typhus fever of Mexico and of Europe.

The conditions under which the disease occurs and under which it spreads most rapidly are such as to suggest that it is carried by some parasitic insect. On epidemiological grounds the insects most open to suspicion are the lice, bed-bugs and fleas.

In 1909, Nicolle, Comte and Conseil, succeeded in transmitting typhus fever from infected to healthy monkeys by means of the body louse (*Pediculus corporis*). Independently of this work, Anderson and Goldberger had undertaken work along this line in Mexico, and in 1910 reported two attempts to transmit the disease to monkeys by means of body lice. The first experiment resulted negatively, but the second resulted in a slight rise in temperature, and in view of later results it seems that this was due to infection with typhus.

Shortly after, Ricketts and Wilder (1910) succeeded in transmitting the disease to the monkey by the bite of body lice in two experiments, the lice in one instance deriving their infection from a man and in another from the monkey. Another monkey was infected by typhus through the introduction of the feces and abdominal contents of infested lice into small incisions. Experiments with fleas and bed-bugs resulted negatively.

Subsequently, Goldberger and Anderson (1912b) indicated that the head louse (*Pediculus humanus*) as well, may become infected with typhus. In an attempt to transmit typhus fever (Mexican virus) from man to monkey by subcutaneous injection of a saline suspension of crushed head lice, the monkeys developed a typical febrile reaction with subsequent resistance to an inoculation of virulent typhus (Mexican) blood. In one of the three experiments to transmit the disease from man to monkey by means of the bite of the head louse, the animal bitten by the presumably infected head lice proved resistant to two successive immunity tests with virulent typhus blood.

In 1910, Ricketts and Wilder reported an experiment undertaken with a view to determining whether the young of infected lice were themselves infected. Young lice were reared to maturity on the bodies of typhus patients, so that if the eggs were susceptible to infection at any stage of their development, they would have every opportunity of being infected within the ovary. The eggs of these infected lice were obtained, they were incubated, and the young lice of the second generation were placed on a normal rhesus monkey. The experimenters were unable to keep the monkey under very close observation during the following three or four weeks, but from the fact that he proved resistant to a subsequent immunity test they concluded that he probably owed this immunity to infection by these lice of the second generation.

Anderson and Goldberger (1912b) object that due consideration was not given to the possibility of a variable susceptibility of the monkey to typhus. Their similar experiment was "frankly negative."

Prophylaxis against typhus fever is, therefore, primarily a question of vermin extermination. A brief article by Dr. Goldberger (1914) so clearly shows the practical application of his work and that of the other investigators of the subject, that we abstract from it the following account:

"In general terms it may be stated that association with a case of typhus fever in the absence of the transmitting insect is no more dangerous than is association with a case of yellow fever in the absence of the yellow fever mosquito. Danger threatens only when the insect appears on the scene."

"We may say, therefore, that to prevent infection of the individual it is necessary for him only to avoid being bitten by the louse. In theory this may readily be done, for we know that the body louse infests and attaches itself almost entirely to the body linen, and that boiling kills this insect and its eggs. Individual prophylaxis is based essentially, therefore, on the avoidance of contact with individuals likely to harbor lice. Practically, however, this is not always as easy as it may seem, especially under the conditions of such intimate association as is imposed by urban life. Particularly is this the case in places such as some of the large Mexican cities, where a large proportion of the population harbors this vermin. Under such circumstances it is well to avoid crowds or crowded places, such as public markets, crowded streets, or public assemblies at which the 'peon' gathers."

"Community prophylaxis efficiently and intelligently carried out is, from a certain point of view, probably easier and more effective in protecting the individual than is the individual's own effort to guard himself. Typhus emphasizes, perhaps better than any other disease, the fact that fundamentally, sanitation and health are economic problems. In proportion as the economic condition of the masses has improved—that is, in proportion as they could afford to keep clean—the notorious filth disease has decreased or disappeared. In localities where it still prevails, its further reduction or complete eradication waits on a further improvement in, or extension of, the improved economic status of those afflicted. Economic evolution is very slow process, and, while doing what we can to hasten it, we must take such precautions as existing conditions permit, looking to a reduction in or complete eradication of the disease."

"When possible, public bath houses and public wash houses, where the poor may bathe and do their washings at a minimum or without cost, should be provided. Similar provision should be made in military and construction camps. Troops in the field should be given the opportunity as frequently as possible to wash and *scald* or *boil* their body linen."

"Lodging houses, cheap boarding houses, night shelters, hospitals, jails and prisons, are important factors in the spread and frequently constitute foci of the disease. They should receive rigid sanitary supervision, including the enforcement of measures to free all inmates of such institutions of lice on admission."

"So far as individual foci of the disease are concerned these should be dealt with by segregating and keeping under observation all exposed individuals for 14 days—the period of incubation—from the last exposure, by disinfecting (boiling or steaming) the suspected bedding, body linen, and clothes, for the destruction of any possible vermin that they may harbor, and by fumigating (with sulphur) the quarters that they may have occupied."

"It will be noted that nothing has been said as to the disposition of the patient. So far as the patient is concerned, he should be removed to 'clean' surroundings, making sure that he does not take with him any vermin. This may be done by bathing, treating the hair with an insecticide (coal oil, tincture of larkspur), and a complete change of body linen. Aside from this, the patient may be treated or cared for in a general hospital ward or in a private house, provided the sanitary officer is satisfied that the new surroundings to which the patient has been removed are 'clean,' that is, free from vermin. Indeed, it is reasonably safe to permit a 'clean' patient to remain in his own home if this is 'clean,' for, as has already been emphasized, there can be no spread in the absence of lice. This is a common experience in native families of the better class and of Europeans in Mexico City."

"Similarly the sulphur fumigation above prescribed may be dispensed with as unnecessary in this class of cases."

# CHAPTER XI

## SOME POSSIBLE, BUT IMPERFECTLY ESTABLISHED CASES OF ARTHROPOD TRANSMISSION OF DISEASE

### Infantile Paralysis or Acute Anterior Poliomyelitis

The disease usually known in this country as infantile paralysis or, more technically, as acute anterior poliomyelitis, is one which has aroused much attention in recent years.

The causative organism of infantile paralysis is unknown, but it has been demonstrated that it belongs to the group of filterable viruses. It gives rise to a general infection, producing characteristic lesions in the central nervous system. The result of the injury to the motor nerves is a more or less complete paralysis of the corresponding muscle. This usually manifests itself in the legs and arms. The fatal cases are usually the result of paralysis of the muscles of respiration. Of the non-fatal cases about 60 per cent remain permanently crippled in varying degrees.

Though long known, it was not until about 1890 that it was emphasized that the disease occurs in epidemic form. At this time Medin reported his observations on an epidemic of forty-three cases which occurred in and around Stockholm in 1887. Since then, according to Frost (1911), epidemics have been observed with increasing frequency in various parts of the world. The largest recorded epidemics have been those in Vermont, 1894, 126 cases; Norway and Sweden, 1905, about 1,500 cases; New York City, 1907, about 2,500 cases. Since 1907 many epidemics have been reported in the United States, and especially in the Northern States east of the Dakotas. In 1912 there were over 300 cases of the disease in Buffalo, N. Y., with a mortality of somewhat over 11 per cent.

In view of the sudden prominence and the alarming spread of infantile paralysis, there have been many attempts to determine the cause, and the manner in which the disease spreads and develops in epidemic form. In the course of these studies, the question of possible transmission by insects was naturally suggested.

C. W. Howard and Clark (1912) presented the results of studies in this phase of the subject. They dealt especially with the house-fly, bedbug, head, and body lice, and mosquitoes. It was found that the house-fly (*Musca domestica*) can carry the virus of poliomyelitis in an active state for several days upon the surface of the body and for several hours within the gastro-intestinal tract. Mosquitoes and lice were found not to take up or maintain the virus. On the other hand, the bedbug (*Cimex lectularius*) was found to take the virus from the infected monkeys and to maintain it in a living state within the body for a period of seven days. This was demonstrated by grinding up in salt solution, insects which had fed on poliomyeletic animals and injecting the filtrate into a healthy monkey. The experimenters doubted that the bedbug is a carrier of the virus in nature.

Earlier in the same year, Brues and Sheppard published the results of an intensive epidemiological study of the outbreak of 1911, in Massachusetts. Special attention had been paid to the possibility of insect transfer and the following conclusion was reached:

"Field work during the past summer together with a consideration of the epidemiology of the disease so far as known, points strongly toward biting flies as possible carriers of the virus. It seems probable that the common stable-fly (*Stomoxys calcitrans* L.) may be responsible to a certain extent for the spread of acute epidemic poliomyelitis, possibly aided by other biting flies, such as *Tabanus lineola*. No facts which disprove such a hypothesis have as yet been adduced, and experiments based upon it are now in progress."

As stated by Brues (1913), especial suspicion fell upon the stable-fly because:

1. The blood-sucking habits of the adult fly suit it for the transfer of virus present in the blood.

2. The seasonal abundance of the fly is very closely correlated with the incidence of the disease, rising rapidly during the summer and reaching a maximum in July and August, then slowly declining in September and October.

3. The geographical distribution of the fly is, so far as can be ascertained, wider, or at least co-extensive with that of poliomyelitis.

4. *Stomoxys* is distinctly more abundant under rural conditions, than in cities and thickly populated areas.

5. While the disease spreads over districts quickly and in a rather erratic way, it often appears to follow along lines of travel, and it is known that *Stomoxys* flies will often follow horses for long distances along highways.

6. In a surprisingly large number of cases, it appeared probable that the children affected had been in the habit of frequenting places where *Stomoxys* is particularly abundant, i.e., about stables, barnyards, etc.

The experiments referred to were carried on during the summer of 1912 and in September Dr. Rosenau announced that the disease was transferred by the bite of the stable-fly.

A monkey infected by inoculation was exposed to the bites of upwards of a thousand of the *Stomoxys* flies daily, by stretching it at full length and rolling it in a piece of chicken wire, and then placing it on the floor of the cage in which the flies were confined. The flies fed freely from the first, as well as later, after paralysis had set in. Alternating with the inoculated monkey, healthy monkeys were similarly introduced into the cage at intervals. New monkeys were inoculated to keep a supply of such infected animals and additional healthy ones were exposed to the flies, which fed willingly and in considerable numbers on each occasion. "Thus the flies were given every opportunity to obtain infection from the monkeys, since the animals were bitten during practically every stage of the disease from the time of the inoculation of the virus till their death following the appearance of paralysis. By the same arrangement the healthy monkeys were likely to be bitten by flies that had previously fed during the various stages of the disease on the infected monkeys. The flies had meanwhile enjoyed the opportunity of incubating the virus for periods varying from the day or two which usually elapses between consecutive feedings, to the two or three-week period for which at least some (although a very small percentage) of the flies lived in the cage."

"In all, twelve apparently healthy monkeys of a small Japan species were exposed to the flies in the manner described for the infected monkeys. Some were placed in the cage only once or twice and others a number of times after varying intervals. These exposures usually lasted for about half an hour, but were sometimes more protracted. No results were apparent until two or three weeks after the experiment was well under way, and then in rather rapid succession six of the animals developed symptoms of poliomyelitis. In three, the disease appeared in a virulent form, resulting in death, while the other three experienced transient tremblings, diarrhœa, partial paralysis and recovery."—Brues, 1913.

Very soon after the announcement of the results of experiments by Rosenau and Brues, they were apparently conclusively confirmed by Anderson and Frost (1912), who repeated the experiments, at Washington. They announced that through the bites of the *Stomoxys* flies that had previously fed on infected monkeys, they had succeeded in experimentally infecting three healthy monkeys.

The results of these experiments gained much publicity and in spite of the conservative manner in which they had been announced, it was widely proclaimed that infantile paralysis was conveyed in nature by the stable-fly and by it alone.

Serious doubt was cast on this theory by the results of further experiments by Anderson and Frost, reported in May of 1913. Contrary to the expectations justified by their first experience, the results of all the later, and more extended, experiments were wholly negative. Not once were these investigators again able to transmit the infection of poliomyelitis through *Stomoxys*. They concluded that it was extremely doubtful that the insect was an important factor in the natural transmission of the disease, not only because of their series of negative results, "but also because recent experiments have afforded additional evidence of the direct transmissibility or contagiousness of poliomyelitis, and because epidemiological studies appear to us to indicate that the disease is more likely transmitted largely through passive human virus carriers."

Soon after this, Kling and Levaditi (1913) published their detailed studies on acute anterior poliomyelitis. They considered that the experiments of Flexner and Clark (and Howard and Clark), who fed house-flies on emulsion of infected spinal cord, were under conditions so different from what could occur in nature that one could not draw precise conclusions from them regarding the epidemiology of the disease. They cited the experiments of Josefson (1912), as being under more reasonable conditions. He sought to determine whether the inoculation of monkeys with flies caught in the wards of the Hospital for Contagious Diseases at Stockholm, where they had been in contact with cases of poliomyelitis, would produce the disease. The results were completely negative.

Kling and Lavaditi made four attempts of this kind. The flies were collected in places where poliomyelitics had dwelt, three, four and twenty-four after the beginning of the disease in the family and one, three, and fifteen days after the patient had left the house. These insects were for the greater part living and had certainly been in contact with the infected person. In addition, flies were used which had been caught in the wards of the Hospital for Contagious Diseases at Söderkoping, when numbers of poliomyelitics were confined there. Finally, to make the conditions as favorable as possible, the emulsions prepared from these flies were injected without previous filtering, since filtration often causes a weakening of the virus. In spite of these precautions, all their results were negative, none of the inoculated animals having contracted poliomyelitis. They also experimented with bedbugs which had fed upon infected patients at various stages of the disease, but the results in these cases also were wholly negative.

Kling and Levaditi considered at length the possibility of transmission of the disease by *Stomoxys*. As a result of their epidemiological studies, they found that infantile paralysis continued to spread in epidemic form in the dead of winter, when these flies were very rare and torpid, or were even completely absent. Numerous cases developed in the northern part of Sweden late in October and November, long after snow had fallen. On account of the rarity of the Stomoxys flies during the period of their investigations they were unable to conduct satisfactory experiments. In one instance, during a severe epidemic, they found a number of the flies in a stable near a house inhabited by an infected family, though none was found in the house itself. These flies were used in preparing an emulsion which, after filtering, was injected into the peritoneal cavity of a monkey. The result was wholly negative.

As for the earlier experiments, Kling and Levaditi believe if the flies were responsible for the transmission of the disease in the cases reported by Rosenau and Brues, and the first experiments of Anderson and Frost, it was because the virus of infantile paralysis is eliminated with the nasal secretions of paralyzed monkeys and the flies, becoming contaminated, had merely acted as accidental carriers.

Still further evidence against the hypothesis of the transmission of acute anterior poliomyelitis by *Stomoxys calcitrans* was brought forward by Sawyer and Herms (1913). Special precautions were used to prevent the transference of saliva or other possibly infectious material from the surface of one monkey to that of another, and to avoid the possibility of complicating the experiments by introducing other pathogenic organisms from wild flies, only laboratory-bred flies were used. In a series of seven carefully performed experiments, in which the conditions were varied, Sawyer and Herms were unable to transmit poliomyelitis from monkey to monkey through the agency of *Stomoxys*, or to obtain any indication that the fly is the usual agent for spreading the disease in nature.

The evidence at hand to date indicates that acute anterior poliomyelitis, or infantile paralysis, is transmitted by contact with infected persons. Under certain conditions insects may be agents in spreading the disease, but their rôle is a subordinate one.

## Pellagra

**Pellagra** is an endemic and epidemic disease characterized by a peculiar eruption or erythema of the skin (figs 144 and 145), digestive disturbances and nervous trouble. Insanity is a common result, rather than a precursor of the disease. The manifestations of pellagra are periodic and its duration indeterminate.

The disease is one the very name of which was almost unknown in the United States until within the past decade. It has usually been regarded as tropical, though it occurs commonly in Italy and in various parts of Europe. Now it is known that it not only occurs quite generally in the United States but that it is spreading. Lavinder (1911) says that "There are certainly many thousand cases of the disease in this country, and the present situation must be looked upon with grave concern."

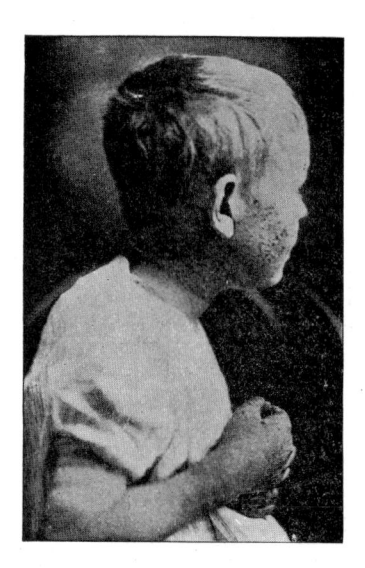

144. Pellagrous eruption on the face. After Watson.

It is not within the scope of this book to undertake a general discussion of pellagra. The subject is of such importance to every medical man that we cannot do better than refer to Lavinder's valuable précis. We can only touch briefly upon the entomological phases of the problems presented.

The most commonly accepted theories regarding the etiology of the disease have attributed it to the use of Indian corn as an article of diet. This supposed relationship was explained either on the basis of, (a) insufficiency of nutriment and inappropriateness of corn as a prime article of food; (b) toxicity of corn or, (c) parasitism of certain organisms—fungi or bacteria—ingested with either sound or deteriorated corn.

In 1905, Sambon proposed the theory of the protozoal origin of pellagra and in 1910 he marshalled an imposing array of objections to the theory that there existed any relationship between corn and the disease. He presented clear evidence that pellagra existed in Europe before the introduction of Indian corn from America, as an article of diet, and that its spread was not *pari passu* with that of the use of corn. Cases were found in which the patients had apparently never used corn, though that is obviously difficult to establish. He showed that preventive measures based on the theory had been a failure. Finally, he believed that the recurrence of symptoms of the disease for successive springs, in patients who abstained absolutely from the use of corn, militated against the theory.

On the other hand, Sambon believed that the periodicity of the symptoms, peculiarities of distribution and seasonal incidence, and analogies of the symptoms to those of other parasitic diseases indi-

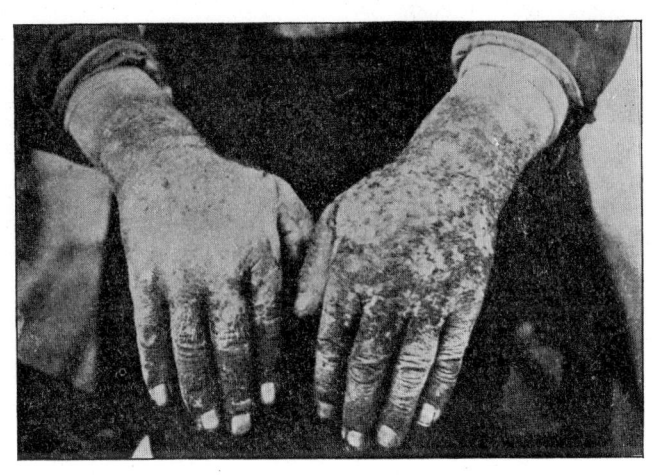

145. Pellagrous eruption on the hand. After Watson.

cated that pellagra was of protozoal origin, and that it was insect-borne.

The insect carriers, he believed to be one or more species of Simuliidæ, or black-flies. In support of this he stated that *Simulium* appears to effect the same topographical conditions as pellagra, that in its imago stage it seems to present the same seasonal incidence, that it has a wide geographical distribution which seems to cover that of pellagra, and that species of the genus are known to cause severe epizootics. Concluding from his studies in Italy, that pellagra was limited almost wholly to agricultural laborers, he pointed out that the Simulium flies are found only in rural districts, and as a rule do not enter towns, villages, or houses.

When Sambon's detailed report was published in 1910, his theory was seized upon everywhere by workers who were anxious to test it

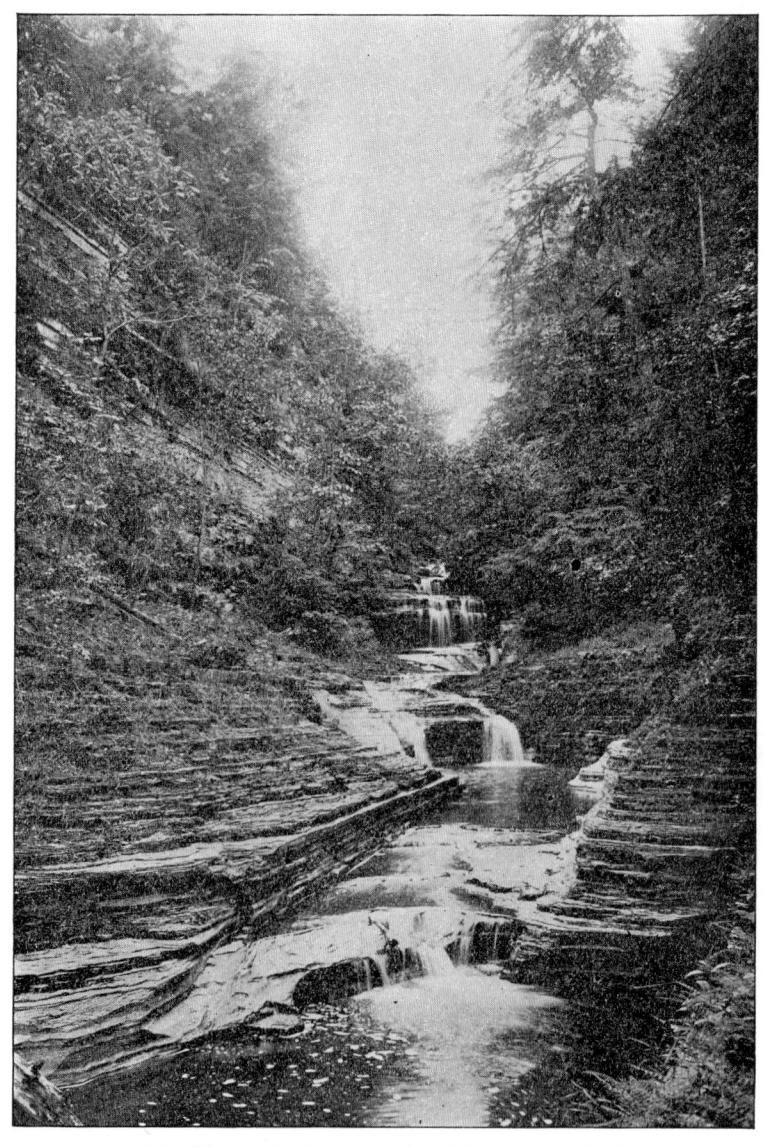

146. A favorite breeding place of Simulium. Ithaca, N. Y.

and who, in most cases, were favorably disposed towards it because of the wonderful progress which had been made in the understanding of other insect-borne diseases. In this country, the entomological aspects of the subject have been dealt with especially by Forbes (1912), and by King and Jennings, under the direction of W. D. Hunter, of the Bureau of Entomology, and in co-operation with the Thompson-McFadden Pellagra Commission of the Department of Tropical Medicine of the New York Post-Graduate Medical School. An important series of experiments with monkeys has been undertaken by S. J. Hunter, of Kansas, but unfortunately we have as yet no satisfactory evidence that these animals are susceptible to the disease—a fact which renders the whole problem difficult.

The accumulated evidence is increasingly opposed to Sambon's hypothesis of the transmission of pellagra by *Simulium*. This has been so clearly manifested in the work of the Thompson-McFadden Commission that we quote here from the report by Jennings (1914):

"Our studies in 1912 convinced us that there was little evidence to support the incrimination of any species of *Simulium* in South Carolina in the transmission of pellagra. Reviewing the group as a whole, we find that its species are essentially "wild" and lack those habits of intimate association with man which would be expected in the vector of such a disease as pellagra. Although these flies are excessively abundant in some parts of their range and are moderately so in Spartanburg County, man is merely an incidental host, and no disposition whatever to seek him out or to invade his domicile seems to be manifested. Critically considered, it is nearer the fact that usually man is attacked only when he invades their habitat."

"As our knowledge of pellagra accumulates, it is more and more evident that its origin is in some way closely associated with the domicile. The possibility that an insect whose association with man and his immediate environment is, at the best, casual and desultory, can be active in the causation of the disease becomes increasingly remote."

"Our knowledge of the biting habits of *Simulium* is not complete, but it is evident, as regards American species at least, that these are sometimes not constant for the same species in different localities. Certain species will bite man freely when opportunity offers, while others have never been known to attack him. To assume that the proximity of a *Simulium*-breeding stream necessarily implies that persons in its vicinity must be attacked and bitten is highly fallacious. In Spartanburg County attacks by *Simulium* seems to be confined to the immediate vicinity of the breeding-places. Our records and observations, exceedingly few in number, refer almost exclusively to such locations. Statements regarding such attacks, secured with much care and discrimination from a large number of persons, including many pellagrins, indicate conclusively that these insects are seldom a pest of man in this county. A certain number of the persons questioned were familiar with the gnats in other localities, but the majority were seemingly ignorant of the existence of such flies with biting habits. This is especially striking, in view of the fact that the average distance of streams from the homes of the pellagra cases studied was about 200 yards, many being at a distance of less than 100 yards, and that 78 per cent of these streams were found to be infested by larval *Simulium*. Such ignorance in a large number of persons cannot be overlooked and indicates strongly that our belief in the negligible character of local attacks by *Simulium* is well founded."

"In localities infested by 'sand-flies,' mosquitoes, etc., these pests are always well known and the ignorance described above is very significant."

"Such positive reports as we received nearly always referred to bites received in the open, along streams, etc., and observations made of their attack were of those on field laborers in similar situations. Males engaged in agricultural pursuits are almost exempt from pellagra in Spartanburg County. During the season of 1913, in some two or three instances, observations were made of the biting of *Simulium* and some additional and entirely creditable reports were received. These observations and reports were under conditions identical with those referred to in the reports of 1912 and confirm the conclusions based on the observations of that year. I would repeat with emphasis that it is inconceivable that a fly of the appearance and habits of the prevalent species of *Simulium* could be present in such a region, especially about the haunts of man and attack him with sufficient frequency and regularity to satisfactorily account for so active and prevalent a disease as pellagra without being a well-known and recognized pest."

"In connection with the conditions in the Piedmont region of South Carolina, it may be well to cite the results of a study of those in the arid region of western Texas."

"In May, 1913, in company with Capt. J. F. Siler of the Thompson-McFadden Pellagra Commission, I visited the region of which Midland in Midland County is the center. This region is very dry and totally devoid of running water for a long distance in every direction. The only natural source of water-supply, a few water holes and ponds, were visited and found to be of such a nature that the survival of *Simulium*, far less its propagation in them, is absolutely impossible. The nearest stream affording possibilities as a source of *Simulium* is 60 miles away, while the average distance of such possibility is not less than 100 miles."

"Artificial sources of water-supply were also investigated carefully and were found to offer no opportunity for the breeding of *Simulium*."

"At Midland the histories of five cases of pellagra were obtained, which gave clear evidence that this place or its immediate vicinity was the point of origin. Persons of long residence in the country were questioned as to the occurrence of such flies as *Simulium* and returned negative answers. These included a retired cattle owner, who is a man of education and a keen observer, an expert veterinarian stationed in the country who has the cattle of the country under constant observation, and a practical cattle man, manager of a ranch and of wide experience. The latter had had experience with 'Buffalo gnats' in other localities (in the East) and is well acquainted with them. His close personal supervision of the cattle under his charge, makes it practically certain that he would have discovered these gnats had they been present in the country."

"At the time the study was made, *Simulium* was breeding and active in the adult state in the vicinity of Dallas, Texas, in the eastern part of the state. We have here a region in which cases of pellagra have originated, yet in which *Simulium* does not and cannot breed."

Other possible insect vectors of pellagra have been studied in great detail and the available evidence indicates that if *any* insect plays a rôle in the spread of the disease, *Stomoxys calcitrans* most nearly fills the conditions. This conclusion was announced by Jennings and King in 1912, and has been supported by their subsequent work.

Yet, after all the studies of the past decade, the old belief that pellagra is essentially of dietary origin is gaining ground. Goldberger, Waring and Willets (1914) of the United States Public Health

Service summarize their conclusions in the statement, (1) that it is dependent on some yet undetermined fault in a diet in which the animal or leguminous protein component is disproportionately large and (2) that no pellagra develops in those who *consume* a mixed, well-balanced, and varied diet, such, for example, as that furnished by the Government to the enlisted men of the Army, Navy, and Marine Corps.

## Leprosy

**Leprosy** is a specific, infectious disease due to *Bacillus lepræ*, and characterized by the formation of tubercular nodules, ulcerations, and disturbances of sensation. In spite of the long time that the disease has been known and the dread with which it is regarded, little is known concerning the method of transfer of the causative organism or the means by which it gains access to the human body.

It is known that the bacilli are to be found in the tubercles, the scurf of the skin, nasal secretions, the sputum and, in fact in practically all the discharges of the leper. Under such conditions it is quite conceivable that they may be transferred in some instances from diseased to healthy individuals through the agency of insects and other arthropods. Many attempts have been made to demonstrate this method of spread of the disease, but with little success.

Of the suggested insect carriers none seem to meet the conditions better than mosquitoes, and there are many suggestions in literature that these insects play an important rôle in the transmission of leprosy. The literature has been reviewed and important experimental evidence presented by Currie (1910). He found that mosquitoes feeding, under natural conditions, upon cases of nodular leprosy so rarely, if ever, imbibe the lepra bacillus that they cannot be regarded as one of the ordinary means of transference of this bacillus from lepers to the skin of healthy persons. He believes that the reason that mosquitoes that have fed on lepers do not contain the lepra bacillus is that when these insects feed they insert their proboscis directly into a blood vessel and thus obtain bacilli-free blood, unmixed with lymph.

The same worker undertook to determine whether flies are able to transmit leprosy. He experimented with five species found in Honolulu,—*Musca domestica, Sarcophaga pallinervis, Sarcophaga barbata, Volucella obesa* and an undetermined species of *Lucilia*. The experiments with *Musca domestica* were the most detailed.

From these experiments he concluded, first, that all of the above-named flies, when given an opportunity to feed upon leprous fluids, will contain the bacilli in their intestinal tracts and feces for several days after such feeding. Second, that considering the habits of these flies, and especially those of *Musca domestica*, it is certain that, given an exposed leprous ulcer, these insects will frequently convey immense numbers of lepra bacilli, directly or indirectly, to the skins, nasal mucosa, and digestive tracts of healthy persons. Additional evidence along this line has recently been brought forward by Honeij and Parker (1914), who incriminate both *Musca domestica* and *Stomoxys calcitrans*. Whether or not such insect-borne bacilli are capable of infecting persons whose skin and mucosa are thus contaminated, Currie was unwilling to maintain, but he concludes that until we have more accurate knowledge on this point, we are justified in regarding these insects with grave suspicion of being one of the means of disseminating leprous infection.

Various students of the subject have suggested that bed-bugs may be the carriers of leprosy and have determined the presence of acid-fast bacilli in the intestines of bed-bugs which had fed on leprous patients. Opposed to this, the careful experiments of Thompson (1913) and of Skelton and Parkham (1913) have been wholly negative.

Borrel has recently suggested that *Demodex*, may play a rôle in spreading the infection in families. Many other insects and acariens have been suggested as possible vectors, but the experimental data are few and in no wise conclusive. The most that can be said is that it is quite possible that under favorable conditions the infection might be spread by any of the several blood-sucking forms or by house-flies.

### Verruga peruviana

**Verruga peruviana** is defined by Castellani and Chalmers as "a chronic, endemic, specific, general disorder of unknown origin, not contagious, but apparently inoculable, and characterized by an irregular fever associated with rheumatoid pains, anemia, followed by granulomatous swellings in the skin, mucous membranes, and organs of the body." It has been generally believed by medical men interested that the comparatively benign eruptive verruga is identical with the so-called Oroya, or Carrion's fever, a malignant type. This view is not supported by the work of Strong, Tyzzer and Brues, (1913).

The disease is confined to South America and to definitely limited areas of those countries in which it does occur. It is especially prevalent in some parts of Peru.

The causative organism and the method of transfer of verruga are unknown. Castellani and Chalmers pointed out in 1910 that the study of the distribution of the disease in Peru would impress one with the similarity to the distribution of the Rocky Mountain fever and would lead to the conclusion that the ætiological cause must in some way be associated with some blood-sucking animal, perhaps an arachnid, and that this is supported by the fact that the persons most prone to the infection are those who work in the fields.

More recently, Townsend (1913), in a series of papers, has maintained that verruga and Carrion's disease are identical, and that they are transmitted to man by the bites of the Psychodid fly, *Phlebotomus verrucarum*. He succeeded in producing the eruptive type of the disease in experimental animals by injecting a physiological salt trituration of wild Phlebotomus flies. A cebus monkey was exposed from October 10 to November 6, by chaining him to a tree in the verruga zone, next to a stone wall from which the flies emerged in large numbers every night. Miliar eruption began to appear on the orbits November 13 and by November 21, there were a number of typical eruptions, with exudation on various parts of the body exactly like miliar eruptive sores commonly seen on legs of human cases.

An assistant in the verruga work, George E. Nicholson, contracted the eruptive type of the disease, apparently as a result of being bitten by the Phlebotomus flies. He had slept in a verruga zone, under a tight net. During the night he evidently put his hands in contact with the net, for in the morning there were fifty-five unmistakable Phlebotomus bites on the backs of his hands and wrists.

Townsend believes that in nature, lizards constitute the reservoir of the disease and that it is from them that the Phlebotomus flies receive the infection.

## Cancer

There are not wanting suggestions that this dread disease is carried, or even caused, by arthropods. Borrel (1909) stated that he had found mites of the genus *Demodex* in carcinoma of the face and of the mammæ. He believed that they acted as carriers of the virus.

Saul (1910) and Dahl (1910) go much further, since they attribute the production of the malignant growth to the presence of mites which Saul had found in cancers. These Dahl described as belonging to a new species, which he designated *Tarsonemus hominis*. These findings have since been confirmed by several workers. Nevertheless, the presence of the mite is so rare that it cannot be regarded as an important factor in the causation of the disease. The theory that cancer is caused by an external parasite is given little credence by investigators in this field.

**In conclusion,** it should be noted that the medical and entomological literature of the past few years abounds in suggestions, and in unsupported direct statements that various other diseases are insect-borne. Knab (1912) has well said "Since the discovery that certain blood-sucking insects are the secondary hosts of pathogenic parasites, nearly every insect that sucks blood, whether habitually or occasionally, has been suspected or considered a possible transmitter of disease. No thought seems to have been given to the conditions and the characteristics of the individual species of blood-sucking insects, which make disease transmission possible."

He points out that "in order to be a potential transmitter of human blood-parasites, an insect must be closely associated with man and normally have opportunity to suck his blood repeatedly. It is not sufficient that occasional specimens bite man, as, for example, is the case with forest mosquitoes. Although a person may be bitten by a large number of such mosquitoes, the chances that any of these mosquitoes survive to develop the parasites in question, (assuming such development to be possible), and then find opportunity to bite and infect another person, are altogether too remote. Applying this criterion, not only the majority of mosquitoes but many other blood-sucking insects, such as Tabanidæ and Simuliidæ, may be confidently eliminated. Moreover, these insects are mostly in evidence only during a brief season, so that we have an additional difficulty of a very long interval during which there could be no propagation of the disease in question." He makes an exception of tick-borne diseases, where the parasites are directly transmitted from the tick host to its offspring and where, for this reason, the insect remains a potential transmitter for a very long period. He also cites the trypanosome diseases as possible exceptions, since the causative organisms apparently thrive in a number of different vertebrate hosts and may be transmitted from cattle, or wild animals, to man.

Knab's article should serve a valuable end in checking irresponsible theorizing on the subject of insect transmission of disease. Nevertheless, the principles which he laid down cannot be applied to the cases of accidental carriage of bacterial diseases, or to those of direct inoculation of pyogenic organisms, or of blood parasites such as the bacillus of anthrax, or of bubonic plague. Accumulated evidence has justified the conclusion that certain trypanosomes pathogenic to man are harbored by wild mammals, and so form an exception. Townsend believes that lizards constitute the natural reservoir of verruga; and it seems probable that field mice harbor the organism of tsutsugamushi disease. Such instances are likely to accumulate as our knowledge of the relation of arthropods to disease broadens.

# CHAPTER XII

## HOMINOXIOUS ARTHROPODS

The following synoptic tables are presented in the hope that they may be of service in giving the reader a perspective of the relationships of the Arthropoda in general and enabling him to identify the more important species which have been found noxious to man. Though applicable chiefly to the arthropods found in the United States, exotic genera and species which are concerned in the transmission of disease are also included. For this reason the keys to the genera of the Muscids of the world are given. As will be seen, the tables embrace a number of groups of species which are not injurious. This was found necessary in order that the student might not be lead to an erroneous determination which would result were he to attempt to identify a species which heretofore had not been considered noxious, by means of a key containing only the noxious forms. The names printed in **bold faced type** indicate the hominoxious arthropods which have been most commonly mentioned in literature.

### CRUSTACEA

Arthropods having two pairs of antennæ which are sometimes modified for grasping, and usually with more than five pairs of legs. With but few exceptions they are aquatic creatures. Representatives are: Crabs, lobsters, shrimps, crayfish, water-fleas, and woodlice. To this class belongs the **Cyclops** (fig. 122) a genus of minute aquatic crustaceans of which at least one species harbors *Dracunculus medinensis*, the Guinea worm (fig. 121).

### MYRIAPODA

Elongate, usually vermiform, wingless, terrestrial creatures having one pair of antennæ, legs attached to each of the many intermediate body segments. This group is divided into two sections, now usually given class rank: the **Diplopoda** or millipeds (fig. 13), commonly known as thousand legs, characterized by having two pairs of legs attached to each intermediate body segment, and the **Chilopoda** or centipeds (fig. 14) having only one pair of legs to each body segment.

## ARACHNIDA

In this class the antennæ are apparently wanting, wings are never present, and the adults are usually provided with four pairs of legs. Scorpions, harvest-men, spiders, mites, etc.

## HEXAPODA (Insects)

True insects have a single pair of antennæ, which is rarely vestigial, and usually one or two pairs of wings in the adult stage. Familiar examples are cockroaches, crickets, grasshoppers, bugs, dragonflies, butterflies, moths, mosquitoes, flies, beetles, ants, bees and wasps.

### ORDERS OF THE ARACHNIDA

a. Abdomen distinctly segmented. A group of orders including scorpions, (fig. 11), whip-scorpions (fig. 10), pseudo-scorpions, solpugids (fig. 12) harvest-men (daddy-long-legs or harvestmen), etc........ **ARTHROGASTRA**
aa. Abdomen unsegmented, though sometimes with numerous annulations ................................................ **SPHÆROGASTRA**
  b. A constriction between cephalothorax and abdomen (fig. 7). True Spiders ................................................ **ARANEIDA**
  bb. No deep constriction between these parts.
    c. Legs usually well developed, body more or less depressed (fig. 49). Mites ................................................ **ACARINA**
    cc. Legs stumpy or absent, body more or less elongate or vermiform, or if shorter, the species is aquatic or semi-aquatic in habit.
      d. Four pairs of short legs; species inhabiting moss or water. Water-bears ................................................ **TARDIGRADA**
      dd. Two pairs of clasping organs near the mouth, instead of legs, in the adult; worm-like creatures parasitic within the nasal passages, lungs, etc. of mammals and reptiles (fig. 148). Tongue worms. ................................................ **LINGUATULINA**

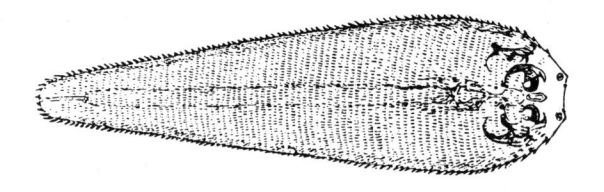

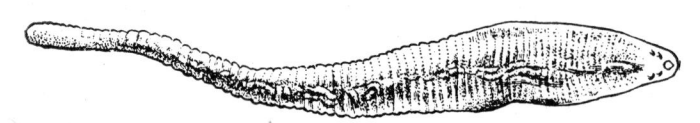

148. Linguatula, (*a*) larva; (enlarged). (*b*) adult; (natural size).

## ACARINA*

a. Abdomen annulate, elongate; very minute forms, often with but four legs (fig. 62).................................................. **DEMODICOIDEA**
  b. With but four legs of five segments each. Living on plants, often forming galls................................................. **ERIOPHYIDÆ**
  bb. With eight legs, of three segments each. Living in the skin of mammals ............................................................. **DEMODICIDÆ**
    To this family belongs the genus **Demodex** found in the sebaceous glands and hair follicles of various mammals, including man. *D. phylloides* Csokor has been found in Canada on swine, causing white tubercles on the skin. *D. bovis* Stiles has been reported from the United States on cattle, upon the skin of which they form swellings. **D. folliculorum** Simon is the species found on man. See page 78.
aa. Abdomen not annulate nor prolonged behind; eight legs in the adult stage.
  b. With a distinct spiracle upon a stigmal plate on each side of the body (usually ventral) above the third or fourth coxæ or a little behind (fig. 50); palpi free; skin often coriaceous or leathery; tarsi often with a sucker.
    c. Hypostome large (fig. 50), furnished below with many recurved teeth; venter with furrows, skin leathery; large forms, usually parasitic ................................................................... **IXODOIDEA**
      d. Without scutum but covered by a more or less uniform leathery integument; festoons absent; coxæ unarmed, tarsi without ventral spurs; pulvilli absent or vestigial in the adults; palpi cylindrical; sexual dimorphism slight................................... **ARGASIDÆ**
        e. Body flattened, oval or rounded, with a distinct flattened margin differing in structure from the general integument; this margin gives the body a sharp edge which is not entirely obliterated even when the tick is full fed. Capitulum (in adults and nymphs) entirely invisible dorsally, distant in the adult by about its own length from the anterior border. Eyes absent......**Argus** Latr.
          f. Body oblong; margin with quadrangular cells; anterior tibiæ and metatarsi each about three times as long as broad. On poultry, southwest United States................**A. persicus miniatus**
           *A. brevipes* Banks, a species with proportionately shorter legs has been recorded from Arizona.
          ff. With another combination of characters. About six other species of *Argas* from various parts of the world, parasitic on birds and mammals.
        ee. Body flattened when unfed, but usually becoming very convex on distention; anterior end more or less pointed and hoodlike; margin thick and not clearly defined, similar in structure to the rest of the integument and generally disappearing on distention; capitulum subterminal, its anterior portions often visible dorsally in the adult; eyes present in some species.
          f. Integument pitted, without rounded tubercles; body provided with many short stiff bristles; eyes absent. On horses, cattle and man (fig. 48)..........................**Otiobius** Banks.
            **O. megnini**, a widely distributed species, is the type of this genus.

---
*Adapted from Banks, Nuttall, Warburton, Stiles, *et. al.*

ff. Integument with rounded tubercles or granules; body without stiff bristles..............................**Ornithodoros** Koch.
  g. Two pairs of eyes; tarsi IV with a prominent subterminal spur above; leg I strongly roughened. On cattle and man.
................................................**O. coriaceus**
  gg. No eyes; no such spur on the hind tarsi.
    h. Tarsi I without humps above..................*O. talaje.*
    hh. Tarsi I with humps above.
      i. Tarsi IV without distinct humps above. On hogs, cattle and man................................**O. turicata**
      ii. Tarsi IV with humps nearly equidistant (fig. 142). Africa.
..........................................**O. moubata**

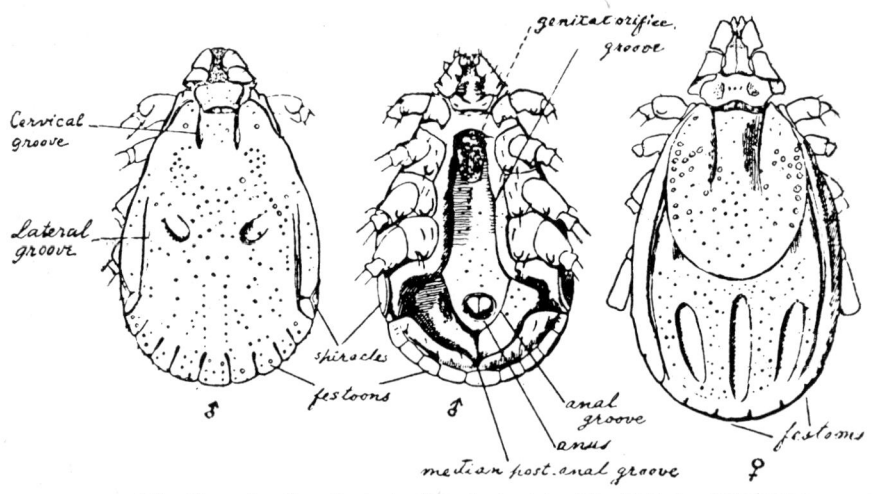

149. Hæmaphysalis wellingtoni. Note short palpi. After Nuttall and Warburton.

dd. With scutum or shield (fig. 50); festoons usually present; coxæ usually armed with spurs, tarsi generally with one or two ventral spurs; pulvilli present in the adults; sexual dimorphism pronounced
................................................**IXODIDÆ**
  e. With anal grooves surrounding anus in front; inornate; without eyes; no posterior marginal festoons; venter of the male with non-salient plates. Numerous species, 14 from the United States, among them **I. ricinus** (fig. 49 and 50), **scapularis, cookei,** *hexagonus, bicornis.*       **Ixodes** Latr. (including Ceratixodes).
  ee. With anal groove contouring anus behind, or groove faint or obsolete.
    f. With short palpi (fig. 149).
      g. Without eyes, inornate, with posterior marginal festoons; male without ventral plates. Numerous species. *H. chordeilis* and *leporis-palustris* from the United States..............
..........................................*Hæmaphysalis* Koch.

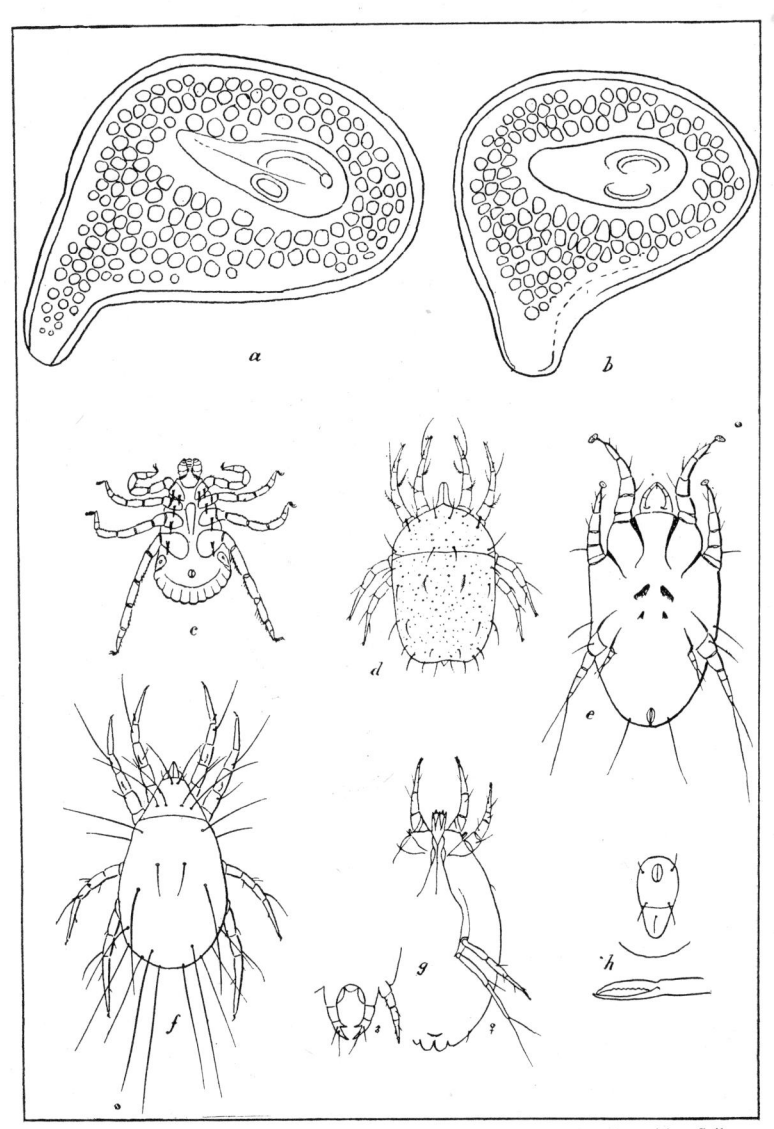

150. Stigmal plate of Dermacentor andersoni; (*a*) of male, (*b*) of female. After Stiles. (*c*) Dermacentor variabilis, male· (*d*) Glyciphagus obesus; (*e*) Otodectes cynotis; (*f*) Tyroglyphus lintneri; (*g*) Tarsonemus pallidus; (*h*) anal plate and mandible of Liponyssus; (*c*) to (*h*) after Banks.

gg. With eyes.
  h. Anal groove distinct; posterior marginal festoons present.
   i. Base of the capitulum (fig. 150c) rectangular dorsally; usually ornate.................**Dermacentor** Koch.
    j. Adults with four longitudinal rows of large denticles on each half of hypostome; stigmal plate nearly circular, without dorso-lateral prolongation, goblets very large, attaining $43\mu$ to $115\mu$ in diameter; not over 40 per plate, each plate surrounded by an elevated row of regularly arranged supporting cells; white rust wanting; base of capitulum distinctly broader than long, its postero-lateral angles prolonged slightly, if at all; coxæ I with short spurs; trochanter I with small dorso-terminal blade. Texas, Arizona, etc. *D. nitens*

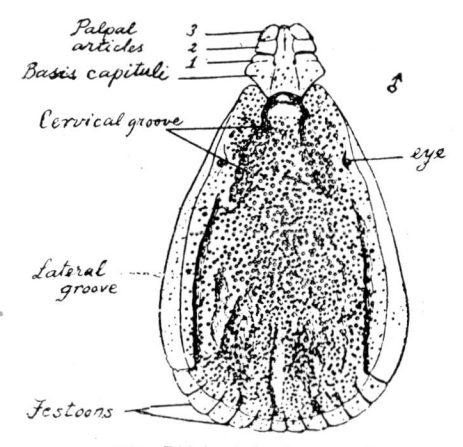

151. Rhipicephalus bursa, male.
After Nuttall and Warburton.

    jj. Adults with three longitudinal rows of large denticles on each half of hypostome; goblet cells always more than 40 per plate; whitish rust usually present.
     k. Dorso-lateral prolongation of stigmal plate small or absent; plates of the adults distinctly longer than broad; goblet cells large, usually $30\mu$ to $85\mu$ in diameter, appearing as very coarse punctations on untreated specimens, but on specimens treated with caustic potash they appear very distinct in outline; base of capitulum distinctly (usually about twice) broader than long, the postero-lateral angles distinctly produced caudad; spurs of coxæ I long, lateral spur slightly longer than median; trochanter I with dorso-terminal spur. *D. albipictus*, (= *variegatus*), *salmoni, nigrolineatus.*

kk. Dorso-lateral prolongation of stigmal plate distinct.
  l. Body of plate distinctly longer than broad; goblet cells of medium size, usually 17.5$\mu$ to 35$\mu$ or 40$\mu$ in diameter, appearing as medium sized punctuations on untreated specimens, but on the specimens treated with caustic potash they appear very distinct in outline, which is not circular; base of capitulum usually less than twice as broad as long, the postero-lateral angles always distinctly prolonged caudad.
    m. Trochanter I with distinct dorso-subterminal retrograde sharp, digitate spur; postero-lateral angles of capitulum pronouncedly prolonged caudal, 112$\mu$ to 160$\mu$ long; goblet cells attain 13$\mu$ to 40$\mu$ in diameter; type locality California ........... **D. occidentalis**
    mm. Trochanter I with dorso-terminal blade; postero-lateral angles of capitulum with rather short prolongations.
      n. Stigmal plate small, goblet cells not exceeding 45 in the male or 100 in the female; scutum with little rust, coxa I with short spurs, the inner distinctly shorter than the outer ............... *D. parumapertus-marginatus*
      nn. Stigmal plate larger; goblet cells over 70 in the male and over 100 in the female; coxa I with longer spurs, inner slightly shorter than the outer; scutum with considerable rust....................... **D. venustus***
  ll. Goblet cells small, rarely exceeding 17.6$\mu$, occasionally reaching 19$\mu$ in diameter; on untreated specimens they appear as very fine granulations, and on specimens treated with caustic potash they may be difficult to see, but their large number can be determined from the prominent stems of the goblets; surface of outline of the goblets distinctly circular; base of the capitulum usually less than twice as broad as long, the postero-lateral angle distinctly prolonged caudad; spurs of coxæ I long.................................
    ...... *D. reticulatus* and *electus* ( = *variabilis?*)
ii. Base of the capitulum (fig. 151) usually hexagonal (except in the male of *puchellus*); and usually inornate.

---

*Dr. C. W. Stiles considers the species which is responsible for spotted fever distinct from the *venustus* of Banks, separating it as follows:
  Goblet cells about 75 in the male or 105 in the female. Texas. *D. venustus.*
  Goblet cells 157 in the male, or 120 in the female; stigmal plate shaped as shown in the figure (figs. 150 a, b). Montana, etc. **D. andersoni.**

j. No ventral plate or shield in either sex (fig. 153). **R. bicornis** from the United States .... **Rhipicentor** Nuttall

jj. Males with a pair of adanal shields, and usually a pair of accessory adanal shields. Numerous species, among them *R. sanguineus* (fig. 154) and *texanus*, the latter from the United States......*Rhipicephalus* Koch

hh. Anal grooves faint or obsolete; no marginal festoons.

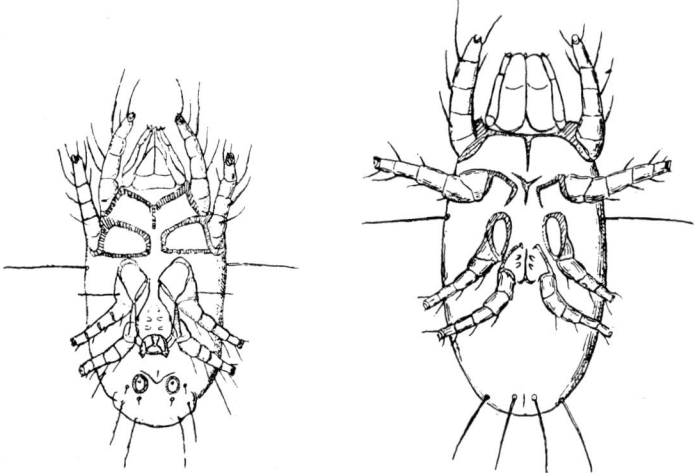

i. Short palpi; highly chitinized; unfed adults of large size; coxæ conical; male with a median plate prolonged in two long spines projecting caudad; segments of leg pair IV greatly swollen (fig. 155, 156). *M. winthemi* .......... ............................. *Margaropus* Karsch

152. Monieziella (Histiogaster) emtomophaga-spermatica, ventral aspect, male and female. After Trouessart,

ii. Very short palpi, ridged dorsally and laterally; slightly chitinized; unfed adults of smaller size; coxæ I bifid; male with adanal and accessory adanal shields (fig. 139). **B. annulatus**........................**Boophilus** Curtis

ff. Palpi longer than broad (fig. 157).

g. Male with pair of adanal shields, and two posterior abdominal protrusions capped by chitinized points; festoons present or absent. Several species, among them **H. ægypticum** (fig. 140) from the old world...................**Hyalomma** Koch

gg. Male without adanal shields but small ventral plaques are occassionally present close to the festoons. Many species, a few from the Unted States (fig. 157).... **Amblyomma** Koch

h. Coxa I with but one spine; metatarsi (except I) with two thickened spurs at tips...............*A. maculatum*

hh. Coxa I with two spines; metatarsi without stout spurs at tips, only slender hairs.

i. Projections of coxa I blunt and short. Large species on the gopher tortoise in Florida.......... *A. tuberculatum*
ii. Projections of coxa I longer, and at least one of them sharp pointed; second segment of palpus twice as long as the third; coxa IV of the male with a long spine.
  j. Porose areas nearly circular; shield of both sexes pale yellowish, with some silvery streaks and marks, and some reddish spots; shield of female as broad as long.
............................**A. cajennense** ( =mixtum).
  jj. Porose areas elongate, shield brown, in the female with an apical silvery mark, in the male with two small and two or four other silvery spots; shield of the female longer than broad (fig 158 e)..**A. americanum.**

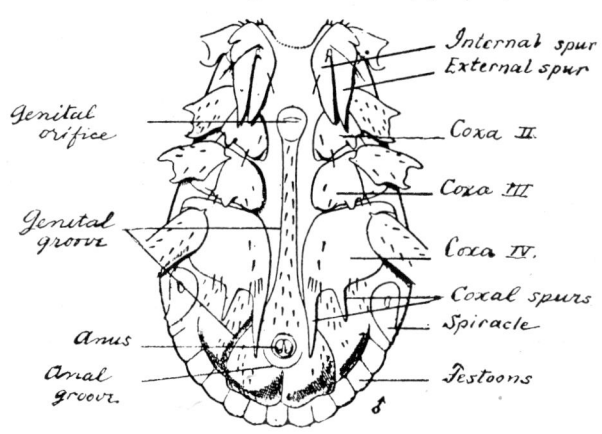

153. Rhipicentor bicornis, ventral aspect, male. After Nuttall and Warburton.

cc. Hypostome small, without teeth, venter without furrows; body often with coriaceous shields, posterior margin of the body never crenulate (i.e. without festoons); no eyes.............GAMASOIDEA.
 d. Parasitic on vertebrates; mandibles fitted for piercing; body sometimes constricted ............................... DERMANYSSIDÆ.
  e. Anal plate present........................... DERMANYSSINÆ.
   f. Body short; legs stout, hind pair reaching much beyond the tip of the body. On bats...................... *Pteroptus* Dufour.
   ff. Body long; hind legs not reaching beyond the tip of the body.
    g. Peritreme on the dorsum, very short; body distinctly constricted................................ *Ptilonyssus* Berl.
    gg. Peritreme on the venter, longer; body not distinctly constricted.
     h. Mandibles in both sexes chelate. Parasitic on bats, mice and birds (fig. 150, h).................. **Liponyssus** Kol.
The species **L.** ( =**Leiognathus**) **sylviarum** frequents the nests of warblers. An instance is on record of these mites attacking man, causing a pruritis.

hh. Mandibles in the male chelate (fig. 158 j), in the female long, styliform. Parasitic on birds......**Dermanyssus** Dug. Two species of importance may be noted, *D. hirundinus* and **D. gallinæ**. The latter (fig. 51) is a serious pest of poultry, sometimes attacking man, causing itching and soreness.

  ee. Anal plate absent. In lungs and air passages of some mammals. .................................... HALARACHNINÆ.

dd. Free or attached to insects, rarely on vertebrates.

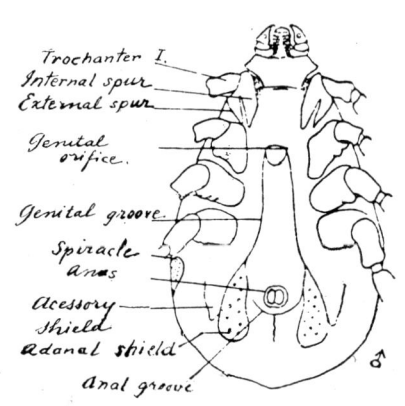

  e. First pair of legs inserted within the same body opening as the oral tube; genital apertures surrounded by the sternum. On insects..........................................UROPODIDÆ.

154. Rhicephalus sanguineus, male. After Nuttall and Warburton.

  ee. First pair of legs inserted at one side of the mouth opening; male genital aperture usually on the anterior margin of the sternal plate ........................................**Gamasidæ**. This family contains a number of genera, some of which are found upon mammals, though the majority affect only other arthopods. One species, **Lælaps stabularis**, frequents the bedding in stables, and in one instance at least, has occasioned irritation and itching, in man.

bb. No distinct spiracle in the stigmal plate on each side of the body.

  c. Body usually coriaceous, with few hairs, with a specialized seta arising from a pore near each posterior corner of the cephalothorax; no eyes; mouth parts and palpi very small; ventral openings of the abdomen large; tarsi without sucker. Not parasitic..........ORIBATOIDEA.

  cc. Body softer; without such specialized seta.

    d. Aquatic species............................HYDRACHNOIDEA.

    dd. Not aquatic.

*Acarina* 267

e. Palpi small, three segmented, adhering for some distance to the lip; ventral suckers at genital opening or near anal opening usually present; no eyes; tarsi often end in suckers; beneath the skin on the venter are seen rod-like epimera that support the legs; body often entire. Adults frequently parasitic....**SARCOPTOIDEA.**
f. With tracheæ; no ventral suckers; legs ending in claws; body divided into cephalothorax and abdomen; the female with a clavate hair between legs I and II. Usually not parasitic on birds and mammals ..................... **TARSONEMIDÆ**
  g. Hind legs of female ending in claw and sucker as in the other pairs.................................**PEDICULOIDINÆ**
    To this sub-family belongs the genus **PEDICULOIDES**
    P. **ventricosus** is described on page 69.

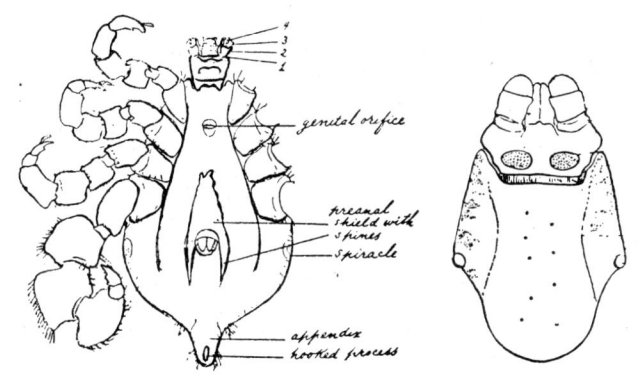

155. Margaropus winthemi, male. After Nuttall and Warburton.

156. Margaropus winthemi, capitulum and scutum. After Nuttall and Warburton.

  gg. Hind legs of the female end in long hairs....... **TARSONEMINÆ**
    **Tarsonemus intectus** Karpelles, normally found upon grain, is said to attack man in Hungary and Russia. Other species of the genus affect various plants (c.f. fig. 150, g).
ff. Without tracheæ; no such clavate hair.
  g. Genital suckers usually present; integument usually without fine parallel lines.
    h. Legs short, without clavate hair on tarsi I and II. On insects............................... **CANESTRINIDÆ.**
    hh. Legs longer, with a clavate hair on tarsi I and II. Not normally parasitic except on bees...... **TYROGLYPHIDÆ**
      i. Dorsal integument more or less granulate; claws very weak, almost invisible; some hairs of the body plainly feathered; ventral apertures large. ............**Glyciphagus** Her.
        This genus occurs in the United States. In Europe the mites have been found feeding on all sorts of substances. They are known as sugar mites and cause the disease

known as grocer's itch. **G. domesticus** and **G. prunorum** are old world species (fig. 150, d).
ii. Dorsal integument not granulate; claws distinct; no prominent feathered hairs; ventral aperture small.
j. Mandibles not chelate; elongate, and toothed below; body without long hairs; palpi enlarged at tip and provided with two divergent bristles. Species feed on decaying substances............*Histiostoma* Kram.
jj. Mandibles chelate; palpi not enlarged at the tip, nor with two bristles.
k. No clavate hair on the base of tarsi I and II; no suture between cephalothorax and abdomen. Live on bees or in their nests..........*Trichotarsus* Can.
kk. A clavate or thickened hair at the base of tarsi I and II.
l. The bristle on the penultimate segment of the legs arises from near the middle; no suture between the cephalothorax and abdomen. The species, some of which occur in the United States, feed on dried fruit, etc.................*Carpoglyphus* Robin.
ll. The bristle on the penultimate segment of the legs arise from near the tip; a suture between cephalothorax and abdomen.
m. Cephalothorax with four distinct and long bristles in a transverse row; tarsi I and II about twice as long as the preceding segment (fig. 150 f) .......................**Tyroglyphus** Latr.
n. Some bristles on tarsi I and II near middle, distinctly spine-like; the sense hair about its length from the base of the segment. Several species in the United States belong to this group.
nn. No spine-like bristles near the middle of the tarsi; sense hair not its length from the base of the segment.
o. Of the terminal abdominal bristles, only two are about as long as the abdomen; leg I of the male greatly thickened and with a spine at apex of the femur below..**T. farinæ.**
oo. Of the terminal abdominal bristles at least six or more are very long, nearly as long as the body.
p. Bristles of the body distinctly plumose or pectinate; tarsi very long..**T. longior.**
pp. Bristles of the body not pectinate.
q. In mills, stored foods, grains, etc. Third and fourth joints of hind legs scarcely twice as long as broad; abdominal bristles not unusually long; legs I

and II of the male not unusually stout.. .............. **T. americanus.**
qq. With other characters and habits. *T. lintneri* (fig. 150 f) the mushroom mite, and several other species.
mm. Cephalothorax with but two long distinct bristles (besides the frontal pair), but sometimes a very minute intermediate pair; tarsi I and II unusually short and not twice as long as the preceding segment.
n. Tarsi with some stout spines. **Rhizoglyphus** Clap. The species of this genus are vegetable feeders. Several occur in the United States. **R. parsiticus** and **R. spinitarsus** have been recorded from the old world, attacking human beings who handle affected plants.
nn. Tarsi with only fine hairs.. **Monieziella** Berl. The species of this genus, as far as known, are predaceous or feed on recently killed animal matter. Several species occur in the United States. **M.** ( = **Histiogaster**) **entomophaga** (fig. 152) from the old world has been recorded as injurious to man.
gg. Genital suckers absent; integument with fine parallel lines. Parasitic on birds and mammals.
h. Possessing a specially developed apparatus for clinging to hairs of mammals.................... LISTROPHORIDÆ.
hh. Without such apparatus.
i. Living on the plumage of birds........ ANALGESIDÆ.
ii. In the living tissues of birds and mammals.
j. Vulva longitudinal. In the skin and cellular tissues of birds ........................... CYTOLEICHIDÆ.
This family contains two species, both occurring in the United States on the common fowl. *Laminosioptes cysticola* occurs on the skin and also bores into the subcutaneous tissue where it gives rise to a calcareous cyst. *Cytoleichus nudus* is most commonly found in the air passages and air cells.
jj. Vulva transverse. In the skin of mammals and birds .................................. SARCOPTIDÆ
k. Anal opening on the dorsum.
l. Third pair of legs in the male without apical suckers. On cats and rabbits.............. **Notœdres** Rail. The itch mite of the cat, **N. cati** (fig. 61) has been recorded on man.
ll. Third leg in the male with suckers. On bats.... ........................ *Prosopodectes* Can.

kk. Anal opening below.
  l. Pedicel of the suckers jointed; mandibles styliform and serrate near the tip........**Psoroptes** Gerv.
    **P. communis ovis** is the cause of sheep scab.
  ll. Pedicel of the suckers not jointed; mandibles chelate.
    m. No suckers on the legs of the females; parasitic on birds, including chickens. *C. mutans* is itch mite of chickens. *Cnemidocoptes* Fürst.
    mm. Suckers at least on legs I and II; parasitic on mammals.
      n. Legs very short; in the male the hind pairs equal in size; body usually short..........
         .........................**Sarcoptes** Latr.
         **S. scabiei** is the itch mite of man (fig. 56).

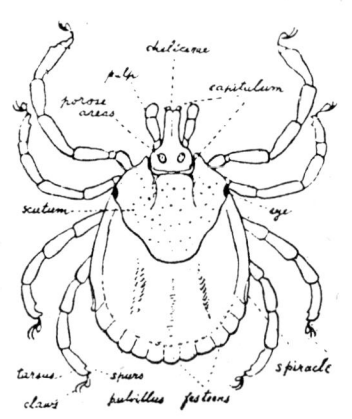

157. Amblyomma, female. After Nuttall and Warburton.

      nn. Legs more slender; in the male the third pair is much larger than the fourth; body more elongate.
        o. Female with suckers on the fourth pair of legs. Species do not burrow in the skin, but produce a scab similar to sheep scab. They occur in the ox, horse, sheep and goat
           ......................**Chorioptes** Gerv.
           **C. symbiotes bovis** of the ox has been recorded a few times on man.
        oo. Female without suckers to the fourth legs.
          p. Hind part of the male abdomen with two lobes. On a few wild animals........
             .....................*Caparinia* Can.

pp. Hind part of the male abdomen without lobes. Live in ears of dogs and cats .................. *Otodectes* Canestr.
*O. cynotis* Hering (fig. 150 e) has been taken in the United States.
ee. Palpi usually of four or five segments, free; rarely with ventral suckers near genital or anal openings; eyes often present; tarsi never end in suckers; body usually divided into cephalothorax and abdomen; rod-like epimera rarely visible; adults rarely parasitic.
f. Last segment of the palpi never forms a thumb to the preceding segment; palpi simple, or rarely formed to hold prey; body with but few hairs....................... **EUPODOIDEA**.
g. Palpi often geniculate, or else fitted for grasping prey; mandibles large and snout like; cephalothorax with four long bristles above, two in front, two behind; last segment of leg I longer than the preceding segment, often twice as long..... ........................................... BDELLIDÆ.
gg. Palpi never geniculate (fig. 158a), nor fitted for grasping prey: beak small; cephalothorax with bristles in different arrangement; last segment of leg I shorter than or but little longer than the preceding joint; eyes when present near posterior border ................................ **EUPODIDÆ**
Moniez has described a species from Belgium (**Tydeus molestus**) which attacks man. It is rose colored; eyeless; its legs are scarcely as long as its body, the hind femur is not thickened; the mandibles are small and the anal opening is on the venter. The female attains a length of about 0.3 mm.
ff. Last segment of the palpus forms a thumb to the preceding, which ends in a claw (with few exceptions); body often with many hairs (fig. 158 k)..................... **TROMBIDOIDEA**.
g. Legs I and II with processes bearing spines; skin with several shields; coxæ contiguous..................... CÆCULIDÆ.
gg. Legs I and II without such processes; few if any shields.
h. Palpi much thickened on the base, moving laterally, last joint often with two pectinate bristles; no eyes; legs I ending in several long hairs; adult sometimes parasitic ............................................ **CHEYLETIDÆ**

**Cheyletus eruditus,** which frequents old books, has once been found in pus discharged from the ear of man.
hh. Palpi less thickened, moving vertically; eyes usually present; leg I not ending in long hairs.
i. Coxæ contiguous, radiate; legs slender, bristly; body with few hairs; no dorsal groove; tarsi not swollen.......... ........................................ ERYTHRÆIDÆ.
ii. Coxæ more or less in two groups; legs less bristly.

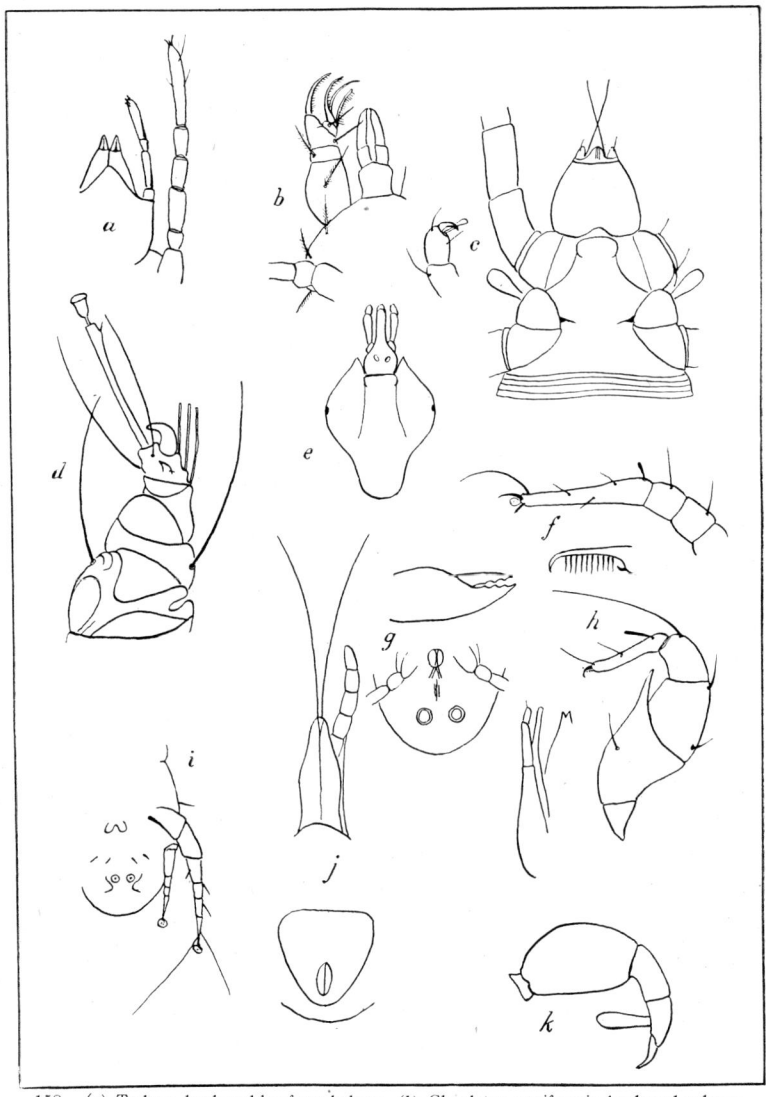

158. (a) Tydeus, beak and leg from below; (b) Cheyletus pyriformis, beak and palpus; (c) beak and claw of Pediculoides; (d) leg of Sarcoptes; (e) scutum of female of Amblyomma americana; (f) leg 1 and tip of mandible of Histiostoma americana; (g) Histiogaster malus, mandible and venter; (h) Aleurobius farinæ, and leg 1 of male; (i) Otodectes cynotis, tip of abdomen of male, (j) beak and anal plate of Dermanyssus gallinæ; (k) palpus of Allothrombium. (a) to (j) after Banks.

j. Body with fewer, longer hairs; often spinning threads; no dorsal groove; tarsi never swollen; mandibles styliform (for piercing).............**TETRANYCHIDÆ**
　The genus **Tetranychus** may be distinguished from the other genera occurring in the United States by the following characters: No scale-like projections on the front of the cephalothorax; legs I as long or longer than the body; palp ends in a distinct thumb; the body is about 1.5 times as long as broad. **T. molestissimus** Weyenb. from South America, and **T. telarius** from Europe and America ordinarily infesting plants, are said also to molest man.

jj. Body with many fine hairs or short spines; not spinning threads; often with dorsal groove; tarsi often swollen.
　k. Mandibles styliform for piercing....**RHYCHOLOPHIDÆ**.
　kk. Mandibles chelate, for biting..........**TROMBIDIDÆ**
　　The genus **Trombidium** has recently been subdivided by Berlese into a number of smaller ones, of which some five or six occur in the United States. The mature mite is not parasitic but the larvæ which are very numerous in certain localities will cause intense itching, soreness, and even more serious complications. They burrow beneath the skin and produce inflammed spots. They have received the popular name of "**red bug,**" The names **Leptus americanus** and **L. irritans** have been applied to them, although they are now known to be immature stages. (Fig. 44.)

## HEXAPODA (Insecta)

The Thysanura (springtails and bristletails), the Neuropteroids (may-flies, stone-flies, dragon-flies, caddis-flies, etc.), Mallophaga (bird lice), Physopoda (thrips), Orthoptera (grasshoppers, crickets, roaches), are of no special interest from our viewpoint. The remaining orders are briefly characterized below.

### SIPHUNCULATA (page 275)

Mouth parts suctorial; beak fleshy, not jointed; insect wingless; parasitic upon mammals. Metamorphosis incomplete. Lice.

### HEMIPTERA (page 275)

Mouth parts suctorial; beak or the sheath of the beak jointed; in the mature state usually with four wings. In external appearance the immature insect resembles the adult except that the immature form (i. e. nymph) never has wings, the successive instars during the process of growth, therefore, are quite similar; and the metamorphosis is thus incomplete. To this order belong the true bugs, the plant lice, leaf hoppers, frog hoppers, cicadas, etc.

### LEPIDOPTERA

The adult insect has the body covered with scales and (with the rare exception of the females of a few species) with four wings also covered with scales. Proboscis, when present, coiled, not segmented, adapted for sucking. Metamorphosis complete, i.e. the young which hatches from the egg is quite unlike the adult, and after undergoing several molts transforms into a quiescent pupa which is frequently enclosed in a cocoon from which the adult later emerges. The larvæ are known as caterpillars. Butterflies and moths.

### DIPTERA (page 285)

The adult insect is provided with two, usually transparent, wings, the second pair of wings of other insects being replaced by a pair of halteres or balancers. In a few rare species the wings, or halteres, or both, are wanting. The mouth parts, which are not segmented, are adapted for sucking. The tarsi are five-segmented. Metamorphosis complete. The larvæ, which are never provided with jointed legs, are variously known as maggots, or grubs, or wrigglers. Flies, midges, mosquitoes.

### SIPHONAPTERA (page 316)

Mouth parts adapted for sucking; body naked or with bristles and spines; prothorax well developed; body compressed; tarsi with five segments; wings absent. Metamorphosis complete. The larva is a wormlike creature. Fleas.

### COLEOPTERA

Adult with four wings (rarely wanting), the first pair horny or leathery, veinless, forming wing covers which meet in a line along the middle of the back. Mouth parts of both immature stages and adults adapted for biting and chewing. Metamorphosis complete. The larvæ of many species are known as grubs. Beetles.

## HYMENOPTERA

Adult insect with four, usually transparent, wings, wanting in some species. Mouth parts adapted for biting and sucking; palpi small; tarsi four or five-segmented. Metamorphosis complete. Parasitic four-winged flies, ants, bees, and wasps.

## SIPHUNCULATA AND HEMIPTERA

a. Legs with claws fitted for clinging to hairs; wings wanting; spiracles of the abdomen on the dorsal surface. (=ANOPLURA=PARASITICA)..... ............................................... SIPHUNCULATA.
   b. Legs not modified into clinging hooks; tibia and tarsus very long and slender; tibia without thumb-like process; antennæ five-segmented .........................................HÆMATOMYZIDÆ Endr. *Hæmatomyzus elephantis* on the elephant.
   bb. Legs modified into clinging hooks; tibia and tarsus usually short and stout; tibia with a thumb-like process; head not anteriorly prolonged, tube-like.
     c. Body depressed; a pair of stigmata on the mesothorax, and abdominal segments three to eight; antennæ three to five-segmented.
       d. Eyes large, projecting, distinctly pigmented; pharynx short and broad; fulturæ (inner skeleton of head) very strong and broad, with broad arms; proboscis short, scarcely attaining the thorax. ............................................. **PEDICULIDÆ**
         e. Antennæ three-segmented. A few species occurring upon old world monkeys...........................*Pedicinis* Gerv.
         ee. Antennæ five-segmented.
           f. All legs stout; thumb-like process of the tibia very long and slender, beset with strong spines, fore legs stouter than the others; abdomen elongate, segments without lateral processes; the divided telson with a conical process posteriorly upon the ventral side.....................**Pediculus** L.
             g. Upon man,
               h. Each abdominal segment dorsally with from one to three more or less regular transverse rows of small setæ; antenna about as long as the width of the head. Head louse (fig. 65).........................**P. humanus**.
               hh. "No transverse rows of abdominal setæ; antenna longer than the width of the head; species larger." Piaget. Body louse of man..................**P. corporis**.
             gg. Upon apes and other mammals..........*P. pusitatus* (?).
           ff. Fore legs delicate, with very long and slender claws; other legs very stout with short and stout claws; thumb-like process of the tibia short and stout; abdomen very short and broad; segment one to five closely crowded, thus the stigmata of segments three to five apparently lying in one segment; segments five to eight with lateral processes; telson without lateral conical appendages (fig. 69). Crab louse of man............ .........................................**Phthirus pubis**.

dd. Eyes indistinct or wanting; pharynx long and slender, fulturæ very slender and closely applied to the pharynx; proboscis very long. Several genera found upon various mammals..... Hæmatopinidæ.
cc. Body swollen; meso- and metathorax, and abdominal segments two to eight each with a pair of stigmata; eyes wanting; antennæ four or five-segmented; body covered with stout spines. Three genera found upon marine mammals..................... Echinophthiriidæ
aa. Legs fitted for walking or jumping; spiracles of abdomen usually ventral; beak segmented.
b. Apex of head usually directed anteriorly; beak arising from its apex; sides of the face remote from the front coxæ; first pair of wings when present thickened at base, with thinner margins.......... **HETEROPTERA**

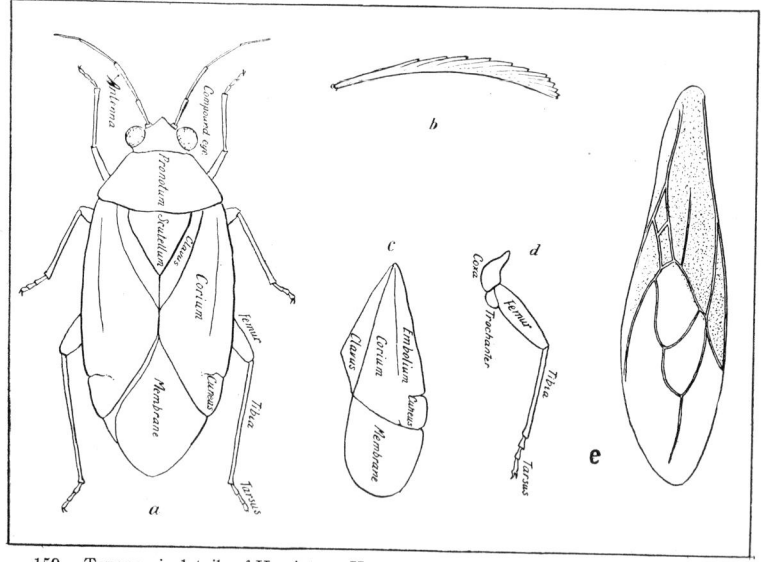

159. Taxonomic details of Hemiptera-Heteroptera. (*a*) Dorsal aspect; (*b*) seta from bedbug; (*c*) wing of Heteropteron; (*d*) leg; (*e*) wing of Sinea.

c. Front tarsi of one segment, spade-form (palæformes); beak short, at most two-segmented; intermediate legs long, slender; posterior pair adapted for swimming............................. Corixidæ
cc. Front tarsi rarely one-segmented, never spade-form; beak free, at least three-segmented.
d. Pulvilli wanting.
e. Hemelytra usually with a distinct clavus (fig. 159), clavus always ends behind the apex of the scutellum, forming the commissure. (Species having the wings much reduced or wanting should be sought for in both sections.)
f. Antennæ very short; meso- and metasternum composite; eyes always present.

g. Ocelli present; beak four-segmented. OCHTERIDÆ and NERTHRIDÆ.
gg. Ocelli wanting; antennæ more or less hidden in a groove.
  h. Anterior coxæ inserted at or near anterior margin of the prosternum; front legs raptorial; beak three-segmented. BELOSTOMIDÆ (with swimming legs), NEPIDÆ, NAUCORIDÆ.
    i. Metasternum without a median longitudinal keel; antennæ always four-segmented.
      j. Beak short, robust, conical; the hairy fleck on the corium elongate, large, lying in the middle between the inner angle of the membrane and the outer vein parallel to the membrane margin; membrane margin S-shaped.
        k. The thick fore femur with a relatively deep longitudinal furrow to receive the tibia. Several American species (fig. 19f.)...**Belostoma** (=Lethocerus Mayer)
        kk. The less thickened fore femur without such a furrow ....................**B. griseus. Benacus** Stal.
      jj. Beak slender, cylindrical; the hairy spot on the corium rounded lying next to the inner angle of the membrane.
        k. Membrane large, furrow of the embolium broadened. *Z. aurantiacum, fluminea*, etc............*Zaitha*
        kk. Membrane very short; furrow of embolium not broadened. Western genus..........*Pedinocoris*
    ii. Metasternum with a long median longitudinal keel. Southwestern forms.....*Abedus ovatus* and *Deniostoma dilatato*
  hh. Anterior coxæ inserted at the posterior margin of the prosternum; legs natatorial. Back swimmers (fig. 19 b.) ..................................NOTONECTIDÆ
    i. Apices of the hemelytra entire; the three pairs of legs similar in shape; beak three-segmented; abdomen not keeled or hairy...........................*Plea* Leach
    ii. Apices of hemelytra notched; legs dissimilar; beak four-segmented; abdomen keeled and hairy.
      j. Hemelytra usually much longer than the abdomen; fourth segment of the antenna longer than the third segment; hind tarsi with claws.........*Bueno* Kirk.
      jj. Hemelytra but little longer than the abdomen; fourth segment of the antenna shorter than the third segment; hind tarsi without claws (fig. 19b)..**Notonecta** L.
ff. Antennæ longer than the head; or if shorter, then the eyes and ocelli absent.
  g. Eyes, ocelli, and scutellum wanting; beak three-segmented; head short; hemelytra always short; membrane wanting. Insects parasitic on bats...................POLYCTENIDÆ
  gg. Eyes present.
    h. First two antennal segments very short, last two long, pilose, third thickened at the base; ocelli present, veins of the hemelytra forming cells. DIPSOCORIDÆ (=CERATOCOMBIDÆ) including SCHIZOPTERIDÆ.

hh. Third segment of the antenna not thickened at the base, second as long or longer than the third, rarely shorter.
  i. Posterior coxæ hinged (cardinate), if rarely rotating, the cuneus is severed, the membrane is one or two-celled, and the meso- and metasternum are composite.
    j. Ocelli absent, clypeus dilated toward the apex; hemelytra always short, membrane wanting. Species parasitic. Bed bugs, etc..........................CIMICIDÆ
    k. Beak short, reaching to about the anterior coxæ; scutellum acuminate at the apex; lateral margin of the elytra but little reflexed, apical margin more or less rounded; intermediate and posterior coxæ very remote.
      l. Body covered with short hairs, only the sides of the pronotum and the hemelytra fringed with longer hairs; antennæ with the third and fourth segments very much more slender than the first and second; pronotum with the anterior margin very *deeply sinuate* ........................ **Cimex** L.
      m. Sides of the pronotum widely dilated, broader than the breadth of one eye, and densely fringed with backward curved hairs; apical margin of the hemelytra nearly straight, rounded toward the interior or exterior angles.
        n. Body covered with very short hairs; second segment of the antenna shorter than the third; sides of the pronotum feebly reflexed, fringed with shorter hairs than the breadth of one eye; hemelytra with the commissural (inner) margin rounded and shorter than the scutellum, apical margin rounded towards the interior angle. The common bed bug (fig. 19h).................**C. lectularius** Linn
        nn. Body covered with longer hairs; second and third segments of the antenna of equal length; side of the pronotum narrowly, but distinctly, reflexed, fringed with longer hairs than the breadth of one eye; hemelytra with the commissural margin straight and longer than the scutellum, apical margin rounded towards the exterior angle. Species found on bats in various parts of the United States................*C. pillosellus* Hov.
      mm. Sides of the pronotum neither dilated, nor reflexed, fringed with less dense and nearly straight hairs; hemelytra with the apical margin distinctly rounded. Parasitic on man, birds and bats. Occurs in the old world, Brazil and the West Indies........ ......**C. hemipterus** Fabr. (=rotundatus)

ll. Body clothed with rather longer silky hairs; third and fourth segments of the antenna somewhat more slender than the first and second; anterior margin of the pronotum *very slightly sinuate* or nearly straight in the middle, produced at the lateral angles. This is the species which in American collections is known as *C. hirundinis*, the latter being an old world form. It is found in swallows nests. **O. vicarius**....**Oeciacus** Stål

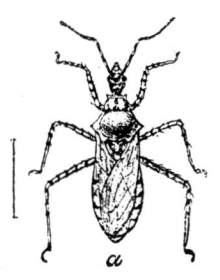

kk. Beak long, reaching to the posterior coxæ; scutellum rounded at the apex; lateral margins of the elytra strongly reflexed, apical margin slightly sinuate toward the middle; intermediate and posterior coxæ sub-contiguous. This species infests poultry in southwest United States and in Mexico. **H. inodorus**................**Hæmatosiphon** Champ.

160. Pselliopsis (Milyas) cinctus. (x2). After C. V. Riley.

jj. Ocelli present, if rarely absent in the female, then the tarsus has two segments; or if with three tarsal segments, the wing membrane with one or two cells.
  k. Beak four-segmented, or with two-segmented tarsi.
    ..IsometopidÆ, MicrophysidÆ and some CapsidÆ.
  kk. Beak three-segmented.
    l. Hemelytra with embolium; head horizontal, more or less conical; membrane with one to four veins, rarely wanting .................**ANTHOCORIDÆ**
      Several species of this family affecting man have been noted, **Anthocoris kingi** and **congolense**, from Africa and **Lyctocoris campestris** from various parts of the world. **Lyctocoris fitchii** Reuter (fig. 19 j), later considered by Reuter as a variety of **L. campestris**, occurs in the United States.
    ll. Hemelytra without embolium. Superfamily Acanthioidea (=SaldÆ Fieber and LeptopodÆ Fieber)

ii. Posterior coxæ rotating.
  j. Claws preapical; aquatic forms. GERRIDÆ and VELIADÆ
  jj. Claws apical.
    k. Prosternum without stridulatory sulcus (notch for beak).
      l. Tarsus with three segments; membrane with two or three longitudinal cells from which veins radiate; rarely with free longitudinal veins (Arachnocoris) or veins nearly obsolete (Arbela); clavus and corium coriaceous; ocelli rarely absent..**NABIDÆ**
**Reduviolus** ( = **Coriscus**) **subcoleoptratus** (fig. 19 g), a species belonging to this family, occurring in the United States, has been accused of biting man. This insect is flat, of a jet black color, bordered with yellow on the sides of the abdomen, and with yellowish legs. It is predaceous, feeding on other insects.
      ll. With other combinations of characters. HYDROMETRIDÆ, HENICOCEPHALIDÆ, NÆOGEIDÆ, MESOVELIADÆ, JOPPEICIDÆ
    kk. Prosternum with stridulatory sulcus (notch for beak); with three segments, short, strong.
      l. Antennæ filiform or sometimes more slender apically, geniculate; wing membrane with two or three large basal cells; scutellum small or moderate ............................. **REDUVIIDÆ**
For a key to the genera and species see next page.
      ll. Last antennal segment clavate or fusiform; wing membrane with the veins often forked and anastomosing; scutellum large; tarsi each with two segments; fore legs strong. ( = PHYMATIDÆ) ........................... MACROCEPHALIDÆ
  ee. Clavus noticeably narrowed towards the apex, never extending beyond the scutellum, the two not meeting to form a commissure; head horizontal, much prolonged between the antennæ, on each side with an antennal tubercle, sometimes acute; ocelli absent; meso- and metasternum simple; tarsi each with two segments; body flattened (fig. 19c). ARADIDÆ, including DYSODIIDÆ.
  dd. Pulvilli present (absent in one Australian family THAUMATOCORIDÆ in which case there is a membranous appendage at the tip of the tibia). **CAPSIDÆ** ( = **MIRIDÆ**),* *Eotrechus* (in family GERRIDÆ), NÆOGAIDÆ, TINGITIDÆ, PIESMIDÆ, MYODOCHIDÆ, CORIZIDÆ, COREIDÆ, ALYDIDÆ, PENTATOMIDÆ, SCUTELLERIDÆ, etc.
bb. Apex of head directed ventrally, beak arising from the hinder part of the lower side of the head; sides of face contiguous to the front coxæ; first

---

*Professor C. R. Crosby who has been working upon certain capsids states that he and his assistant have been bitten by **Lygus pratensis**, the tarnished plant bug, by **Chlamydatus associatus** and by **Orthotylus flavosparsus**, though without serious results.

pair of wings, when present, of uniform thickness. Cicadas, scale insects, plant lice (Aphids), spittle-insects, leaf hoppers, etc........... .............................................. HOMOPTERA

## REDUVIIDÆ OF THE UNITED STATES
(Adapted from a key given by Fracker).

a. Ocelli none; wings and hemelytra always present in the adults; no discodial areole in the corium near the apex of the clavus. *Orthometrops decorata, Oncerotrachelus acuminatus*, etc., Pennsylvania and south...... *Sarcinæ*
aa. Ocelli present in the winged individuals; anterior coxæ not as long as the femora.
  b. Hemelytra without a quadrangular or discoidal areole in the corium near the apex of the clavus.
    c. Ocelli not farther cephalad than the caudal margins of the eyes; segment two of the antenna single.
      d. Thorax usually constricted caudad of the middle; anterior coxæ externally flat or concave............................. **PIRATINÆ**
        e. Middle tibiæ without spongy fossa, head long, no lateral tubercle on neck. *S. stria*, Carolina, Ill., Cal........ *Sirthenia* Spinola
        ee. Middle tibiæ with spongy fossa; fore tibiæ convex above; neck with a small tubercle on each side.
          f. Apical portion of anterior tibiæ angularly dilated beneath, the spongy fossa being preceded by a small prominence.......... ....................................... **Melanolestes** Stål
            g. Black, with piceous legs and antennæ. N. E. States (fig. 19a) ......................................... **M. picipes**
            gg. Sides, and sometimes the whole dorsal surface of the abdomen red. Ill., and southward.................. **M. abdominalis**
          ff. Tibiæ not dilated as in "f"; spongy fossa elongate; metapleural sulci close to the margin. **R. biguttatus** (fig. 22). South ..................................... **Rasahus** A. and S.
      dd. Thorax constricted in the middle or cephalad of the middle; anterior tarsi each three-segmented.
        e. Apex of the scutellum narrow, without spines or with a single spine ............................................. **REDUVIINÆ**
          f. Antennæ inserted in the lateral or dorso-lateral margins of the head; antenniferous tubercles slightly projecting from the sides of the head; head produced strongly cephalad; ocelli at least as far apart as the eyes.
            g. Antennæ inserted very near the apex of the head; segments one and three of the beak short, segment two nearly four times as long as segment one. **R. prolixus.** W. I......... ......................................... **Rhodnius** Stål
            gg. Antennæ inserted remote from the vertex of the head.
              h. Body slightly hairy; pronotum distinctly constricted; angles distinct; anterior lobe four-tuberculate, with the middle tubercles large and conical. *M. phyllosoma*, large species the southwest....................... ......... **Meccus** Stål

hh. Body smooth, margin of the pronotum sinuous, scarcely constricted; anterior lobe lined with little tubercles
..................................Conorhinus Lap.
i. Surface of the pronotum and prosternum more or less grandular.
j. Eyes small, head black; body very narrow, a fifth as wide as long; beak reaches the middle of the prosternum. California......................C. protractus
jj. Eyes large, head fuscous; body at least a fourth as wide as long. Southern species........ C. rubrofasciatus
ii. Pronotum and prosternum destitute of granules.
j. Border of abdomen entirely black except for a narrow yellowish spot at the apex of one segment. Texas
.................................. C. gerstaeckeri
jj. Border of abdomen otherwise marked.
k. Beak slender, joints one and two slightly pilose, two more than twice as long as one; tubercles at the apical angles of the pronotum slightly acute, conical. Md. to Ill. and south. The masked bed bug hunter (fig. 71)..........................C. sanguisugus
kk. Beak entirely pilose, joint two a third longer than joint one; joint one much longer than three; tubercles at the apical angles of pronotum slightly elevated, obtuse. Ga., Ill., Tex., Cal. .. C. variegatus
ff. Antenna inserted on top of the head between margins, close to the eyes; antenniferous tubercles not projecting from the side of the head.
g. Anterior lobe of the pronotum with a bispinous or bituberculate disc; femora unarmed. *S. arizonica, S. bicolor*. Southwestern species..........................*Spiniger* Burm.
gg. Disc of pronotum unarmed; apex of scutellum produced into a spine; ocelli close to the eyes; eyes large and close together.............................Reduvius Lamarck
h. Color piceous. Widely distributed in the United States. (Fig. 20) ............................. R. personatus
hh. More or less testaceous in color. Southwestern states
..........................................R. senilis
ee. Apex of scutellum broad, with two or three spines. . ECTRICHODIINÆ
f. First segment of the antenna about as long as the head. *E. cruciata* Pa. and south; E. *cinctiventris*, Tex. and Mex ................
......................................*Ectrichodia* L. et S.
ff. First segment of the antennæ short. *P. æneo-nitens.* South
..............................................*Pothea* A. et S.
cc. Ocelli cephalad of the hind margins of the eyes; first segment of the antennæ stout, second segment divided into many smaller segments. South and west. *Homalocoris maculicollis*, and *Hammatocerus purcis*........................................ HAMMATOCERINÆ

bb. Hemelytra with a quadrangular or discoidal areole in the corium near the apex of the clavus (fig. 159e).
  c. Anal areole of the membrane not extending as far proximad as the costal areole; basal segment of the antenna thickened, porrect; the other segments slender, folding back beneath the head and the first segment .................................................... STENOPODINÆ
    d. Head armed with a ramous or furcate spine below each side, caudad of the eyes.
      e. First segment of the antenna thickened, apex produced in a spine beyond the insertion of the second segment. Species from Va., Ill. and south............................... *Pnirontis* Stål.
      ee. First segment of the antenna not produced beyond the insertion of the second segment. *Pygolampis*, N. E. states and south; *Gnathobleda*, S. W. and Mex.
    dd. Head unarmed below or armed with a simple spine; rarely with a subfurcate spine at the side of the base. Carolina, Missouri and south. *Stenopoda, Schumannia, Diaditus, Narvesus, Oncocephalus*
  cc. Anal areole of membrane extending farther proximad than the costal areole.
    d. Ocelli farther apart than the eyes. *A. crassipes*, widely distributed in the United States; other species occur in the southwest...... ........................................... *Apiomerus* Hahn.
    dd. Ocelli not so far apart as the eyes..................... ZELINÆ
      e. Sides of mesosternum without a tubercle or fold in front.
        f. Fore femur as long as or longer than the hind femur; first segment of the beak much shorter than the second. *Z. audax*, in the north eastern states; other species south and west..*Zelus* Fabr.
        ff. Fore femur shorter than the hind femur, rarely of equal length, in this case the first segment of the beak as long or longer than the second.
          g. First segment of the beak shorter than the second; fore femur a little shorter than the hind femur; the first segment of the beak distinctly longer than the head before the eyes. *P. cinctus* a widely distributed species (fig. 160). *P. punctipes, P. spinicollis*, Cal., Mex.....(= *Milyas*) *Pselliopus* Berg.
          gg. First segment of the beak as long or longer than the second.
            h. Pronotum armed with spines on the disc.
              i. Juga distinctly prominent at the apex and often acute or subacute; fore femur distinctly thickened; hemelytra usually not reaching the apex of the abdomen. *Fitchia aptera*, N. Y., south and west; *F. spinosula*, South; *Rocconata annulicornis*, Texas, etc.
              ii. Juga when prominent, obtuse at apex; eyes full width of the head; fore femur not thickened; pronotum with four spines on posterior lobe. *R. taurus*, Pa., south and west ........................................*Repipta* Stål.
            hh. Pronotum unarmed on the disc.

i. Spines on each apical angle of the penultimate abdominal segment. *A. cinereus*, Pa., and south..*Atrachelus* A. et S.
ii. Apical angle of the penultimate abdominal segment unarmed. *Fitchia* (in part); *Castolus ferox*, Arizona.

ee. Sides of the mesosternum with a tubercle of fold in front at the hind angles of the prosternum; first segment of the beak longer than the part of the head cephalad of the eyes.

f. Fore femur thickened, densely granulated; hind femur unarmed.

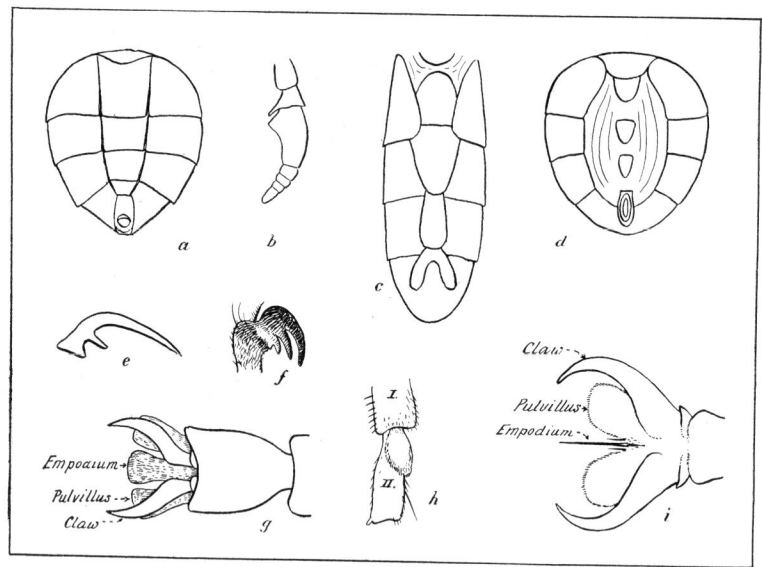

161. Taxonomic details of Diptera. (*a*) Ventral aspect of abdomen of Cynomyia; (*b*) antenna of Tabanus; (*c*) ventral aspect of abdomen of Chortophila; (*d*) ventral aspect of abdomen of Stomoxys; (*e*) claw of Aedes (Culex) sylvestris, male; (*f*) claw of Hippoboscid; (*g*) foot of dipterous insect showing empodimm developed pulviliform; (*h*) hind tarsal segment of Simulium vittatum, female; (*i*) foot of dipterous insect showing bristle-like empodium.

g. Fore tibiæ each with three long spines on the ventral side. *S. diadema* (fig. 159e), a widely distributed species; and several southwestern species................*Sinea* A. et S.
gg. Fore tibiæ unarmed. *A. multispinosa*, widely distributed; *A. tabida*, Cal..........................*Acholla* Stäl.

ff. Fore femur unarmed, rarely a little thickened, a little granulated.
g. Pronotum produced caudad over the scutellum, with a high mesal tuberculate ridge (fig. 19e). **A. cristatus**. N. Y. to Cal. and south......................**Arilus** Hahn.
gg. Caudal lobe of the pronotum six sided, neither elevated nor produced caudad. *H. americanus*, Southwest; also several W. I. and Mexican genera..............**Harpactor** Lap.

## DIPTERA (Mosquitoes, Midges, Flies)

a. Integument leathery, abdominal segments indistinct; wings often wanting; parasitic forms....................................**PUPIPARA**
b. Head folding back on the dorsum of the thorax; wingless flies parasitic on bats. Genus *Nycteribia*............................NYCTERIBIIDÆ
bb. Head not folding back upon the dorsum of the thorax; flies either winged or wingless; parasitic on birds and on bats and other mammals.
  c. Antennæ reduced, wings when present, with distinct parallel veins and outer crossveins; claws simple; palpi leaf-like, projecting in front of the head. Flies chiefly found on bats. Several genera occur in North America ...........................................STREBLIDÆ

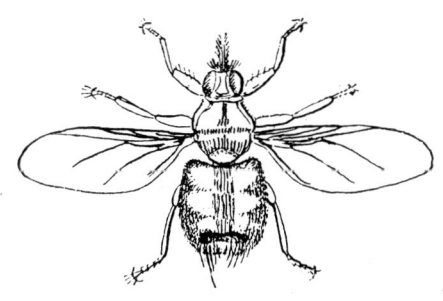

162. Hippobosca equina. x4. After Osborn.

  cc. Antennæ more elongate, segments more or less distinctly separated; head sunk into an emargination of the thorax; wings when present with the veins crowded toward the anterior margin; palpi not leaf-like.......................................**HIPPOBOSCIDÆ**
    d. Wings absent or reduced and not adapted for flight.
      e. Wings and halteres (balancers) absent. *M. ovinus*, the sheep tick ....................................*Melophagus* Latr.
      ee. Wing reduced (or cast off), halteres present.
        f. Claw bidentate; ocelli present. On deer after the wings are cast off. *L. depressa*........................*Lipoptena* Nitsch
        ff. Claw tridentate (fig. 161 f). ....On *Macropis*. *B. femorata* ...............................*Brachypteromyia* Will.
    dd. Wings present and adapted for flight.
      e. Claws bidentate.
        f. Ocelli present; head flat; wings frequently cast off. On birds before casting of the wing..............*Lipoptena* Nitsch.
        ff. Ocelli absent; head round; wings present. The horse tick **H. equina** may attack man (fig. 162)........**Hippobosca** L.
      ee. Claws tridentate (fig. 161 f.).
        f. Anal cell closed at apical margin by the anal crossvein.
          g. Ocelli absent.........................*Stilbometopa* Coq.
          gg. Ocelli present.

      h. R$_{4+5}$ does not form an angle at the crossvein. On birds. There is a record of one species of this genus attacking man .................................**Ornithomyia** Latr.
      hh. R$_{4+5}$ makes an angle at the crossvein. *O. confluens*. ........................................*Ornithoica* Rdi.
   ff. Anal cell not closed by an anal crossvein. *Lynchia, Pseudolfersia*, and *Olfersia* are chiefly bird parasites. The first mentioned genus is said to be the intermediate host of *Hæmoproteus columbæ*.
aa. Abdominal segments chitinous; not parasitic in the adult stage.
  b. Antennæ with six or more segments and empodium not developed pulvilliform; palpi often with four segments.
    c. Ocelli present. **BLEPHAROCERIDÆ**, RHYPHIDÆ, BIBIONIDÆ, MYCETOPHILIDÆ, besides some isolated genera of other families.
    cc. Ocelli absent.
      d. Dorsum of the thorax with a V-shpaed suture; wings usually with numerous veins; legs often very long and slender. Crane flies. ................................................ TIPULIDÆ
      dd. Dorsum of the thorax without a V-shaped suture.
        e. Not more than four longitudinal veins ending in the wing margin; wing usually hairy: antennæ slender; coxæ not long; tibiæ without spurs, legs long and slender. Small, delicate flies often called Gall gnats....................................CECIDOMYIIDÆ
        ee. More than four longitudinal veins ending in the wing margin.
          f. The costal vein is not produced beyond the tip of the wing; radius with not more than three branches.
            g. Antennæ short, composed of ten or eleven closely united segments; legs stout; body stout; abdomen oval; anterior veins stout, posterior ones weak (fig. 163 b); eyes of the male contiguous over the antennæ. Black flies, buffalo flies, turkey gnats. Many North American species, several of them notorious for their blood sucking propensities......
..............................................SIMULIIDÆ
              h. Second joint of the hind tarsus with basal scale-like process and dorsal excision (fig. 161 h); radial sector not forked; no small cell at the base of the wing. *S. forbesi, jenningsi, johannseni, meridionale, piscicidium,* **venustum, vittatum,** etc. Widely distributed species........................
........................(=**Eusimulium**) **Simulium** Latr.
              hh. No basal scale-like process on the second joint of the hind tarsus; radial sector usually forked (fig. 163 b).
                i. Face broad, small basal cell of the wing present. *P. fulvum*, **hirtipes,** *mutatum,* **pecuarum,** *pleurale*..**Prosimulium** Roub.
                ii. Face linear; small basal cell of the wing absent. One species, *P. furcatum*, from California...............
...............................*Parasimulium* Malloch
          gg. Flies of a different structure.
            h. Antennæ composed of apparently two segments and a terminal arista formed of a number of closely united segments. Rare flies with aquatic larvæ........ORPHNEPHILIDÆ

hh. Antennæ of six to fifteen segments, those of the male usually plumose; legs frequently slender and wings narrow ................................... **CHIRONOMIDÆ**

i. Media forked (except in the European genus *Brachypogon*); thorax without longitudinal fissure and not produced over the head (except in four exotic genera); antennæ usually fourteen-jointed in both sexes; fore tibia with a simple comb of setulæ, hind tibia with two unequal combs, middle tibia without comb.......... **CERATOPOGONINÆ**

j. Thorax produced cap-like over the head, wing narrow and very long. *Jenkinsia, Macroptilum* and *Calyptopogon*, eastern hemisphere; *Paryphoconus*, Brazil.

jj. Thorax not produced over the head.

k. Eyes pubescent, empodium well developed, or if short then $R_{2+3}$ distinct and crossvein-like or the branches of R coalescent; r-m crossvein present; fore femora not thickened; wing either with appressed hairs or with microscopic erect setulæ ............................. *Dasyhelea* Kieff.

kk. Eyes bare, or otherwise differing from the foregoing.

l. Empodium well developed, nearly as long as the claws and with long hairs at the base; femora and fifth tarsal segments unarmed, i.e. without spines or stout setæ; fourth tarsal segment cylindrical.

m. Wing with erect and microscopic setulæ. Widely distributed..............................
........(=Atrichopogon) *Ceratopogon* Meig.

mm. Wing with long and depressed hairs. Widely distributed................... *Forcipomyia*

n. Hind metatarsus shorter or not longer than the following (i.e. the second tarsal) segment .................Subgenus *Prohelea* Kieff

nn. Hind metatarsus longer than the following segment....Subgenus *Forcipomyia* Meig.

ll. Empodium short, scarcely reaching the middle of the claws, or vestigial.

m. R-m crossvein wanting.

n. Palpi four segmented; inferior fork of the media **obliterated** at the base. Australia.........
......................*Leptoconops* Skuse

nn. Palpi three-segmented.

o. Legs spinulose, tarsal claws of the female with a basal tooth or strong bristle, those of the male unequal, the anterior with a long sinuous tooth, the posterior with a short arcuate tooth. Italy............
......................**Mycterotypus** Noé

oo. Legs unarmed; no crossvein between the branches of the radius (fig. 163e). New Mexico............**Tersesthes** Townsend
mm. R-m crossvein present.
n. Fore femora very much swollen, armed with spines below, fore tibia arcuate and applied closely to the inferior margin of the femur.
o. $R_{2+3}$ present, therefore cell $R_1$ and $R_2$ both present; wing usually fasciate. United States.................*Heteromyia* Say.
oo. $R_{2+3}$ not distinct from $R_{4+5}$, hence cell $R_3$ obliterated. South America........
............*Pachyleptus* Arrib. (Walker)
nn. Fore femur not distinctly swollen.
o. $R_{2+3}$ present therefore cells $R_1$ and $R_3$ both present, or if not, then the branches of the radius more or less coalescent, obliterating the cells.
p. At least the tip of the wing with erect setulæ; tip of $R_{4+5}$ scarcely attaining the middle of the wing, empodium rather indistinct, not reaching the middle of the claws, the claws not toothed, equal, with long basal bristle; legs without stout setæ. Widely distributed............
.....................**Culicoides** Latr.
**Hæmatomyidium** and **Oecacta** are probable synonyms of this.
pp. Wings bare, if rarely with hair, then the radius reaches beyond two-thirds the length of the wing, or the femur or fifth tarsal segment with stout black spines.
q. Media unbranched. Europe..........
.................*Brachypogon* Kieff
qq. Media branched.
r. Hind femur much swollen and spined. America and Europe. *Serromyia* Meg.
rr. Hind femur not distinctly swollen.
s. Cell $R_1$ not longer than high; fork of the media distad of the crossvein; wing with microscopic setulæ..............*Stilobezzia* Kieff
ss. Cell $R_1$ elongate.
t. Femora unarmed. Widely distributed. ( = Sphaeromias Kieff. 1913 not Curtis?)...........
..........**Johannseniella** Will.

*Diptera*

   tt. Femora, at least in part, with strong black spines. Widely distributed. *Palpomyia* Megerle
  oo. $R_{2+3}$ coalescent with $R_{4+5}$ hence cell $R_3$ is obliterated.
   p. In the female the lower branch of the media with an elbow near its base projecting proximad, the petiole of the media coalescent with the basal section of the radius, wing long and narrow, radial sector ending near the tip of the wing; venation of the male as in *Bezzia*; front concave. United States........ ..................... *Stenoxenus* Coq.
  pp. Venation otherwise, front not concave.
   q. Subcosta and $R_1$ more or less coalescent with the costa; wing pointed at the apex, much longer than the body; antennæ fourteen segmented, not plumose. India........*Haasiella* Kieff.
  qq. Subcosta and radius distinct from the costa.
   r. Abdomen petiolate...*Dibezzia* Kieff.
   rr. Abdomen not petiolate.
    s. Head semi-globose; hind tarsi unusually elongate in the female; antennæ of the male not plumose. Europe......*Macropeza* Meigen.
    ss. Head not globose, more or less flattened in front; antennæ of the male plumose. Widely distributed..........*Bezzia* Kieff.
     t. Fore femora, at least, armed with stout spines below............ ......Subgenus *Bezzia* Kieff.
     tt. Femora unarmed.............. ....Subgenus *Probezzia* Kieff.
  ii. Media of the wing simple, and otherwise not as in "i". To this group belong numerous Chironomid genera, none of which are known to be noxious to man.
 ff. The costal vein apparently is continued around the hind margin of the wing; radius with at least four branches.
  g. Wing ovate pointed, with numerous veins; crossveins, if evident, before the basal third of the wing; veins very hairy; very small moth-like flies................... **PSYCHODIDÆ**
  h. With elongate biting proboscis; the petiole of the anterior forked cell of the wing ($R_2$) arises at or beyond the middle of the wing (fig. 163d).................... **Phlebotomus** Rdi.

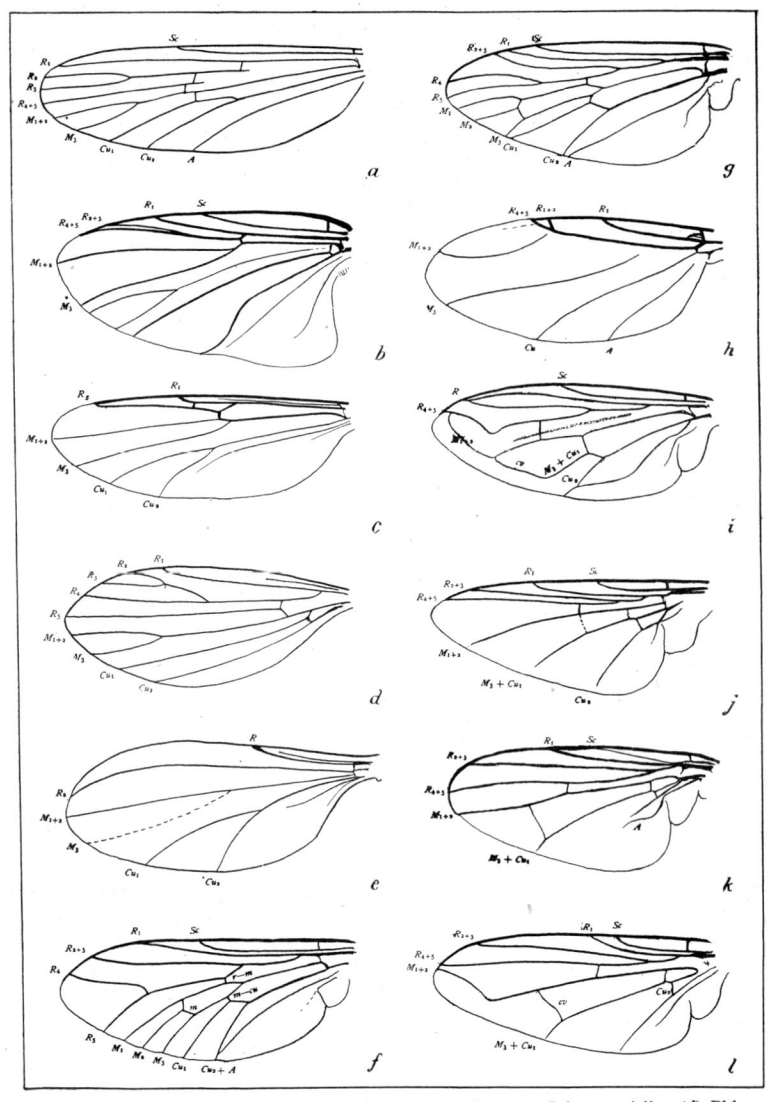

163. Wings of Diptera. (a) Anopheles; (b) Prosimulium; (c) Johannseniella; (d) Phlebotomus (After Doerr and Russ); (e) Tersesthes (after Townsend); (f) Tabanus; (g) Symphoromyia; (h) Aphiochaeta; (i) Eristalis; (j) Gastrophilus; (k) Fannia; (l) Musca.

hh. With shorter proboscis; the petiole of the anterior forked cell arises near the base of the wing..................
..........................*Psychoda, Pericoma*, etc.
gg. The r-m crossvein placed at or beyond the center of the wing; wings not folded roof-like over the abdomen.
  h. Proboscis short, not adapted for piercing; wings bare (DIXIDÆ); or wings scaled (CULICIDÆ, Subf. CORETHRINÆ).
  hh. Proboscis elongate, adapted for piercing; wings scaled, fringed on the hind margin; antennæ of the male bushy plumose. Mosquitoes......................  ............
.................CULICIDÆ (exclusive of CORETHRINÆ)
   i. Metanotum without setæ.
    j. Proboscis strongly decurved; body with broad, appressed, metalescent scales; cell $R_2$ less than half as long as its petiole; claws of female simple, some of the claws of the male toothed. Several large southern species believed to feed only on nectar of flowers
..............................*Megarhinus* R. D.
    jj. Proboscis straight or nearly so, or otherwise different.
     k. Scutellum evenly rounded, not lobed; claws simple in both sexes....................**Anopheles** Meig.
      l. Abdomen with clusters of broad outstanding scales along the sides; outstanding scales on the veins of the wing rather narrow, lanceolate; upper side of the thorax and scutellum bearing many appressed lanceolate scales. Florida and southward (**Cellia**).
       m. Hind feet from the middle of the second segment largely or wholly snow white.
        n. With a black band at the base of the last segment of each hind foot..................
..........**A. albimanus\*** and **tarsimaculata\***
        nn. Without such a band....**A. argyritarsis\***
       mm. Hind feet black, mottled with whitish and with bands of the same color at the sutures of the segments. W. I............ **A. maculipes**
      ll. Abdomen without such a cluster of scales; outstanding scales of the wing veins rather narrow, lanceolate; tarsi wholly black.
       m. Deep black, thorax obscurely lined with violaceous, especially posteriorly; head, abdomen and legs black; no markings on the pleura; abdomen without trace of lighter bandings; wing scales outstanding, uniform, not forming spots, though little thicker at the usual points indicating the spottings. Florida..**A. atropus**

---

\*Species marked with an \* are known to transmit malaria. Species found only in tropical North America and not known to carry malaria have been omitted from this table, but all found in the United States are included.

mm. Otherwise marked when the wings are unspotted.
n. Wings unspotted.
o. Petiole of the first forked cell ($R_2$) more than a third the length of the cell. Mississippi valley......................**A. walkeri**
oo. Petiole of the first forked cell a third the length of the cell. Md......**A. barberi**
nn. Wings spotted.
o. Front margin of the wings with a patch of whitish and yellow scales at a point about two-thirds or three-fourths of the way from base to apex of wing.
p. Veins of the wing with many broad obovate outstanding scales; thorax with a black dot near the middle of each side. W. I. .......................**A. grabhami***
pp. The outstanding scales of the wings rather narrow, lanceolate.
q. Scales of the last vein of the wings white, those at each end black; $R_{4+5}$ black scaled, the extreme apex white scaled. Widely distributed north and south (fig. 131)..........**A. punctipennis** A dark variety from Pennsylvania has been named **A. perplexens.**
qq. Scales of the last vein of the wing white, those at its apex black; $R_{4+5}$ white scaled and with two patches of black scales. South and the tropics. **A. franciscanus** and **pseudopunctipennis***
oo. Front margin of the wings wholly black scaled.
p. Last (anal) vein of the wings white scaled with three patches of black scales (fig. 132). New Jersey to Texas..**A. crucians***
pp. Last vein of the wings wholly black scaled.
q. Widely distributed north and south (fig. 130), ( =**maculipennis**)..........
............**A. quadrimaculatus***
qq. Distributed from Rocky Mountains westward............**A. occidentalis**
kk. Scutellum distinctly trilobed.
l. Cell $R_2$ less than half as long as its petiole; thorax with metallic blue scales; median lobe of the scutellum not tuberculate; few small species which are not common..............**Uranotænia** Arrib.

ll. Cell $R_2$ nearly or quite as long as its petiole, or otherwise distinct.
   m. Femora with erect outstanding scales; occiput broad and exposed. Large species. **P. ciliata. P. howardi**................**Psorophora** R. D.
   mm. Femora without erect scales.
      n. Clypeus bearing several scales or hairs, scutellum with broad scales only; back of head with broad scales; scales along the sides of the mesonotum narrow; some or the claws toothed; thorax marked with a pair of silvery scaled curved stripes; legs black with white bands at the bases of some of the segments (fig. 134). Yellow Fever mosquito ..............**Aedes** (=**Stegomyia**) **calopus.**
      nn. With another combination of characters. Numerous species of mosquitoes belonging to several closely related genera, widely distributed over the country. (*Culex, Aedes, Ochlerotatus,* etc.). **Culex** in the wide sense.
  ii. Metanotum with setæ. *Wyeomyia* (found in the United States); and related tropic genera.
bb. Antennæ composed of three segments with a differentiated style or bristle; third segment sometimes complex or annulate, in which case the empodium is usually developed like the pulvilli, i.e., pad-like (fig. 161 g).
  c. Empodium developed pad-like (pulvilliform) i.e., three nearly equal membranous appendages on the underside of the claws (fig. 161g).
    d. Squamæ, head, and eyes large; occiput flattened or concave; third segment of the antennæ with four to eight annuli or segments, proboscis adapted for piercing; body with fine hairs, never with bristles; middle tibia with two spurs; wing venation as figured (fig. 163f); marginal vein encompasses the entire wing. Horse flies, greenheads, deer flies, gad flies.................**TABANIDÆ***
    e. Hind tibia with spurs at tip; ocelli usually present (**PANGONINÆ**)
    f. Third joint of the antennæ with seven or eight segments; probocis usually prolonged.
      g. Each section the the third antennal segment branched. Central American species, *P. festæ*................*Pityocera* G. T.
      gg. Sections of the third antennal segment not branched.
        h. Upper corner of the eyes in the female terminating in an acute angle; wings of both sexes dark anteriorly. *G. chrysocoma,* a species from the eastern states..........*Goniops* Ald.
        hh. Upper corner of the eye in the female not so terminating; wings nearly uniform in color, or hyaline.
          i. Proboscis scarcely extending beyond the palpi; front of the female wide; much wider below than above. S. W. States............................*Apatolestes* Will.

---
*This table to the North American genera of the Tabanidæ is adapted from one given by Miss Ricardo.

ii. Proboscis extending beyond the palpi.
j. Wing with cell M₃ closed. Tropic America ..........
.........................(=*Diclisa*) *Scione* Wlk.
jj. Cell M₃ open; ocelli present or absent. Two or three eastern species; many south and west..**Pangonia** Rdi.
ff. Third segment of the antenna with five divisions; ocelli present.
g. First and second segments of the antenna short, the second only half as long as the first, three western species....**Silvius** Rdi.
gg. First and second segments of the antenna long, the second distinctly over half as long as the first. Deer flies. Many species, widely distributed..............**Chrysops** Meig.
ee. Hind tibia without spurs; ocelli absent.
f. Third segment of antenna with four divisions, no tooth or angulation; wings marked with rings and circles of darker coloring; front of the female very wide. Widely distributed. *H. americana, H. punctulata*..................**Hæmatopota** Meig.
ff. Third segment of the antenna with five divisions (fig. 161b).
g. Third segment of the antenna not furnished with a tooth or distinct angular projection.
h. Body covered with metallic scales; front of female of normal width; front and middle tibiæ greatly dilated. *L. lepidota*........................... *Lepidoselaga* Macq.
hh. Body without metallic scales; antennæ not very long, the third segment not cylindrical, not situated on a projecting tubercle; front of the female narrow. South. *D. ferrugatus.* ..............(=*Diabasis*) *Diachlorus* O. S.
gg. Third segment of the antenna furnished with a tooth or a distinct angular projection.
h. Hind tibiæ ciliate with long hairs. S. W. and tropics. ............................*Snowiella* and *Stibasoma*.
hh. Hind tibiæ not ciliate.
i. Species of slender build, usually with a banded thorax and abdomen; third segment of the antenna slender, the basal prominence long; wings mostly with brownish markings. Tropic America........*Dichelacera* Macq.
ii. Species of a stouter build; third segment of the antenna stout, its basal process short (fig. 161b). Many species, widely distributed......................**Tabanus** L.
dd. With another group of characters.
e. Squamæ small, antennæ variable, thinly pilose or nearly bare species, without distinct bristles; wing veins not crowded anteriorly, R₄ and R₅ both present, basal cells large; middle tibiæ at least with spurs ..............................................**LEPTIDÆ**
f. Flagellum of the antenna more or less elongated, composed of numerous more or less distinct divisions......................
...................... XYLOPHAGINÆ and ARTHROCERATINÆ.
ff. Antennæ short, third segment simple, with arista or style; face small, proboscis short .......................... **LEPTINÆ**

g. Front tibiæ each with one or two spurs, or if absent, then no discal cell. *Triptotricha, Pheneus, Dialysis, Hilarimorpha.*
gg. Front tibæ without terminal spurs, discal cell present.
   h. Hind tibæ each with a single spur.
      i. Anal cell open (fig. 163g); third antennal segment kidney-shaped with dorsal or subdorsal arista; first antennal segment elongate and thickened. About a dozen species have been described from the United States, of which at least one (**S. pachyceras**) is known to be a vicious blood sucker......................**Symphoromyia** Frauenf.
      ii. Anal cell closed; third antennal segment not kidney-shaped............... *Chrysopila, Ptiolina, Spania.*
   hh. Hind tibiæ each with two spurs.
      i. Third segment kidney-shaped, the arista subdorsal; anal cell closed............................*Atherix* Meig.
      ii. Third segment of the antenna short and with terminal arista; anal cell open...................*Leptis* Fabr. Two European species of this genus have been accused of blood sucking habits, but the record seems to have been based upon error in observation.
ee. With another combination of characters........................
.............................. STRATIOMYIIDÆ, CYRTIDÆ, etc.
cc. Empodium bristlelike or absent.
  d. Antennæ apparently two-segmented, with three-segmented arista, wings (rarely wanting) with several stout veins anteriorly, the weaker ones running obliquely across the wing (fig. 163h); small, quick running, bristly, humpbacked flies. Several genera; **Aphiochæta, Phora, Trineura,** etc........................... PHORIDÆ
  dd. Flies with other characters.
    e. No frontal lunule above the base of the antennæ; both $R_4$ and $R_5$ often present; third segment of the antenna often with a terminal bristle. ASILIDÆ, MYDAIDÆ, APIOCERIDÆ, THEREVIDÆ, SCENOPINIDÆ, BOMBYLIIDÆ, EMPIDIDÆ, DOLICHOPODIDÆ, LONCHOPTERIDÆ.
    ee. A frontal lunule above the base of the antennæ; third segment of the antenna always simple, i.e., not ringed, usually with a dorsal arista; $R_4$ and $R_5$ coalesced into a simple vein.
      f. A spurious vein or fold between the radius and the media, rarely absent; the cell $R_{4+5}$ closed at the apex by vein $M_1$; few or no bristles on the body, none on the head; flies frequently with yellow markings. **Eristalis** (fig. 163i), **Helophilus,** and many other genera..................................SYRPHIDÆ
      ff. No spurious vein present.
         g. Body without bristles; proboscis elongate and slender, often folding; front of both male and female broad....CONOPIDÆ
         gg. Bristles almost always present on head, thorax, abdomen and legs.

h. Arista terminal; hind metatarsus enlarged, sometimes ornamented, hind tarsus more or less flattened beneath...... ................................ PLATYPEZIDÆ
hh. Flies having a different combination of characters.
   i. Head large, eyes occupying nearly the entire head; cell $R_{4+5}$ narrowed in the margin; small flies..PIPUNCULIDÆ
   ii. Head and eyes not unusually large.
      j. Squamæ (tegulæ, or calyptræ, or alulæ) not large, often quite small, the lower one lacking, or at most barely projecting from below the upper one (antisquama); front of both male and female broad, the eyes therefore widely separated; posthumeral and intraalar macrochæta not simultaneously present; thorax usually without a complete transverse suture; postalar callus usually absent; the connectiva adjoining the ventral sclerites always visible; hypopleural macrochætæ absent; last section of $R_{4+5}$ and $M_{1+2}$ with but few exceptions nearly parallel; subcostal vein often wanting or vestigial or closely approximated to $R_1$; the latter often short, basal cells small, the posterior ones often indistinct or wanting; vibrissæ present or absent ........................ ACALYPTRATE MUSCOIDEA
         k. Subcosta present, distinctly separated from $R_1$ at the tip; $R_1$ usually ends distad of the middle of the wing; the small basal cells of the wing distinct.
            l. A bristle (vibrissa) on each side of the face near the margin of the mouth. CORDYLURIDÆ, SEPSIDÆ, PHYCODROMIDÆ, HETERONEURIDÆ, HELOMYZIDÆ.
            ll. No vibrissæ present.
               m. Head nearly spherical, cheeks broad and retreating; proboscis short; the cell $R_5$ closed or narrowed in the margin; legs very long; tarsi shorter than the tibiæ. **Calobata** and other genera..................... MICROPEZIDÆ
               mm. Flies with another combination of characters. RHOPALOMERIDÆ, TRYPETIDÆ, ORTALIDÆ, SCIOMYZIDÆ.
         kk. Subcosta absent or vestigial, or if present, then apparently ending in the costa at the point where $R_1$ joins it; $R_1$ usually ends in the costa at or before the middle of the wing.
            l. Arista long plumose, or pectinate above; oral vibrissæ present; anal cell complete; costa broken at the apex of $R_1$. **Drosophila, Phortica,** and other genera....................... DROSOPHILIDÆ
            ll. With another combination of characters.
               m. The cell M and first $M_2$ not separated by a crossvein; anal cell absent; front bare or only

bristly above; usually light colored flies. **Hippelates, Oscinus,** and other genera. (See also m m m ..................... OSCINIDÆ

mm. Cell M and cell first M₂ often separated by a crossvein; anal cell present, complete, though frequently small; scutellum without spines or protuberances; oral vibrissæ present; arista bare or short plumose; front bristly at vertex only; small dark flies. **Piophila** (fig. 99), **Sepsis** and other genera... SEPSIDÆ

mmm. The GEOMYZIDÆ, AGROMYZIDÆ, PSILIDÆ, TRYPETIDÆ, RHOPALOMERIDÆ, BORBORIDÆ and DIOPSIDÆ differ in various particulars from either the OSCINIDÆ and the SEPSIDÆ noted above.

jj. Squamæ well developed, usually large, the lower one frequently projecting from below the upper one; both posthumeral and intraalar macrochætæ present; thorax with a complete transverse suture; postalar callus present and separated by a distinct suture from the dorsum of the thorax; front of the female broad, of the male frequently narrow, the eyes then nearly or quite contiguous; the connectiva adjoining the ventral sclerites either visible or not; hypopleural macrochætæ present or absent; subcosta always distinct in its whole course, $R_1$ never short...................
.................... CALYPTRATE MUSCOIDEA*

k. Oral opening small, mouth parts usually much reduced or vestigial. This family is undoubtedly of polyphyletic origin but for convenience it is here considered as a single family.............. OESTRIDÆ.

l. The costal vein ends at the tip of $R_{4+5}$, $M_{1+2}$ straight, not reaching the wing margin, hence cell $R_5$ wide open (fig. 163j); squamæ small; arista bare; ovipositor of the female elongate. Larvæ in the alimentary canal of horses, etc.
............................. **Gastrophilus**

m. Posterior crossvein (m-cu) wanting; wings smoky or with clouds. Europe.. **G. pecorum**

mm. Posterior crossvein (m-cu) present, at least in part.

---

*The classification of the Muscoidea as set forth by Schiner and other earlier writers has long been followed, although it is not satisfactory, being admittedly more or less artificial. Within the last two or three decades several schemes have been advanced, that of Brauer and Bergenstamm and of Girschner, with the modifications of Schnabl and Dziedzicki having obtained most favor in Europe. Townsend, in 1908, proposed a system which differs from Girschner's in some respects, but unfortunately it has not yet been published in sufficient detail to permit us to adopt it. From considerations of expediency we use here the arrangement given in Aldrich's Catalogue of North American Diptera, though we have drawn very freely upon Girschner's most excellent paper for taxonomic characters to separate the various groups.

It may sometimes be found that a species does not agree in all the characters with the synopsis; in this case it must be placed in the group with which it has the most characters in common.

n. Wing hyaline with smoky median cross band, and two or three spots; posterior trochanters with hook in the male and a prominence in the female. World wide distribution. **G. equi.**
nn. Wings without spots.
    o. Posterior crossvein (m-cu) distad of the anterior crossvein (r-m); legs, particularly the femora, blackish brown. Europe and North America........**G. hæmorrhoidalis**
    oo. Posterior crossvein opposite or proximad of the anterior crossvein. Europe and North America....................**G. nasalis**
ll. The costal vein ends at the tip of $M_1$ $_2$, $M_{1+2}$ with a bend, the cell $R_5$ hence much narrowed in the margin, or closed.
    m. Proboscis geniculate, inserted in a deep slit; female without extricate ovipositor; arista either bare or plumose; squamæ large; facial grooves approximated below.
        n. Arista bare, short. Larvæ in rodents. Tropic America. *B. princeps*......*Bogeria* Austen
        nn. Arista pectinate above.
            o. Tarsi broadened and flattened, hairy, anal lobe of the wing large. Larvæ in rodents. A number of American species. *Cuterebra.*
            oo. Tarsi slender, not hairy; anal lobe of the wing moderate. Larvæ in man and other mammals. Tropic America. **D. cyaniventris** ....................**Dermatobia** Br.
    mm. Mouth parts very small, vestigial; arista bare.
        n. Facial grooves approximated below, leaving a narrow median depression or groove.
            o. Cell $R_5$ closed and petiolate, body nearly bare. Larvæ in the nasal cavities of the smaller Ungulates. The sheep bot fly. **O. ovis.** Widely distributed..**Oestrus** L.
            oo. Cell $R_5$ narrowly open, body hairy. Larvæ parasitic on deer. Europe and America ..................... *Cephenomyia* Latr.
        nn. Facial grooves far apart, enclosing between them a broad shield-shaped surface; squamæ large; female with elongate ovipositor. Larvæ hypodermatic on Ungulates...... ....................**Hypoderma** Clark
            o. Palpi wanting; tibiæ thickened in the middle.
                p. Hair at apex of the abdomen yellow; legs including femora yellowish brown.... ........................ **H. diana**

pp. Hair at the apex of the abdomen reddish yellow. Europe and America.
q. Tibiæ and tarsi yellow; femora black .........................**H. lineata**
qq. Legs black with black hair; tips of hind tibia and tarsi yellowish brown ......................... **H. bovis**
oo. Palpi small, globular; tibiæ cylindrical, straight. On reindeer. ....*O. tarandi* ..................... *Oedemagena* Latr.
kk. Oral opening of the usual size; mouth parts not vestigial.
l. Hypopleurals wanting; if three sternopleurals are present the arrangement is 1:2; conjunctiva (fig. 161c) of the venter usually present; if the terminal section of $M_{1+2}$ is bent it has neither fold nor appendage (**ANTHOMYIIDÆ** of Girschner).
m. Sternopleurals wanting; $M_{1+2}$ straight toward the apex, costa ends at or slightly beyond the tip of $R_{4+5}$; mouth parts vestigial.........
.......... **GASTROPHILINÆ**. See **OESTRIDÆ**
mm. Sternopleurals present, if rarely absent then differing in other characters.
n. Caudal margin of the fifth ventral abdominal sclerite of the male deeply notched on the median line usually to beyond the middle; abdomen often cylindrical or linear; abdomen often with four to eight spots; eyes of the male usually widely separated; sternopleurals three, arranged in an equilateral triangle; subapical seta of the hind tibia placed very low; $M_{1+2}$ straight; anal vein abbreviated; wings not rilled. *Cænosia, Caricea, Dexiopsis, Hoplogaster, Schœnomyia*, etc. (CŒNOSINÆ)*..................
..................... ANTHOMYIIDÆ in part
nn. Caudal margin of the fifth ventral abdominal sclerite of the male incurved, rarely deeply cleft, rarely entire, in a few genera deeply two or three notched; $M_{1+2}$ straight

---

*There are several genera of flies of the family *Cordyluridæ* (i.e. *Acalyptratæ*) which might be placed with the *Anthomyiidæ* (i.e. *Calyptratæ*), owing to the relatively large size of their squamæ. As there is no single character which will satisfactorily separate all doubtful genera of these two groups we must arbitrarily fix the limits. In general those forms on the border line having a costal spine, or lower squama larger than the upper, or the lower surface of the scutellum more or less pubescent, or the eyes of the male nearly or quite contiguous, or the eyes hairy, or the frontal setæ decussate in the female; or any combination of these characters may at once be placed with the *Anthomyiidæ*. Those forms which lack these characteristics and have at least six abdominal segments (the first and second segments usually being more or less coalescent) are placed with the Acalyptrates. There are other acalyptrates with squamæ of moderate size which have either no vibrissæ, or have the subcosta either wholly lacking or coalescent in large part with $R_1$, or have spotted wings; they, therefore will not be confused with the calyptrates.

or curved; abdomen usually short or elongate oval; sternopleurals, if three are present, arranged in the order 1:2 in a right triangle. ....(MUSCINÆ-ANTHOMYIINÆ of Girschner)
 o. $M_{1+2}$ straight, hence cell $R_5$ not narrowed in the margin........**ANTHOMYIIDÆ** in part
 p. Underside of the scutellum more or less sparsely covered with fine hairs; anal vein nearly always reaches the hind margin of the wing; extensor surface of the hind tibiæ with a number of stout setæ; squamæ often small and equal. **Anthomyia,** *Chortophila, Eustalomyia, Hammomyia, Hylemyia, Prosalpia, Pegomyia,* etc.... **HYLEMYINÆ-PEGOMYINÆ**
 pp. Underside of the scutellum bare; anal vein does not reach the wing margin.
  q. First anal vein short, second anal suddenly flexed upwards; hind tibiæ each with one or two strong setæ on the extensor surface. **Fannia** (=**Homalomyia**), *Cœlomyia, Choristoma, Euryomma, Azelia,* etc. **FANNINÆ-AZELINÆ**
  qq. Anal veins parallel or divergent.
   r. Setæ on the exterior surface of the hind tibiæ wanting (except in *Limnaricia* and *Cœnosites*), lower squama not broadened to the margin of the scutellum. *Leucomelina, Limnophora, Limnospila, Lispa, Mydaea, Spilogaster,* etc. ................
........ MYDÆINÆ-LIMNOPHORINÆ
   rr. One (rarely more) seta on the extensor surface of the hind tibia; squamæ usually large and unequal. **Hydrotaea,** *Aricia, Drymeia, Ophyra, Phaonia* (=*Hyetodesia*), *Pogonomyia, Trichophthicus,* etc. **ARICINÆ**
 oo. $M_{1+2}$ curved or bent, hence the cell $R_5$ more or less narrowed in the margin. (**MUSCINÆ**). **MUSCIDÆ** in part. See page 303 for generic synopsis.
ll. Hypopleurals present; when three sternopleurals are present the arrangement is 2:1 or 1:1:1. ....................(TACHINIDÆ of Girschner)
 m. Conjunctiva of the ventral sclerites of the abdomen present, frequently well developed, surrounding the sclerites.

## Diptera

n. Mouth parts vestigial. **OESTRIDÆ.** See page 297 for generic synopsis.

nn. Mouth parts well developed.

   o. $M_{1+2}$ straight, hence cell $R_5$ wide open in the margin; costa ending at the tip of $R_5$; three sternopleurals present; antennal arista plumose. *Syllegoptera.* Europe.
....(SYLLEGOPTERINÆ)..DEXIIDÆ in part

   oo. $M_{1+2}$ bent, hence cell $R_5$ narrowed in the margin; sternopleurals rarely wanting, usually 1:1 or 0:1; facial plate strongly produced below vibrissal angle like the bridge of the nose; antennal arista bare. Parasitic on Hemiptera and Coleoptera. *Allophora, Cistogaster, Clytia, Phasia,* etc. (PHASIINÆ)..TACHINIDÆ in part.

mm. Conjunctiva of the ventral sclerites invisible (fig. 161a).

  n. Second ventral sclerite of the abdomen lying with its edges either upon or in contact with the ventral edges of the corresponding dorsal sclerite.

   o. Outermost posthumeral almost always lower (more ventrad) in position than the presutural macrochæta; fifth ventral abdominal sclerite of the male cleft beyond the middle, often strongly developed; body color very frequently metallic green or blue, or yellow; arista plumose. (**CALLIPHORINÆ**) ............**MUSCIDÆ** in part. See page 303 for generic synopsis.

   oo. Outermost posthumeral macrochæta on level or higher (more dorsad) than the presutural macrochæta; arista bare, pubescent, or plumose only on the basal two-thirds; body coloring usually grayish (fig. 106)..............**SARCOPHAGIDÆ**

    p. Fifth ventral sclerite of the male either wanting or with the caudal margin straight; presutural intraalar rarely present.............(**SARCOPHAGINÆ**)

    q. Fifth ventral abdominal sclerite of the male much reduced, the remaining segments with straight posterior margin, overlapping scale-like; in the female only segment one and two scale-like, the others wholly or in part covered; sternopleurals usually three or more. **Sarcophaga** and related genera.

qq. Fifth ventral sclerite of the male plainly visible; sternopleurals usually two. **Sarcophila, Wohlfahrtia,** *Brachycoma, Hilarella, Miltogramma, Metopia, Macronychia,, Nyctia, Paramacronychia, Pachyphthalmus,* etc.

pp. Fifth ventral abdominal sclerite of the male cleft to beyond the middle; ventral sclerites usually visible, shield-like. *Rhinophora, Phyto, Melanophora....* .................... RHINOPHORINÆ

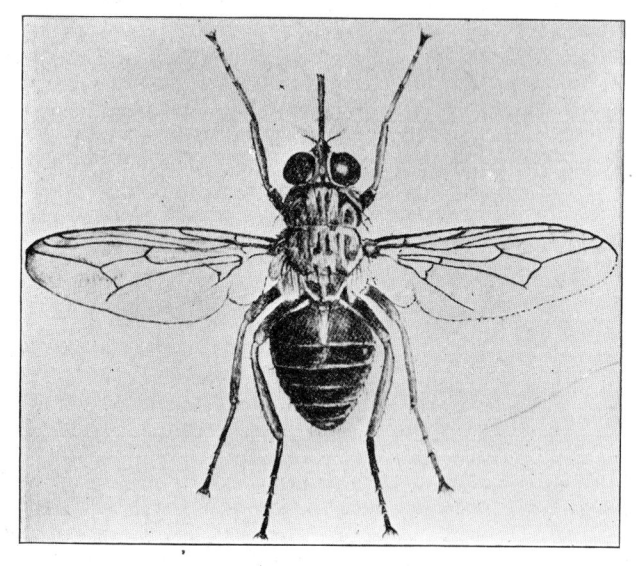

164. Glossina palpalis. (x4.) After Austen.

nn. Second ventral abdominal sclerite as well as the others more or less covered, sometimes wholly, by the edges of the dorsal sclerite.

o. The presutural intraalar wanting; ventral sclerites two to five nearly or quite covered by the edges of the corresponding dorsal sclerites; base of the antennæ usually at or below the middle of the eye; arista usually plumose; legs usually elongate; abdominal segments with marginal and often discal macrochætæ............DEXIIDÆ

oo. Presutural intraalar present, if absent, then the ventral sclerites broadly exposed or the fifth ventral sclerite vestigial;

## Muscidæ

base of the antennæ usually above the middle of the eye; arista bare; at least two posthumerals and three posterior intraalars present. Parasitic on caterpillars, etc................TACHINIDÆ

**SYNOPSIS OF THE PRINCIPAL GENERA OF THE MUSCIDÆ OF THE WORLD**

a. Proboscis long, directed forward, adapted for piercing, or oral margin much produced, snout-like.
 b. Oral margin produced snout-like; vibrissa placed high above the oral margin; antennal arista either pectinate or more or less plumose.
  c. Antennal arista short or long-plumose; neither sex with distinct orbital bristles.
   d. No facial carina between the antennæ ............ RHYNCHOMYIINÆ
    e. Arista short-plumose. *R. speciosa.* Europe....*Rhynchomyia* R. D.
    ee. Arista long-plumose. *I. phasina.* Europe and Egypt. *Idiopsis.* B. B.
   dd. With flattened carina, the bases of the antennæ separated; no abdominal macrochætæ.......................................COSMININÆ
    *C. fuscipennis.* South Africa......................*Cosmina*
  cc. Antennal arista pectinate; bases of the antennæ separated by a flattened carina.....................................RHINIINÆ R. D.
   d. Cell $R_5$ open, or closed at the margin.
    e. Third segment of the antenna twice as long as the second; claws of both sexes short; cell $R_5$ open. *I. lunata.* Eastern Hemisphere. ............................................*Idia* Meigen
    ee. Third segment of the antenna three times as long as the second; cell $R_5$ open or closed; claws of the male long and slender, of the female shorter than the last tarsal joint. *I. mandarina,* China. ............................................*Idiella* B. B.
   dd. Cell $R_5$ petiolate...................*Rhinia;* and *Beccarimyia* Rdi.
 bb. Proboscis long, directed forward, adapted for piercing....... **STOMOXINÆ**
  c. Arista flat, pectinate above with plumose rays; sternopleurals 1:2; bases of the veins $R_1$ and $R_{4+5}$ without setæ; base of the media bowed down; apical cell opens before the apex of the wing. African species ............................................**Glossina** Wied.
   d. Species measuring over twelve mm. in length. *G. longipennis* and **fusca**.
   dd. Species less than twelve mm. in length.
    e. All segments of the hind tarsi black.
     f. The fourth and fifth segments of the fore tarsi black; antennæ black (fig. 164).....................**G. palpalis** R. D.
     ff. Otherwise marked. ............ *G. bocagei, tachinoides, pallicera.*
    ee. First three segments of the hind tarsi are yellow, the fourth and fifth segments are black.
     f. Fourth and fifth segments of the first and second pair of tarsi are black.
      g. The yellow bands of the abdominal segments occupy a third of the segment (fig. 165)............**G. morsitans** Westw.
      gg. The yellow band on each segment of the abdomen occupies a sixth of the segment..................**G. longipalpis** Wied.

ff. Tarsi of the first and second pairs of legs wholly yellow..........
.....................................G. pallidipes Austen
cc. Rays of the arista not plumose; only one or two sternopleurals; base of the media not strongly bowed down; apical cell opens at or very near the apex of the wing.
　d. Vein $R_{4+5}$ without setæ at the base; palpi about as long as the proboscis.
　　e. Arista pectinate (i. e. rays on one side only), the rays often undulate; two yellow sternopleurals often difficult to detect; vein $M_{1+2}$ only slightly bent, the apical cell hence wide open. The horn fly, **H. irritans** ($=Lyperosia\ serrata$) and related species. Widely distributed (figs. 167, 168) ............**Hæmatobia** R. D. not B. B.

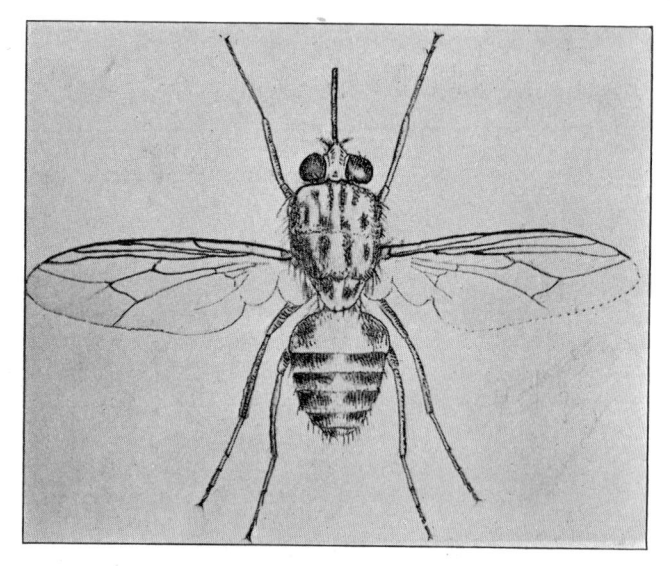

165. Glossina morsitans. (x4.) After Austen.

　　ee. Arista also with rays below; vein $M_{1+2}$ more strongly bent, the apical cell hence less widely open.
　　　f. Palpi strongly spatulate at the tips, lower rays of the arista about six in number, **B. sanguinolentus.** South Asia..............
.....................................**Bdellolarynx** Austen
　　　ff. Palpi feebly spatulate; apical cell of the wing narrowly open slightly before the tip; sternopleurals black, anterior bristle sometimes absent. **H. atripalpis.** Europe................
.....................................**Hæmatobosca** Bezzi
　dd. Vein $R_{4+5}$ with setæ at the base.*

---

*Pachymyia* Macq. is closely related to *Stomoxys*. It differs in having the arista rayed both above and below. *P. vexans*, Brazil.

## Muscidæ

 e. Veins $R_1$ and $R_{4+5}$ with setæ at the base; two equally prominent sternopleural macrochætæ; arista with rays both above and below; palpi as long as the proboscis; apical cell of the wing wide open. **L. tibialis.** (*Hæmatobia* B. B. not R. D.)................................................**Lyperosiops** Town.
 ee. Only vein $R_{4+5}$ with basal setæ; anterior sternopleural macrochæta wanting; arista pectinate.
   f. Palpi as long as the proboscis, the latter stout, with fleshy terminal labellæ; apical cell narrowly open; sternopleural macrochætæ black. **S. maculosa** from Africa and related species from Asia............................**Stygeromyia** Austen
   ff. Palpi much shorter than the proboscis, the latter pointed at the apex, without fleshy labellæ; apical cell of the wing wide open. **S. calcitrans**, the stable fly and related species. Widely distributed in both hemispheres (fig. 110)........**Stomoxys** Geof.
aa. Proboscis neither slender nor elongate, the labellæ fleshy and not adapted for piercing.
 b. Hypopleuræ without a vertical row of macrochætæ............**MUSCINÆ**
  c. Arista bare; distal portion of $R_{4+5}$ broadly curved at the end; hypopleurae with a sparse cluster of fine hairs. *S. braziliana*, Southern States and southward........................ *Synthesiomyia* B. B.
  cc. Arista pectinate or plumose.
   d. Arista pectinate. *H. vittigera*, with the posterior half of the abdomen metallic blue. Mexico....................*Hemichlora* V. d. W.
   dd. Arista plumose.
    e. Middle tibia with one or more prominent setæ on the inner (flexor) surface beyond the middle, or inner surface very hairy.
     f. $R_1$ ends distad of the m-cu crossvein; $R_{4+5}$ with a broad curve near its apical end. (=*Neomesembrina* Schnabl, =*Metamesembrina* Town). *M. meridiana.* Europe.... *Mesembrina* Meigen
     ff. $R_1$ ends proximad of the m-cu crossvein.
      g. Eyes pilose, sometimes sparsely in the female.
       h. Female with two or three stout orbital setæ; the hind metatarsus of the male thickened below at the base and penicillate. *D. pratorum.* Europe ............ *Dasyphora* R. D.*
       hh. Neither sex with orbital setæ.
        i. Abdomen without macrochætæ; arista plumose. *C. asiatica.* Eastern Hemisphere.... *Cryptolucilia* B. B.
        ii. Abdomen with strong macrochætæ; arista very short-plumose, nearly bare. *B. tachinina.* Brazil..........................................*Reinwardtia* B. B.
      gg. Eyes bare.
       h. Body densely pilose; thoracic macrochætæ wanting; middle tibiæ much elongate and bent; last section of $R_{4+5}$ with a gentle curve. H. (*Mesembrina*) *mystacea, et al.*, Europe and *H. solitaria*, N. America....*Hypodermodes* Town.
       hh. Body not densely pilose.

---

*The genus *Eudasyphora* Town. has recently been erected to contain *D. lasiophthalma*.

i. Dorsocentrals six; last section of $R_{4+5}$ with a gentle curve.
   j. Inner dorsocentrals ("acrostichals") wanting; sternopleurals arranged 1:3.  *P. cyanicolor, cadaverina*, etc. Europe and America.................*Pyrellia* R. D.
   jj. Inner dorsocentrals ("acrostichals") present; sternopleurals arranged 1:2. *E. latreillii.* North America.
   ..........................*Eumesembrina* Town.
  ii. Dorsocentrals five; inner dorsocentrals present; last section of $R_{4+5}$ with a rounded angle; sternopleurals arranged 1:2. *P. cornicina* Europe and America. (*Pseudopyrellia* Girsch.)................*Orthellia* R. D.
ee. Middle tibia without a prominent bristle on the inner surface beyond the middle.

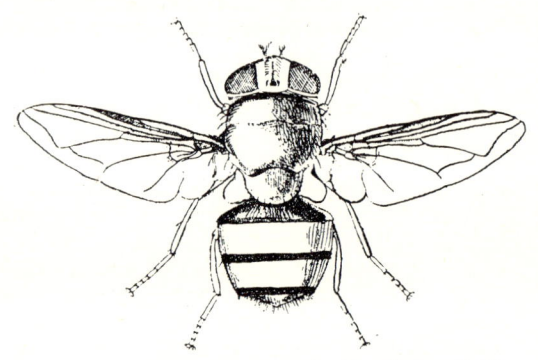

166. Pycnosoma marginale. (x4.)   After Graham-Smith.

 f. Squamula thoracalis broadened mesad and caudad as far as the scutellum.
  g. Sternopleural macrochætæ arranged in an equilateral triangle; front of both sexes broad; genæ bare; dorsocentrals six, small; wing not rilled. (To COENOSINÆ). *Atherigona* Rdi.
  gg. Sternopleural macrochætæ when three are present, arranged in a right triangle.
   h. Last section of $R_{4+5}$ with a more or less rounded angle (fig. 163l).
    i. Eyes of the male pilose or pubescent, of the female nearly bare; m-cu crossvein usually at or proximad of the mid-distance between the r-m crossvein and the bend of $R_{4+5}$. P. (= *Placomyia* R. D.) *vitripennis*............
    ..............................*Plaxemyia* R. D.
    ii. Eyes bare; the m-cu crossvein always nearer to the bend of $R_{4+5}$ than to the r-m crossvein.
     j. Apex of the proboscis when extended reveals a circlet of stout chitinous teeth. **P. insignis** Austen, of India, bites both man and animals. (= *Pristirhynchomyia*) ......................**Philæmatomyia** Austen

jj. Apex of the proboscis without black teeth.
  k. Eyes of male separated by a distance equal to a fourth the width of the head. House or typhoid fly. **M. domestica** L. Widely distributed..**Musca** L.
  kk. Eyes of the male contiguous. **E. corvina.** Europe. ............................**Eumusca** Town
hh. Last section of $R_{4+5}$ with a gentle curve (fig. 102).
  i. Eyes pilose.
    j. Claws in the male somewhat elongated; no orbitals in either sex; antennæ separated at the base by a flat carina; abdomen marked with red or yellow. *G. maculata.* Europe and America....*Graphomyia* R. D.
    jj. Claws short and equal in the two sexes; two or three stout orbital macrochætæ in the female; $R_1$ scarcely produced beyond the r-m crossvein; eyes contiguous in the male. *P. obsoleta.* Brazil ..*Phasiophana* Br.
  ii. Eyes bare; fronto-orbital macrochætæ in a double row, antennæ contiguous at the base.
    j. One or more pairs of well developed anterior inner dorso-central (acrostichal) macrochætæ; seta on extensor surface of hind tibia. **M. assimilis, stabulans,** etc. Europe and America..............**Muscina** R. D.
    jj. Anterior inner dorsocentrals and the setæ on the extensor surface of the hind tibia wanting. *M. micans,* etc. Europe and North America....*Morellia* R. D.
ff. Squamula thoracalis not broadened mesad and caudad, not reaching the margin of the scutellum; macrochætæ on extensor surface of the hind tibia wanting.
  g. Eyes pubescent. *M. meditabunda.* Europe and America. ..................................*Myiospila* Rdi.
  gg. Eyes bare; $R_1$ ends before the middle of the wing. A number of species from the tropics of both hemispheres. .......... .................................*Clinopera* V. d. W.
bb. Hypopleuræ with a vertical row of macrochætæ.
  c. Eyes pubescent.
    d. $R_1$ ends about opposite the r-m crossvein; basal section of $R_{4+5}$ bristly nearly to the crossvein; *S. enigmatica.* Africa. *Somalia* Hough
    dd. $R_1$ ends distad of the r-m crossvein.
      e. Eastern hemisphere. Australasia. *N. ochracea, dasypthalma.* ......................................*Neocalliphora* Br.
      ee. Western Hemisphere. *T. muscinum.* Mexico..*Tyreomma* V. d. W.
  cc. Eyes bare.
    d. The vibrissal angle situated at a noticeable distance above the level of the margin of the mouth.
      e. Sternopleural macrochætæ arranged in the order 1:1.
        f. Genæ with microchætæ.
          g. Body grayish, with depressed yellow woolly hair among the macrochætæ; wings folded longitudinally over the body when

at rest. Cluster flies. *P. rudis* and related species, widely distributed............................ *Pollenia* R. D.*
gg. Body metallic blue or green. Eastern Hemisphere.
  h. Vibrissal angle placed very high above the oral margin; a carina between the antennæ; outer posthumeral wanting; anterior intraalar present. *T. viridaurea.* Java ......
................................................ *Thelychæta* Br.

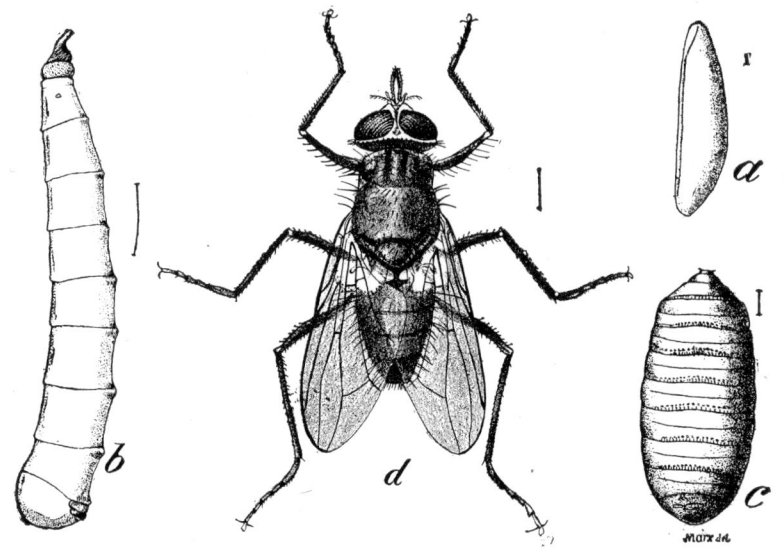

167. Horn fly. (*a*) egg; (*b*) larva; (*c*) puparium; (*d*) adult. (x4). Bureau of Entomology

  hh. Vibrissal angle moderately high above the oral margin; carina small or wanting; no post humeral macrochæta; lower squamæ hairy above. (=*Paracompsomyia* Hough) (fig. 166)...................... *Pycnosoma* Br.
  ff. Genæ bare. *S. terminata.* Eastern Hemisphere.............
...................................... *Strongyloneura* Bigot
ee. Sternopleurals arranged 2:1.
  f. Body metallic green or blue, with gray stripes; genæ hairy to the lower margin; post humerals often wanting; lower squamæ bare above. (=*Compsomyia* Rdi.) ............ **Chrysomyia** R. D.
    g. With one or two orbitals; height of bucca less than half the height of the eye. South and east U. S. (fig. 107).........
.............................................**C. marcellaria**
    gg. No orbitals; height of bucca about a third less than height of eye. West U. S.................... *C. wheeleri* Hough

---

*\**Nitellia*, usually included in this genus has the apical cell petiolate. *Apollenia* Bezzi, has recently been separated from *Pollenia* to contain the species *P. nudiuscula.* Both genera belong to the Eastern hemisphere.

ff. Body black or sordidly metallic greenish gray, usually yellow pollinose or variegate; genæ at most hairy above. *N. stygia*. Eastern Hemisphere........................*Neopollenia* Br.
dd. Vibrissal angle situated nearly on a level of the oral margin.
  e. Species wholly blackish, bluish, or greenish metallic in color.
    f. First section of $R_{4+5}$ with at most three or four small bristles at the immediate base.
      g. The bend of $R_{4+5}$ a gentle curve; costal spine present; cell $R_5$ closed, ending before the apex of the wing. *S. cuprina*. Java..............................*Synamphoneura* Bigot
      gg. Bend of $R_{4+5}$ angular; or the insect differs in other characters; dorsal surface of the squamula thoracalis hairy (except in *Melinda*); arista plumose only on the basal two-thirds (except usually in *Calliphora* and *Eucalliphora*).

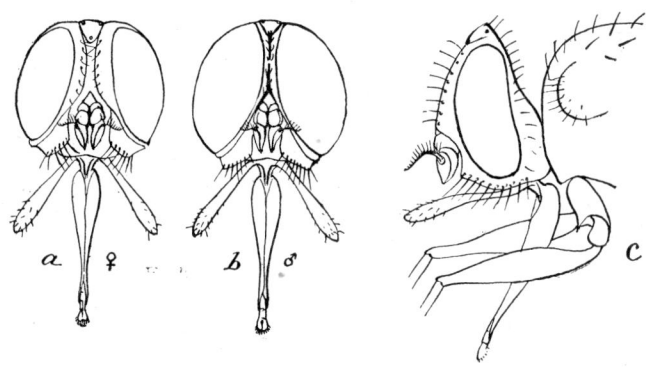

168. Head of horn-fly (Lyperosia irritans); (*a*) female; (*b*) male; (*c*) lateral aspect of female.

    h. Arista plumose only on the basal two-thirds.
      i. Base of the antennæ ventrad of the middle of the eye; eyes of the male nearly contiguous; genæ hairy; second abdominal segment with median marginal macrochætæ; two, rarely three, postsutural intraalar macrochætæ.
        j. Squamula thoracalis dorsally with long black hairs; male hypopgium two-segmented, large, projecting; claws and pullvilli of the male elongate; three strong sternopleural macrochætæ; genæ at least half the width of the eye; buccæ (cheeks) half the height of the eyes; oviviparous. *O. sepulcralis*. Europe......*Onesia* R. D.
        jj. Dorsal surface of the squamula thoracalis bare; male hypopygium small, scarcely projecting below; claws and pulvilli not elongate; two stout sternopleural macrochætæ, sometimes with a delicate one below the anterior; genæ nearly linear in the male; buccæ about a third of the eye height; oviparous. *M. cærulea*. Europe.........................*Melinda*. R. D.

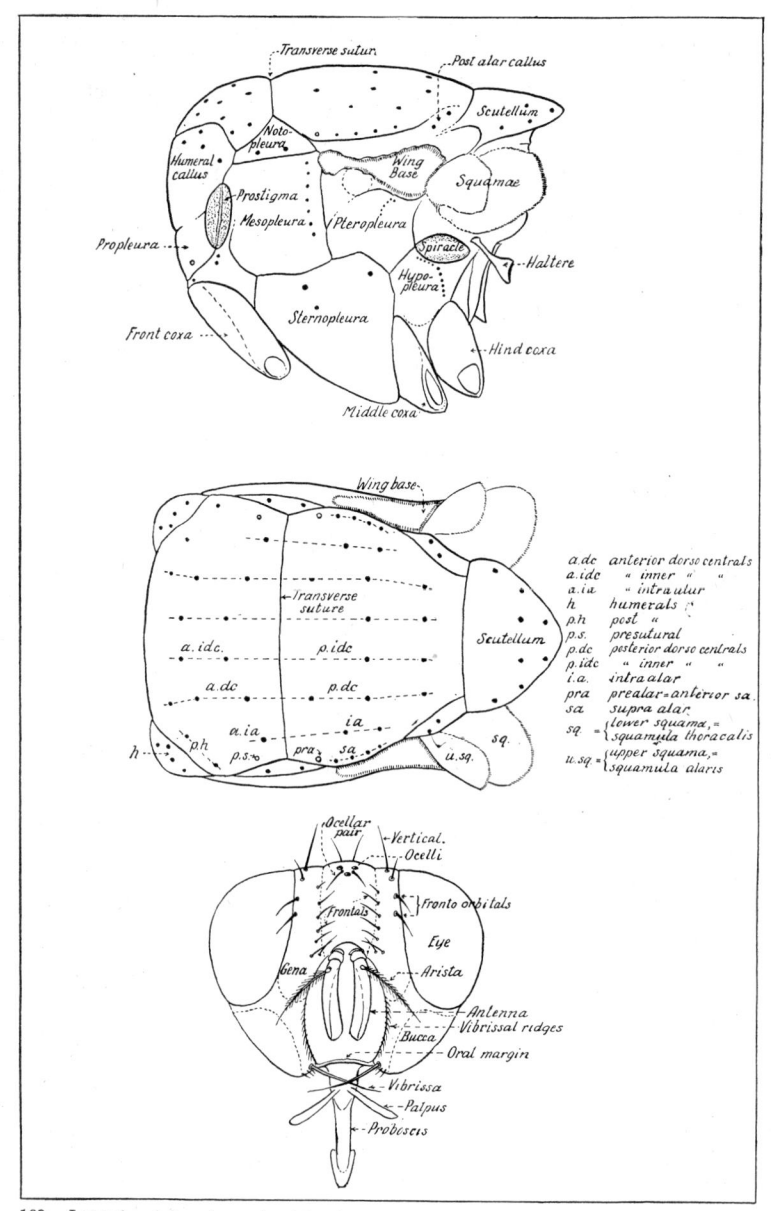

169. Lateral and dorsal aspects of the thorax, and frontal aspect of the head of a muscoidean fly, with designations of the parts commonly used in taxonomic work.

*Muscidæ* 311

ii. Base of the antennæ dorsad of the middle of the eye; eyes of both sexes distinctly separated; dorsal surface of the squamula thoracalis with black hairs; two post sutural intraalar macrochætæ.

j. Hypopygium of the male large, with a pair of slightly curved forceps whose ends are concealed in a longitudinal slit in the fifth ventral sclerite; third posterior inner dorso-central (acrostichal) macrochætæ absent; anterior intraalar rarely present; abdomen usually not pollinose; the second segment without median marginal macrochætæ; face yellow. *C. mortuorum, cadaverina,* and related species. Both hemispheres.
..................................*Cynomyia* R. D.*

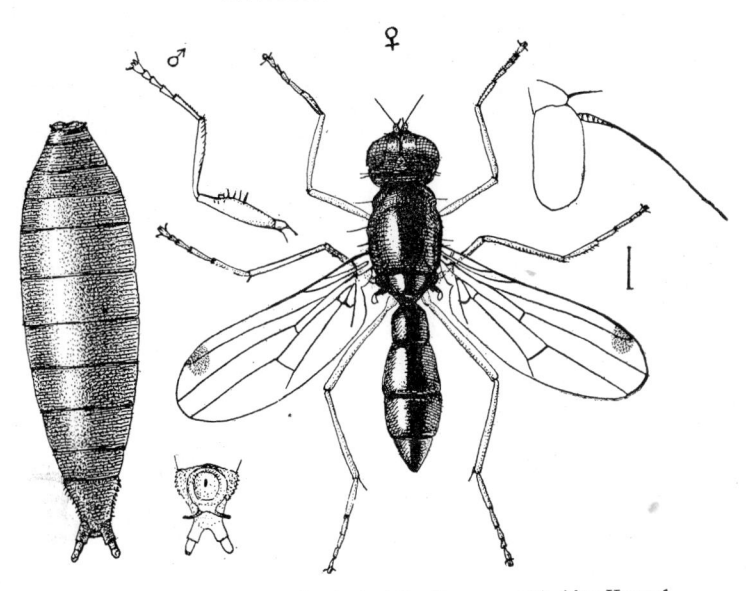

170. Sepsis violacea; puparium and adult. (See page 297.) After Howard.

jj. Three pairs of posterior inner dorsocentrals (acrostichals) present; second abdominal segment with a row of marginal macrochætæ; genæ hairy, at least above.

k. Hypopygium of the male with a projecting style. *S. stylifera.* Europe............*Steringomyia* Pok.

---

*The following three genera are not sufficiently well defined to place in this synopsis. In color and structural characters they are closely related to *Cynomyia* from which they may be distinguished as follows. *Catapicephala* Macq., represented by the species *C. splendens* from Java, has the setæ on the facial ridges rising to the base of the antennæ and has median marginal macrochætæ on the abdominal segments two to four: *Blepharicnema* Macq., represented by *B. splendens* from Venezuela has bare genæ, oral setæ not ascending; tibiæ villose; claws short in both sexes; *Sarconesia* Bigot with the species *S. chlorogaster* from Chile, setose genæ; legs slender, not villose; claws of the male elongate.

           kk. Hypopygium of the male without style.  A. *stelviana*
              B. B...........................*Acrophaga* B. B.
       hh. Arista usually plumose nearly to the tip; posterior dorso-
           centrals and inner dorsocentrals (acrostichals) well
           developed; dorsal surface of the squamula thoracalis
           hairy; abdomen metallic and usually pollinose; genæ
           hairy.
           i. With one pair of ocellar macrochætæ. **C. vomitoria,
              erythrocephala, viridescens**, and related species. Both
              hemispheres........................**Calliphora** R. D.
           ii. With two strong pairs of ocellar macrochætæ..*E. latifrons*.
              Pacific slope of the U. S........*Eucalliphora* Town.
    ff. First section of $R_{4+5}$ bristly near or quite half way to the small
        crossvein; dorsal surface of the squamula thoracalis is bare;
        the hypopygium of the male is inconspicuous.
        g. Genæ bare; posterior inner and outer dorsocentrals distinct
           and well developed. *L. cæsar, sericata, sylvarum*, and
           related species. Widely distributed in both hemispheres
           (fig. 103)..............................*Lucilia* R. D.
        gg. Genæ with microchætæ, at least down to the level of the base
            of the arista.
            h. Mesonotum flattened behind the transverse suture.
               i. Posterior dorsocentrals inconstant and unequally developed;
                  one pair of posterior inner dorsocentrals. *P. terraenovæ*.
                  North America.................*Protophormia* Town.
               ii. Posterior dorsocentrals well developed, the inner dorso-
                   centrals (acrostichals) unequally developed. *P. azurea,
                   chrysorrhœa*, etc. Europe and America..............
                   ............................*Protocalliphora* Hough
            hh. Mesonotum not flattened behind the transverse suture;
                posterior inner and outer dorsocentrals inconstant
                and unequally developed. *P. regina*. Europe and
                America............................**Phormia** R. D.
  ee. Species more or less rufous or yellow in color.
    f. Anterior dorsocentrals wanting; first section of the $R_{4+5}$ at most
       only bristly at the base, bend near apex rectangular, $R_1$ ends over
       the crossvein; fronto-orbital macrochæta absent; eyes of the
       male contiguous. *C. semiviridis*. Mexico..*Chloroprocta* V. d. W
    ff. With another combination of characters.
        g. Body robust, of large size, abdomen elongate, not round; genæ
           with several ranges of microchætæ; vibrissal ridges strongly
           convergent; abdomen with well developed macrochætæ;
           costal spine usually absent; eyes of the male widely separated.
           h. Peristome broad, pteropleural macrochætæ distinct; one or
              two sternopleurals; in the female a single orbital macro-
              chæta; last abdominal segment without discal macro-
              chætæ; hypopygial processes of the male with a long
              stylet; second abdominal segment of the female sometimes

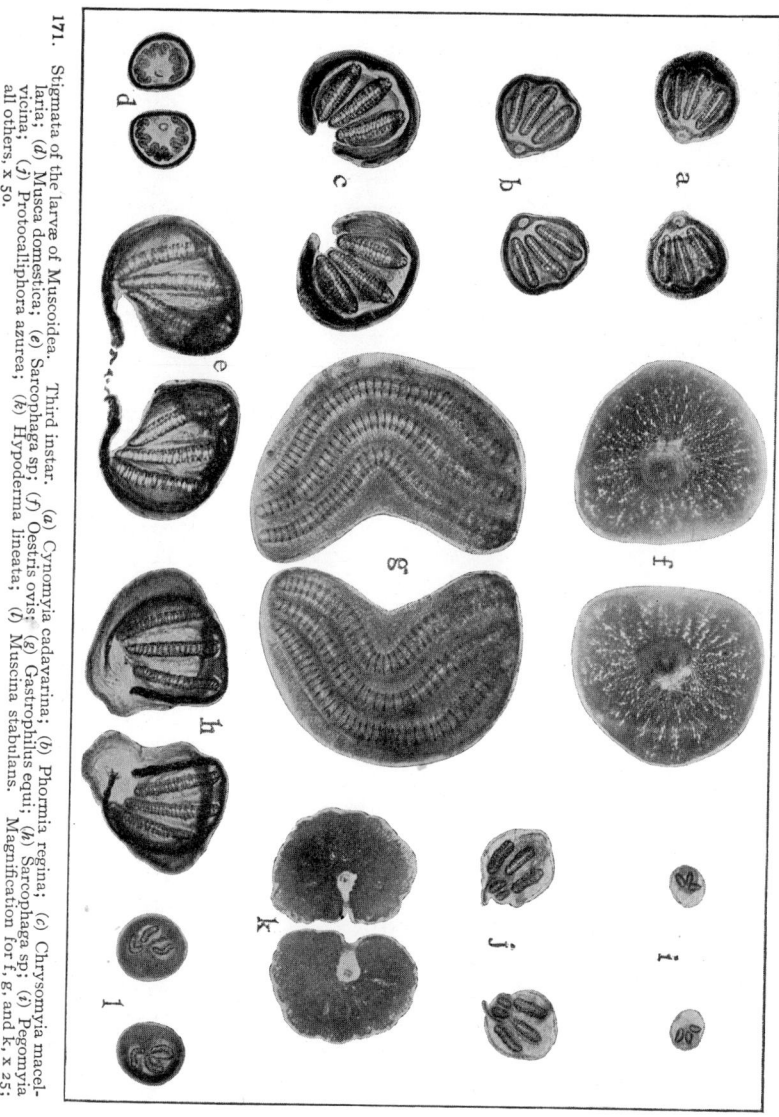

171. Stigmata of the larvæ of Muscoidea. Third instar. (*a*) Cynomyia cadavarina; (*b*) Phormia regina; (*c*) Chrysomyia macellaria; (*d*) Musca domestica; (*e*) Sarcophaga sp; (*f*) Oestris ovis; (*g*) Gastrophilus equi; (*h*) Sarcophaga sp; (*i*) Pegomyia vicina; (*j*) Protocalliphora azurea; (*k*) Hypoderma lineata; (*l*) Muscina stabulans. Magnification for f, g, and k, x 25; all others, x 50.

much elongate. **A. luteola** (fig. 86). Africa. The subgenus *Chæromyia* Roub. is included here. **Auchmeromyia** B.B.

hh. Peristome narrow; no pteropleurals, two sternopleurals; two orbitals in the female; second segment not elongate; the fourth with two well developed discal macrochætæ. **B. depressa.** Africa.................**Bengalia** R. D

gg. With another combination of characters.

h. Costal spine present; body in part black; antennæ noticeably shorter than the epistome, inserted above the middle of the eye and separated from each other by a carina; abdominal segments with marginal macrochætæ; sternopleurals 2:1 or 1:1...................*Paratricyclea* Villen.

hh. Costal spine not distinct, or if present, insect otherwise different.

i. Genæ with several ranges of microchætæ; vibrissal ridges strongly converging; peristome broad; arista moderately plumose; sternopleurals usually 1:1; color entirely testaceous. **C. anthropophaga** (fig. 87) and **grunbergi.** Africa...........................**Cordylobia** Grünb.

ii. Genæ bare or with but one range of setæ; vibrissal ridges less converging; peristome narrow; arista long plumose.

j. Genæ with a single row of microchætæ.

k. Sternopleurals 2:1; color entirely testaceous......... ............................*Ochromyia* Macq.*

kk. Sternopleurals 1:1. *P. varia* Hough. Africa....... ......................*Parochromyia* Hough.

jj. Genæ bare.

k. Basal section of $R_{4+5}$ bristly only at the immediate base, distal section with a broad curve; distal portion of the abdomen metallic; sternopleurals usually 1:1, rarely 2:1. *M. æneiventris* Wd. Tropic America...................*Mesembrinella*. G. T.

kk. $R_{4+5}$ bristly at least nearly half way to the small crossvein; sternopleurals 1:1.

l. Macrochætæ of the abdomen marginal; neither sex with orbitals; no carina between the base of the antennæ; three pairs of presutural inner dorsocentrals. Eastern hemisphere. *T. ferruginea. Tricyclea* V. d. W. ( = *Zonochroa* B. B. according to Villeneuve 1914).

ll. Abdomen without macrochætæ; wing usually with a marginal streak and gray markings. Brazil ............................*Hemilucilia* B. B.

---

*Plinthomyia* Rdi. and *Hemigymnochæta* Corti are related to *Ochromyia*, though too briefly described to place in the key.

*Muscoidea* 315

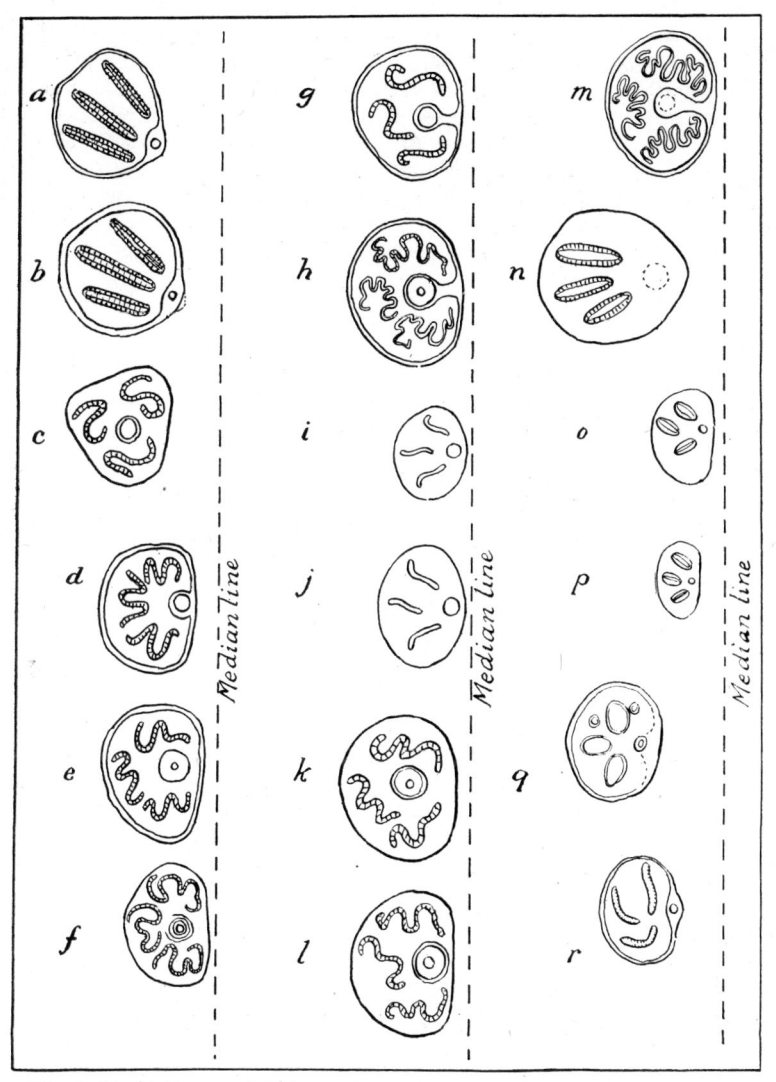

172. Left hand stigmata of the larvæ of muscoidea. Third instar. (*a*) Lucilia cæsar; (*b*) Calliphora vomitoria; (*c*) Stomoxys calcitrans; (*d*) Pseudopyrellia cornicina; (*e*) Pyrellia cadavarina; (*f*) Lyperosia irritans; (*g*) Mesembrina mystacea; (*h*) Mesembrina meridiana; (*i*) Myospila meditabunda; (*j*) Mydæa umbana; (*k*) Polietes albolineata; (*l*) Polietes lardaria; (*m*) Morellia hortorum; (*n*) Hydrotæa dentipes; (*o*) Hebecnema umbratica; (*p*) H. vespertina; (*q*) Limnophora septemnotata; (*r*) Muscina stabulans. (*a* and *b*) after MacGregor; (*d*) after Banks; all others after Portchinsky. Magnification varies. The relative distance to the median line is indicated in each figure.

## SIPHONAPTERA. Fleas
### Adapted from a table published by Oudemans.

a. Elongated fleas, with jointed (articulated) head, with combs (ctenidia) on head and thorax; with long, oval, free-jointed flagellum of the antenna (fig. 92d).................................Suborder FRACTICIPATA
  b. With ctenidia in front of the antennæ and on the genæ (cheeks); maxillæ with acute apices; labial palpi five-segmented, symmetrical; eyes poorly developed or wanting. On rodents..............HYSTRICHOPSYLLIDÆ
    c. Abdominal segments without ctenidia.
      d. Post-tibial spines in pairs and not in a very close set row; head with ctenidia.................................*Ctenophthalmus* Kol.
      dd. Post-tibial spines mostly single and in a close set row. *Ctenopsyllus* and *Leptopsyllus*. The last genus has recently been erected for *L. musculi*, a widely distributed species occurring on rats and mice.
    cc. Abdominal segments with one or more ctenidia; post-tibial spines in numerous, short, close-set transverse rows on posterior border with about four spines in each row. *H. americana*..*Hystrichopsylla* Taschenb.
  bb. With only two pairs of subfrontal ctenidia; labial palpi five-segmented, symmetrical; eyes vestigial or wanting. On bats. (=ISCHNOPSYLLIDÆ).........................................NYCTERIDIPSYLLIDÆ
With more or less blunt maxilla; all tibiæ with notch; a single antepygidial bristle; metepimeron without ctenidium. *N. crosbyi* from Missouri was found on bats. Rothschild suggests that this is probably the same as *N. insignis*.
    .................. (=*Ischnopsyllus* = *Ceratopsyllus*), *Nycteridiphilus*
aa. Head not jointed, i.e. the segments coalescent, traces of the segmentation still being visible in the presence of the vertex tubercle, the falx (sickle-shaped process), and a suture............Suborder INTEGRICIPITA
  b. Flagellum of the antennæ long and oval.
    c. Usually elongate fleas, with a free-segmented flagellum of the antenna; thorax not shorter than the head, longer than the first tergite.
      d. Genæ of the head and the pronotum with ctenidia....NEOPSYLLIDÆ
        e. Labial palpi four or five-segmented; symmetrical; hind coxæ with patch of spines inside; row of six spatulate spines on each side in front of the antennæ. *C. ornata* found on a California mole .............................................. *Corypsylla*
        ee. Labial palpi two-segmented, transparent, membranous. On hares...................................*Spilopsyllus* Baker
      dd. No ctenidium on the head.
        e. Pronotum with ctenidium....................**DOLICHOPSYLLIDÆ**
          f. Labial palpi five-segmented, symmetrical.
            g. Antepygidial bristles one to three; eyes present.
              h. Inner side of hind coxæ distally with a comb of minute teeth; falx present. On rodents and carnivores................
                ..................................*Odontopsyllus* Baker
              hh. Inner side of hind coxæ without comb or teeth. Many North American species on rodents....................
                ................................**Ceratophyllus** Curtis

gg. Antepygidial bristles five on each side; eyes absent; suture
white. *D. stylosus* on rodents......,.. *Dolichopsyllus* Baker
ff. Labial palpi four or five-segmented; asymmetrical (membranous
behind), apex acute. *Hoplopsyllus anomalus* found on Spermophiles in Colorado........................HOPLOPSYLLIDÆ
ee. Pronotum without ctenidium. *Anomiopsyllus californicus* and
*nudatus* on rodents........................ANOMIOPSYLLIDÆ
cc. Very short fleas; flagellum of the antenna with pseudo-segments coalescent; thorax much shorter than the head and than the first tergite
............................................. HECTOPSYLLIDÆ
Flagellum of the antenna with six coalescent pseudo-segments; maxilla
blunt. The chigger on man (fig. 93). **D. penetrans**................
............ ( = **Rhynchoprion** = **Sarcopsylla**) **Dermatophilus** Guérin
bb. Flagellum short, round, free portion of the first segment shaped like a
mandolin.
c. Thorax not shorter than the head, longer than the first tergite; flagellum
either with free segments or in part with the segments coalescent.
d. Head and pronotum with ctenidium; labial palpi asymmetrical....
........................................ ARCHÆOPSYLLIDÆ
With four subfrontal, four genal, and one angular ctenidia. Widely
distributed ............................. **Ctenocephalus** Kol.
e. Head rounded in front (fig. 92a). Dog flea ..............**C. canis**
ee. Head long and flat (fig. 92b). Cat flea..................**C. felis**
dd. Neither head nor pronotum with ctenidium. Labial palpi asymmetrical, membranous behind........................ PULICIDÆ
e. Mesosternite narrow, without internal rod-like thickening from the
insertion of the coxæ upwards. Human flea, etc...... **Pulex** L.
ee. Mesosternite broad with a rod-like internal thickening from the
insertion of the coxæ upwards (fig. 89). **X.** (**Lœmopsylla**) **cheopis**,
plague or rat flea ................................ **Xenopsylla**
cc. Thorax much shorter than the head and than the first tergite. **Echidnophagidæ. E. gallinacea,** the hen flea also attacks man (fig. 96).
..................( = **Argopsylla** = **Xestopsylla**) **Echidnophaga** Olliff.

# APPENDIX

## HYDROCYANIC ACID GAS AGAINST HOUSEHOLD INSECTS

The following directions for fumigating with hydrocyanic acid gas are taken from Professor Herrick's circular published by the Cornell Reading Course:

Hydrocyanic acid gas has been used successfully against household insects and will probably be used more and more in the future. It is particularly effective against bed-bugs, and cockroaches, but because *it is such a deadly poison it must be used very carefully.*

The gas is generated from the salt potassium cyanid, by treating it with sulfuric acid diluted with water. Potassium cyanid is a most poisonous substance and the gas emanating from it is also deadly to most, if not all, forms of animal life. The greatest care must always be exercised in fumigating houses or rooms in buildings that are occupied. Before fumigation a house should be vacated. It is not necessary to move furniture or belongings except brass or nickel objects, which may be somewhat tarnished, and butter, milk, and other larder supplies that are likely to absorb gas. If the nickel and brass fixtures or objects are carefully covered with blankets they will usually be sufficiently protected.

There may be danger in fumigating one house in a solid row of houses if there is a crack in the walls through which the gas may find its way. It also follows that the fumigation of one room in a house may endanger the occupants of an adjoining room if the walls between the two rooms are not perfectly tight. It is necessary to keep all these points in mind and to do the work deliberately and thoughtfully. The writer has fumigated a large college dormitory of 253 rooms, once a year for several years, without the slightest accident of any kind. In order to fumigate this building about 340 pounds of cyanid and the same amount of sulfuric acid were used each time. In addition to this, the writer has fumigated single rooms and smaller houses with the gas. In one instance the generating jars were too small; the liquid boiled over and injured the floors and the rugs. Such an accident should be avoided by the use of large jars and by placing old rugs or a quantity of newspapers beneath the jars.

## The Proportions of Ingredients

Experiments and experience have shown that the potassium cyanid should be ninety-eight per cent pure in order to give satisfactory results. The purchaser should insist on the cyanid being of at least that purity, and it should be procurable at not more than forty cents per pound. The crude form of sulfuric acid may be used. It is a thickish, brown liquid and should not cost more than four or five cents a pound. If a room is made tight, one ounce of cyanid for every one hundred cubic feet of space has been shown to be sufficient. It is combined with the acid and water in the following proportions:

| | |
|---|---|
| Potassium cyanid | 1 ounce |
| Commercial sulfuric acid | 1 fluid ounce |
| Water | 3 fluid ounces |

### A Single Room as an Example

Suppose a room to be 12 by 15 by 8 feet. It will contain 12 x 15 x 8, or 1440 cubic feet. For convenience the writer always works on the basis of complete hundreds; in this case he would work on the basis of 1500 cubic feet, and thus be sure to have enough. The foregoing room, then, would require 15 ounces of cyanid, 15 ounces of sulfuric acid, and 45 ounces of water. The room should be made as tight as possible by stopping all the larger openings, such as fireplaces and chimney flues, with old rags or blankets. Cracks about windows or in other places should be sealed with narrow strips of newspaper well soaked in water. Strips of newspaper two or three inches wide that have been thoroughly soaked in water may be applied quickly and effectively over the cracks around the window sash and elsewhere. Such strips will stick closely for several hours and may be easily removed at the conclusion of the work.

While the room is being made tight, the ingredients should be measured according to the formula already given. The water should be measured and *poured first* into a stone jar for holding at least two gallons. The jar should be placed in the middle of the room, with an old rug or several newspapers under it in order to protect the floor.

The required amount of sulfuric acid should then be poured rather slowly into the water. *This process must never be reversed;* that is, *the acid must never be poured into the jar first.* The cyanid should be weighed and put into a paper bag beside the jar. All hats, coats, or other articles that will be needed before the work is over should be removed from the room. When everything is ready the operator should drop the bag of cyanid gently into the jar, holding his breath, and should walk quickly out of the room. The steam-like gas does not rise immediately under these conditions, and ample time is given for the operator to walk out and shut the door. If preferred, however, the paper bag may be suspended by a string passing through a screw eye in the ceiling and then through the keyhole of the door. In this case the bag may be lowered from the outside after the operator has left the room and closed the door.

The writer has most often started the fumigation toward evening and left it going all night, opening the doors in the morning. The work can be done, however, at any time during the day and should extend over a period of five or six hours at least. It is said that better results will be obtained in a temperature of 70° F., or above, than at a lower degree.

At the close of the operation the windows and doors may be opened from the outside. In the course of two or three hours the gas should be dissipated enough to allow a person to enter the room without danger. The odor of the gas is like that of peach kernels and is easily recognized. The room should not be occupied until the odor has disappeared.

## Fumigating a Large House

The fumigation of a large house is merely a repetition, in each room and hall, of the operations already described for a single room. All the rooms should be made tight, and the proper quantities of water and sulfuric acid should be measured and poured into jars placed in each room with the cyanid in bags besides the jars. When all is ready, the operator should *go to the top floor and work downward* because the gas is lighter than air and tends to rise.

## Precautions

The cyanid should be broken up into small pieces not larger than small eggs. This can best be done on a cement or brick pavement. It would be advantageous to wear gloves in order to protect the hands, although the writer has broken many pounds of cyanid without any protection on the hands. Wash the hands thoroughly at frequent intervals in order to remove the cyanid.

The operations of the work must be carried out according to directions.

The work should be done by a calm, thoughtful and careful person—best by one who has had some experience.

Conspicuous notices of what has been done should be placed on the doors, and the doors should be locked so that no one can stray into the rooms.

The gas is lighter than air, therefore one should always begin in the rooms at the top of the house and work down.

After fumigation is over the contents of the jar should be emptied into the sewer or some other safe place. The jars should be washed thoroughly before they are used again.

*It must be remembered that cyanid is a deadly poison;* but it is very efficient against household insects, if carefully used, and is not particularly dangerous when properly handled.

## LESIONS PRODUCED BY THE BITE OF THE BLACK-FLY

While this text was in press there came to hand an important paper presenting a phase of the subject of black fly injury so different from others heretofore given that we deem it expedient to reproduce here the author's summary. The paper was published in *The Journal of Cutaneous Diseases*, for November and December, 1914, under the title of "A Clinical, Pathological and Experimental Study of the Lesions Produced by the Bite of the Black Fly" (*Simulium venustum*)," by Dr. John Hinchman Stokes, of the University of Michigan.

### Resume and Discussion of Experimental Findings

The principal positive result of the work has been the experimental reproduction of the lesion produced by the black-fly in characteristic histological detail by the use of preserved flies. The experimental lesions not only reproduced the pathological pictures, but followed a clinical course, which in local symptomatology especially, tallied closely with that of the bite. This the writer interprets as satisfactory evidence that the lesion is not produced by any living infective agent. The experiments performed do not identify the nature of the toxic agent. Tentatively they seem to bring out, however, the following characteristics.

1. The product of alcoholic extraction of flies do not contain the toxic agent.
2. The toxic agent is not inactivated by alcohol.
3. The toxic agent is not destroyed by drying fixed flies.
4. The toxic agent is not affected by glycerin, but is, if anything, more active in pastes made from the ground fly and glycerin, than in the ground flies as such.

5. The toxic agent is rendered inactive or destroyed by hydrochloric acid in a concentration of 0.25%.

6. The toxic agent is most abundant in the region of the anatomical structures connected with the biting and salivary apparatus (head and thorax).

7. The toxic agent is not affected by a 0.5 % solution of sodium bicarbonate.

8. The toxic agent is not affected by exposure to dry heat at 100° C. for two hours.

9. The toxic agent is destroyed or rendered inactive in alkaline solution by a typical hydrolytic ferment, pancreatin.

10. Incomplete experimental evidence suggests that the activity of the toxic agent may be heightened by a possible lytic action of the blood serum of a sensitive individual, and that the sensitive serum itself may contain the toxic agent in solution.

These results, as far as they go (omitting No. 10), accord with Langer's except on the point of alcoholic solubility and the effect of acids. The actual nature of the toxic agent in the black-fly is left a matter of speculation.

The following working theories have suggested themselves to the writer. First, the toxin may be, as Langer believes in the case of the bee, an alkaloidal base, toxic as such, and neutralized after injection by antibodies produced for the occasion by the body. In such a case the view that a partial local fixation of the toxin occurs, which prevents its immediate diffusion, is acceptable. Through chemotactic action, special cells capable of breaking up the toxin into harmless elements are attracted to the scene. Their function may be, on the other hand, to neutralize directly, not by lysis. This would explain the rôle of the eosinophiles in the black-fly lesion. If their activities be essential to the destruction or neutralization of the toxin, one would expect them to be most numerous where there was least reaction. This would be at the site of a bite in an immune individual. A point of special interest for further investigation, would be the study of such a lesion.

Second, it is conceivable that the injected saliva of the fly does not contain an agent toxic as such. It is possible, that like many foreign proteins, it only becomes toxic when broken down. The completeness and rapidity of the breaking down depends on the number of eosinophiles present. In such a case immunity should again be marked by intense eosinophilia.

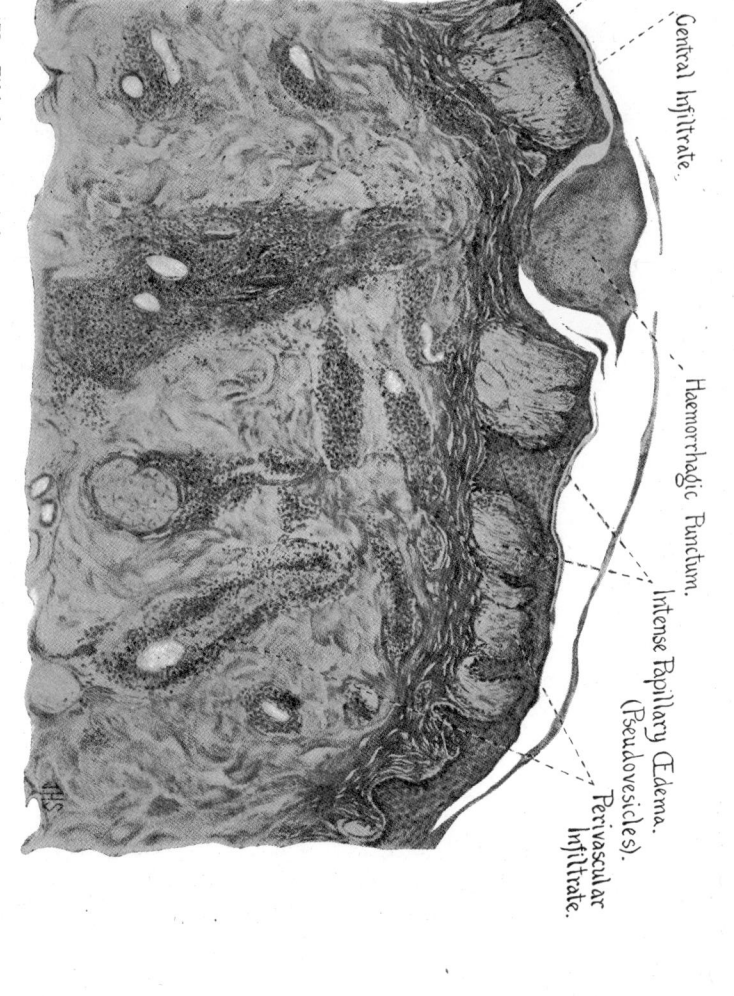

173. Fifth day mature lesion. Lower power drawing showing papillary œdema and infiltrate in the region of the puncture.

Labels: Central Infiltrate. — Haemorrhagic Punctum. — Intense Papillary Œdema (Pseudovesicles). — Perivascular Infiltrate.

Third, lytic agents in the blood serum may play the chief rôle in the liberation of the toxic agent from its non-toxic combination. An immune individual would then be one whose immunity was not the positive one of antibody formation, but the negative immunity of failure to metabolize. An immune lesion in such a case might be conceived as presenting no eosinophilia, since no toxin is liberated. If the liberation of the toxin is dependent upon lytic agents present in the serum rather than in any cellular elements, a rational explanation would be available for the apparent results (subject to confirmation) of the experiment with sensitive and immune sera. In this experiment it will be recalled that the sensitive serum seemed to bring out the toxicity of the ground flies, and the serum itself seemed even to contain some of the dissolved or liberated toxin. The slowness with which a lesion develops in the case of the black-fly bite supports the view of the initial lack of toxicity of the injected material. The entire absence of early subjective symptoms, such as pain, burning, etc., is further evidence for this view. It would appear as if no reaction occurred until lysis of an originally non-toxic substance had begun. Regarding the toxin itself as the chemotactic agent which attracts eosinophiles, its liberation in the lytic process and diffusion through the blood stream attracts the cells in question to the point at which it is being liberated. Arriving upon the scene, these cells assist in its neutralization.

The last view presented is the one to which the author inclines as the one which most adequately explains the phenomena.

A fourth view is that the initial injection of a foreign protein by the fly (i.e., with the first bite) sensitizes the body to that protein. Its subsequent injection at any point in the skin gives rise to a local expression of systematic sensitization. Such local sensitization reactions have been described by Arthus and Breton, by Hamburger and Pollack and by Cowie. The description of such a lesion given by the first named authors, in the rabbit, however, does not suggest, histopathologically at least, a strong resemblance to that of the black-fly. Such an explanation of many insect urticariæ deserves further investigation, however, and may align them under cutaneous expressions of anaphylaxis to a foreign protein injected by the insect. Depending on the chemical nature of the protein injected, a specific chemotactic reaction like eosinophilia may or may not occur. Viewed in this light the development of immunity to insect bites assumes a place in the larger problem of anaphylaxis.

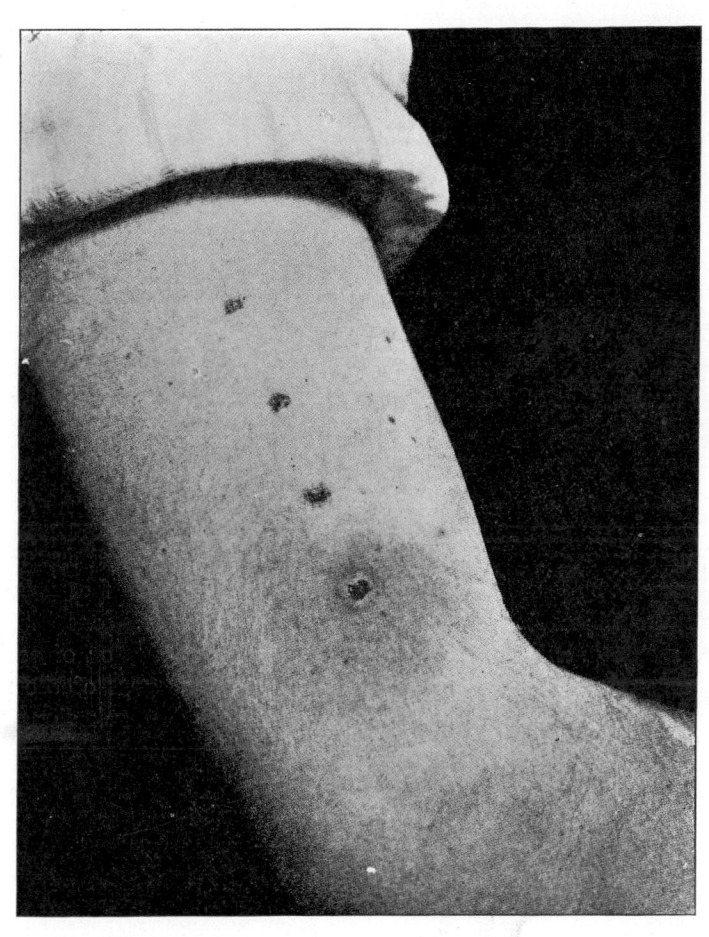

174. Experimental lesion produced from alcohol-fixed flies, dried and ground into a paste with glycerin.

## Summary

In order to bring the results of the foregoing studies together, the author appends the following résumé of the clinical data presented in the first paper.

The black-fly, *Simulium venustum*, inflicts a painless bite, with ecchymosis and hæmorrhage at the site of puncture. A papulovesicular lesion upon an urticarial base slowly develops, the full course of the lesion occupying several days to several weeks. Marked differences in individual reaction occur, but the typical course involves four stages. These are, in chronological order, the papular stage, the vesicular or pseudovesicular, the mature vesico-papular or weeping papular stage and the stage of involution terminating in a scar. The papule develops in from 3 to 24 hours. The early pseudovesicle develops in 24 to 48 hours. The mature vesico-papular lesion develops by the third to fifth day and may last from a few days to three weeks. Involution is marked by cessation of oozing, subsidence of the papule and scar-like changes at the site of the lesion. The symptoms accompanying this cycle consist of severe localized or diffused pruritus, with some heat and burning in the earlier stages if the œdema is marked. The pruritus appears with the pseudovesicular stage and exhibits extraordinary persistence and a marked tendency to periodic spontaneous exacerbation. The flies tend to group their bites and confluence of the developing lesions in such cases may result in extensive œdema with the formation of oozing and crusted plaques. A special tendency on the part of the flies to attack the skin about the cheeks, eyes and the neck along the hair line and behind the ears, is noted. In these sites inflammation and œdema may be extreme.

A distinctive satellite adeonpathy of the cervical glands develops in the majority of susceptible persons within 48 hours after being bitten in the typical sites. This adenopathy is marked, discrete and painful, the glands often exquisitely tender on pressure. It subsides without suppuration.

Immunity may be developed to all except the earliest manifestations, by repeated exposures. Such an immunity in natives of an infested locality is usually highly developed. There are also apparently seasonal variations in the virulence of the fly and variations in the reaction of the same individual to different bites.

Constitutional effects were not observed but have been reported.

# BIBLIOGRAPHY

**Aldrich, J. M.** 1905. A catalogue of North American Diptera. Washington, D. C. 1–680.

**Alessandri, G.** 1910. Studii ed esperienze sulle larve della Piophila casei. Arch. Parasit. xiii, p. 337–387.

**Anderson, J. F.** and **Frost, W. H.** 1912. Transmission of poliomyelitis by means of the stable-fly (Stomoxys calcitrans). Public Health Reports. Washington. xxvii, p. 1733–1735.

────── 1913. Further attempts to transmit the disease through the agency of the stable-fly (Stomoxys calcitrans). Public Health Repts., Washington. xxviii, p. 833–837.

**Anderson, J. F.** and **Goldberger, J.** 1910. On the infectivity of tabardillo or Mexican typhus for monkeys, and studies on its mode of transmission. Public Health Repts., Washington. xxv, p. 177.

**Annandale, N.** 1910. The Indian species of papataci fly (Phlebotomus). Records of Indian Mus. iv, p. 35–52, pls. iv–vi.

**Austen, E. E.** 1903. Monograph of the tsetse-flies. 8vo. London, British Mus. (ix+319 p.).

**Bacot, A. W.** and **Martin, C. J.** 1914. Observations of the mechanism of the transmission of plague by fleas. Journ. Hygiene, xiii, Plague supplement, p. 423–439. Pls. xxiv–xxvi.

**Bacot, A. W.** and **Ridewood, W. G.** 1914. Observations on the larvæ of fleas. Parasitology, vii, p. 157–175.

**Baker, C. F.** 1904. A revision of American Siphonaptera. Proc. U. S. Nat. Mus. xxviii, p. 365–469.

────── 1905. xxix, The classification of the American Siphonaptera. ibid p. 121–170.

**Balfour, A.** 1911. The rôle of the infective granules in certain protozoal diseases. British Med. Journ. 1911, p. 1268–1269.

────── 1912. The life-cycle of *Spirochæta gallinarum*. Parasitology, v, p. 122–126.

**Bancroft, Th.** 1899. On the metamorphosis of the young form of *Filaria bancrofti* in the body of *Culex ciliaris*. Proc. Roy. Soc. N. S. Wales. xxxiii, p. 48–62.

**Banks, N.** 1904. A treatise on the Acarina, or mites. Proc. U. S. Nat. Mus. xxviii, p. 1–114.

────── 1908. A revision of the Ixodoidea, or ticks, of the United States. U. S. Dept. Agric., Bur. Ent. tech. ser. xv, 61p.

────── 1912. The structure of certain dipterous larvæ with particular reference to those in human foods. U. S. Dept. Agr. Bur. Ent. Bul. tech. ser. No. 22.

**Basile, C.** 1910. Sulla Leishmaniosi del cane sull' ospite intermedio del Kala-Azar infantile, Rendiconti Reale Accad. Lincei xix (2) p. 523–527.

────── 1911. Sulla transmissione delle Leishmaniosa. ibid, xx (1) p. 50–51.

────── 1911. Sulla leishmaniosi e sul suo modo di transmissione. ibid, xx (1) p. 278–282, 479–485, 955–959.

────── 1914. La meteorologia della leishmaniosi interna nel Mediterraneo. ibid, xxiii (1) p. 625–629.

**Bayon, H.** 1912. The experimental transmission of the spirochæte of European relapsing fever to rats and mice. Parasitology v, p. 135–149.

**Beauperthuy, L. D.** 1853. (Cited by Boyce, 1909.)

**Berlese, A.** 1899. Fenomeni che accompagnano la fecondazione in talun Insetti. Revista di Patologia veg., vi, p. 353–368; vii, p. 1–18.

**Bertkau, P.** 1891. Ueber das Vorkommen einer Giftspinne (Chiracanthium nutrix) in Deutschland. Sitzungsb. niederrheinischen Gesellschaft in Bonn, 1891, p. 89–93.

**Bezzi, M.** 1907. Die Gattungen der blutsaugenden Musciden. Zeitsch. Syst. Hymenopterologie und Dipt. vii, p. 413–416.
**Bishopp, F. C.** 1914. The stable–fly. U. S. Dept. Agric., Farmers' Bul. 540, p. 1–28.
**Blackwell, J.** 1855. Experiments and observations on the poison of animals of the order Araneidea. London, Trans. Linn. Soc. xxi, p. 31–37.
**Blaizot, L., Conseil, E.,** and **Nicolle, C.** 1913. Etiologie de la fièvre récurrente, son mode de transmission par les poux. Ann. Inst. Pasteur xxvii, p. 204–225.
**Blanchard, R.** 1892. Sur les Oestrides américains dont la larve vit dans la peau de l'homme. Ann. Soc. Ent. France, lxi, p. 109–150.
──────── 1898. Sur le pseudo-parasitisme des Myriapodes chez l'Homme. Arch. Parasit. 1, p. 452–490.
──────── 1902. Nouvelles observations sur le pseudo-parasitisme des Myriapodes chez l'homme. Arch. parasit. vi, p. 245–256.
──────── 1905. Les moustiques. Histoire naturelle et médicale. 8vo. Paris, Rudeval. (xiii + 673 p.).
──────── 1907. Parasitisme du *Dipylidium caninum* dans l'espéce humanine, á propos d'un cas nouveau. Arch. Parasit. xi, p. 439–471.
**Blankmeyer, H. C.** 1914. Intestinal myiasis; with report of case. Journ. Amer. Med. Assoc. lxiii, p. 321.
**Bordas, M. L.** 1905. Recherches anatomiques, histologiques et physiologiques sur les glandes venimeuses ou glandes des chélicères des malmignattes (*Lactrodectus 13–guttatus* Rossi.) Ann. Sci. Nat. (ix ser) i, 147–164, 1 pl. 4 text fig.
**Borrell, A.** 1910. Parasitisme et Tumeurs. Ann Inst. Pasteur, xxiv, p. 778–788.
**Boyce, R.** 1909. Mosquito or man? The conquest of the tropical world. 8vo. London, Murray. (xvi + 267 p.).
**Brauer, F.** 1899. Beiträge zur Kenntniss der Muscaria schizomatopa. Sitzungsb. kais. Akad. Wissensch. Math.-Naturwiss. Klasse. cviii, p. 495–529.
**Brauer, F.** and **Bergenstamm, J.** 1889–1894. Die Zweiflügler des Kaiserl. Museum zu Wien. Denkschr. Kais. Akad. Wissensch. Math.-Naturwiss Klasse. lvi, p. 69–180; lviii, p. 305–446; lx, p. 89–240; lxi, p. 537–624.
**Braun, M.** 1908. Die tierischen Parasiten des Menschen. 4 Aufl. 8vo. Würzburg, Kabitzsch. (ix + 623 p.). Also, Eng. Trans. of 3d ed., with additions by Sambon and Theobald.
**Briot, A.** 1904. Sur le venin de scolopendres. C. R. Soc. Biol. Paris. lvi, p. 476–477.
**Bruce, D.** 1907. Trypanosomiases. Osler's Modern Med. Philadelphia, Lea Bros. & Co. i, p. 460–487.
**Bruck, C.** 1911. Ueber das Gift der Stechmücke. Deutsche medizin. Wochenschr. 28 Sept. 1911, p. 1787–1790.
**Brues, C. T.** 1913. The relation of the stable-fly (*Stomoxys calcitrans*) to the transmission of infantile paralysis. Journ. Econ. Ent. vi, p. 101–109.
**Brues, C. T.** and **Sheppard, P. A. E.** 1912. The possible etiological relation of certain biting insects to the spread of infantile paralysis. Journ. Econ. Ent. v, p. 305–324.
**Brumpt, E.** 1905. Maladie du sommeil. Distribution géographique, étiologie, prophylaxie. Arch. Parasit. ix, p. 205–224.
──────── 1913. Précis de parasitologie. 2 ed. 8°. Paris, Masson & Cie. (xxviii + 1011 p.).
**Brunetti, E.** 1912. Description of Apiochæta ferruginea, a hitherto undescribed species of Phoridæ that causes myasis in man. Rec. Indian Mus. vii p. 83–86.
**Bugnion, E.** and **Popoff, N.** 1908. L'appareil salivaire des hémiptères. Arch. d'anatomie micr. x, p. 227–456.
──────── 1911. Les piéces buccales des Hémipteres. Arch. Zool. Exper. (5) vii, p. 643–674.

**Calandruccio, S.** 1899. Sul pseudo-parassitismo delle larve dei Ditteri nell' intestino umano. Arch. Parasit. ii, p. 251–257.
**Calkins, G. N.** 1909. Protozoology. New York. Lea and Febiger (349 p.).
**Castellani, A.** and **Chalmers, A. J.** 1910. Manual of tropical medicine 4°. New York. Wm. Wood & Co. (xxv + 1242p.). 2 ed., 1914.
**Celli, A.** 1886. Acque potabile e malaria. Giornale della Società italiana di igiene.
——— 1900. Malaria according to the new researches. Eng. trans. 2 ed. 8vo. London, Longmans, Green & Co. (xxiv + 275 p.).
**Chevril, R.** 1909. Sur la myiase des voies urinaires. Arch. Parasit. xii, p. 369–450.
**Chittenden, F. H.** 1906. Harvest mites or "chiggers". U. S. Dept. Agric. Bur. Ent. Circ. No. 77, p. 1–6.
**Cholodkovsky, N.** 1904. Zur Kentniss der Mundwerkzeuge und Systematik der Pediculiden. Zool. Anz. xxviii, p. 368–370.
——— 1905. Noch ein Wort über die Mundeile der Pediculiden. ibid., xxix p. 149.
**Christophers, S. R.** 1907. *Piroplasma canis* and its life cycle in the tick. Sci. Mem. Med. Ind., Calcutta. n. s. xxix, p. 1–83.
——— 1912. The development of *Leucocytozoon canis* in the tick, with a reference to the development of *Piroplasma*. Parasitology, v, p. 37–48.
**Coates, G. M.** 1914. A case of myasis aurium accompanying the radical mastoid operation. Journ. Amer. Med. Assoc. lxiii, p. 479.
**Comstock, J. H.** 1912. The spider book. A manual for the study of the spiders and their near relatives found in America north of Mexico. Large 8vo. New York, Doubleday, Page & Co. (xv + 721 p., 771 figs.)
**Comstock, J. H.** and **A. B.** 1914. A manual for the study of insects. 12th ed. 8°. Ithaca, N. Y. (x + 701 p., 797 text figs. and 6 pls.).
**Cook, F. C.**, **Hutchison, R. H.** and **Scales, F. M.** 1914. Experiments in the destruction of fly larvæ in horse manure. U. S. Dept. Agric. Bul. 118, p. 1–26.
**Copeman, S. M.**, **Howlett, F. M.** and **Merriman, G.** 1911. An experimental investigation on the range of flight of flies. Rept. to the Local Gov't Board on Publ. Health. n. s. liii, p. 1–9.
**Coquillett, D. W.** 1906. A classification of the mosquitoes of North and Middle North America. U. S. Dept. Agric. Bur. Ent. Tech. Bul. xi, p. 1–31.
——— 1907. Discovery of blood-sucking Psychodidæ in America. Ent. News xviii, p. 101–102.
**Cox, G. L.**, **Lewis, F. C.** and **Glynn, E. F.** 1912. The numbers and varieties of bacteria carried by the common housefly in sanitary and insanitary city areas. Journ. Hygiene, xii, p. 290–319.
**Crampton, G. C.** 1914. On the misuse of the terms parapteron, hypopteron, tegula, squamula, patagium and scapula. Journ. N. Y. Ent. Soc. xxii, p. 248–261.
**Currie, D. H.** 1910. Mosquitoes in relation to the transmission of leprosy. Flies in relation to the transmission of leprosy. Public Health Bul. Washington, No. 39, p. 1–42.
**Dahl, Fr.** 1910. Milben als Erzeuger von Zellwucherungen. Centralbl. Bakt. Jena. Abt. 1, liii, Originale, p. 524–533.
**Dalla Torre, Dr. K. von.** 1908. Anoplura. Genera Insectorum. Fasc. 81, p. 1–22.
**Darling, S. T.** 1913. The part played by flies and other insects in the spread of infectious diseases in the tropics, with special reference to ants and to the transmission of Tr. hippicum by *Musca domestica*. Trans. 15th Intern. Congress on Hygiene and Demography, Washington, iv, p. 182–185.
**Doane, R. W.** 1910. Insects and disease. 8vo. New York, Holt & Co. (xiv+227 p.).
**Doerr, H.** and **Russ, V.** 1913. Die Phlebotomen. In Mense's Handbuch der Tropenkrankheiten, i, p. 263–283, pls. 11–12.
**Doflein, F.** 1911. Lehrbuch der Protozoenkunde, 3 ed. 4°. Jena. G. Fischer (xii+1043 p.).

**Dufour, L.** 1833. Recherches anatomiques et physiologiques sur les Hémiptères. Mém d. savant etrang. à l'Acad. d. Sc. iv, p. 129–462.
**Duges, A.** 1836. Observations sur les Aranéides. Ann. sci. nat. (zool.) Paris. (Sér 2) vi, 159–218.
**Dutton, J. E.** and **Todd, J. L.** 1905. The nature of human tick fever in the eastern part of the Congo Free State, with notes on the distribution and bionomics of the tick. Liverpool School Trop. Med. Mem. xvii, p. 1–18.
**Dyar, H. G.** 1906. Key to the known larvæ of the mosquitoes of the United States U. S. Dept. Agric. Bur. Ent. Circ. 72, p. 1–6.
**Dyar,** See Howard, Dyar and Knab.
**Dziedzicki.** See Schnabl.
**Enderlein, G.** 1901. Zur Kenntniss der Flöhe und Sandflöhe. Zool. Jahrb. (Syst.) xiv, p. 548–557, pl. 34.
——— 1904. Lause-Studien. Ueber die Morphologie, Klassifikation und systematische Stellung der Anopluren, nebst Bemerkungen zur Systematik der Insektenordnungen. Zool. Anz. xxviii, p. 121–147.
**Esten, W. M.** and **Mason, C. J.** 1908. Sources of bacteria in milk. Storrs Agric. Exp. Sta. Bul. li, p. 65–109.
**Ewing, H. E.** 1912. The origin and significance of parasitism in the Acarina. Trans. Acad. Sci. of St. Louis. xxi, p. 1-70. pls. i–vii.
**Eysell, A.** 1913. Die Krankheitsereger und Krankheitsüberträger unter den Arthropoden. See, Mense (1913).
**Felt, E. P.** 1904. Mosquitoes or Culicidæ of New York State. N. Y. State Museum. Bul. 79. p. 241–391. 57 plates.
——— 1913. Queen blow-fly. Georgian flesh-fly. 28th rept. of the State Entomologist. p. 75–92.
**Finlay, Charles J.** 1881 et seq. Trabajos selectos. Selected papers. Republica de Cuba. Secretaria de Sanidad y Beneficencia. Havana 1912. xxxiv + 657 p.
**Forbes, S. A.** 1912. On black-flies and buffalo-gnats, (*Simulium*), as possible carriers of pellagra in Illinois. 27th Rept. of the State Entomologist of Illinois, p. 21–55.
**Forel, A.** 1878. Der Giftapparat und die Analdrüsen der Ameisen. Zeitschr. wiss. Zool. xxx, p. 28–68.
**Fox, G. H.** 1880. Photographic illustrations of skin disease. 4°. New York, E. B. Treat.
**Fracker, S. B.** 1914. A systematic outline of the Reduviidæ of North America. Iowa Acad. Sci. p. 217–252.
**French, G. H.** 1905. *Nitidula bipustulata* in a new rôle. Canadian Entomologist, xxxvii, p. 420.
**Frost, W. H.** 1911. Acute anterior poliomyelitis (*Infantile paralysis*). A précis. Public Health Bul. Washington. No. 44, p. 1–52.
**Fuller, C.** 1914. The skin maggot of man. S. African Agric. Journ. vii, p. 866–874.
**Galli-Valerio, B.** 1908. Le rôle des arthropodes dans la dissemination des maladies. Centralbl. Bakt. 1 Abt. Ref. xli, p. 353–360.
**Gerhardt, C.** 1884. Ueber Intermittensimpfungen. Zeitschr. f. klin. Med. vii, p. 372.
**Girault, A. A.** 1905–06. The bed-bug, *Clinocoris*, ( = *Cimex* = *Acanthia* = *Klinophilos*) *lectularia* Linnæus. Psyche xii, p. 61–74, vol. xiii, p. 42–58.
——— 1910–14 Preliminary studies on the biology of the bed-bug, *Cimex lectularius*, Linn. Jour. Econ. Biol. v, p. 88–91; vii, p. 163–188; ix, p. 25–45.
**Girault, A. A.** and **Strauss, J. F.** 1905. The bed-bug, *Clinocoris lectularius* (Linnæus) and the fowl bug, *Clinocoris columbarius* (Jenyns): host relations. Psyche, xii, p. 117–123.
**Girschner, E.** 1893. Beitrag zur Systematik der Musciden. Berliner Ent. Zeitschr. xxxviii, p. 297–312.
——— 1896. Ein neues Musciden-System auf Grund der Thoracalbeborstung und der Segmentierung des Hinterleibes. Wochenschr. für Entom. i, p.12–16, 30–32, 61–64, 105–112.

**Goeldi, E. A.** 1913. Die sanitarisch-pathologische Bedeutung der Insekten und verwandten Gliedertiere 8°. Berlin. Friedländer & Sohn. (155 p.).

**Goldberger, J.** 1910. The straw itch. (Dermatitis Schambergi). Public Health Repts., Washington, xxv, p. 779-784.

**Goldberger, J. and Anderson, J. F.** 1912. The transmission of typhus fever, with especial reference to transmission by the head-louse (*Pediculus capitis*). Public Health Repts., Washington, xxvii, p. 297-307.

**Goldberger, J., Waring, C. H., and Willets, D. G.** 1914. The treatment and prevention of pellagra. Public Health Repts., Washington, xxix, p. 2821-2826.

**Graham-Smith, G. S.** 1913. Flies in relation to disease: non-bloodsucking flies. 8vo. Cambridge Univ. Press. (xiv + 292 p.)

**Grassi, B.** 1907. Ricerche sui Flebotomi. Memorie della Società ital. della Scienze, ser. 3 a, xiv, p. 353-394, pls. i-iv.

**Grassi, B. and Noe, G.** 1900. Propagation of the filariæ of the blood exclusively by means of the puncture of peculiar mosquitoes. British Med. Journ. ii, p. 1306—1307.

**Griffith, A.** 1908. Life history of house-flies. Public Health, xxi, p. 122-127.

**Grünberg, K.** 1907. Die blutsaugenden Dipteren. 8vo. Jena, Fischer. (vi + 188 p).

**Hadwen, S.** 1913. On "tick paralysis" in sheep and man following bites of *Dermacentor venustus*. Parasitology, vi, p. 283-297.

**Hawden, S. and Nuttall, G. H. F.** 1913. Experimental "tick paralysis" in the dog. Parasitology, vi, p. 298-301.

**Hall, M. C. and Muir, J. F.** 1913. A critical study of a case of myasis due to *Eristalis*. Arch. Int. Med., Chicago, xi, p. 193-203.

**Hamilton, J.** 1893. Medico-entomology. Entom. News iv, p. 217-219.

**Hart, C. A.** 1895. On the entomology of the Illinois river and adjacent waters. Bul. Ill. State Lab. Nat. Hist., iv, p. 149-273.

**Headlee, T. J.** 1914. Anti-mosquito work in New Jersey. Jour. Econ. Ent. vii, p. 260-268.

**Hecker, J. F. C.** 1885. The dancing mania of the Middle Ages. Transl. by B. G. Bahington. 8vo. New York, Humboldt Library. (53p.).

**Hendel.** 1901. Beitrag zur Kenntniss der Calliphorinen. Wiener Ent. Zeitung. xx, p. 28-33.

**Herms, W. B.** 1911. The house-fly in its relation to public health. Cal. Agric. Exp. Sta. Bul. 215, p. 511-548.

—— 1913. Malaria: cause and control. 8°. New York, Macmillan Co. (xi + 163 p.).

**Herrick, G. W.** 1903. The relation of malaria to agriculture and other industries of the South. Pop. Sci. Mo. lxii, p. 521-525.

—— 1913. Household insects and methods of control. Cornell Reading Course, (N. Y. State College of Agric.), iii, 47 p.

—— 1914. Insects injurious to the household and annoying to man. 8vo. New York, Macmillan Co. (xvii + 470).

**Hewitt, C. G.** 1910. The house-fly. A study of its structure, development, bionomics, and economy. 8vo. Manchester Univ. Press. (xiv + 196 p.).

—— 1912. *Fannia (Homalomyia) canicularis* Linn. and *F. scalaris* Fab. Parasitology, v. p. 161-174.

**Heymons, R.** 1901. Biologische Beobachtungen an asiatischen Solifugen, nebst Beiträge zur Systematik derselben. Abl. Ak. Berlin, 1901, Anh. i, 1-65 p.

**Higgins, F. W.** 1891. Dipterous larvæ vomited by a child. Insect Life, Washington. iii, p. 396-397.

**Hindle, E.** 1911 a. The relapsing fever of tropical Africa. A Review. Parasitology, iv, p. 183-203.

—— 1911 b. On the life cycle of *Spirochæta gallinarum*. ibid, iv. p. 463-477.

**Hindle, E. and Merriman, G.** 1914. The range of flight of *Musca domestica*. Journ. of Hygiene, xiv. p. 23-45.

**Hine, J. S.** 1903. Tabanidæ of Ohio. Papers Ohio Acad. Sci. No. 5, 55 p.
——— 1906. Habits and life-histories of some flies of the family Tabanidæ. U. S. Dept. Agric. Bur. Ent. tech. bul, 12, p. 19-38.
——— 1907. Second report upon the horse-flies of Louisiana. La. Stat. Exp. Bul. 93, p. 1-59.
**Hodge, C. F.** 1910. A practical point in the study of the typhoid, or filth-fly. Nature Study Review, vi. p. 195-199.
——— 1913. The distance house-flies, blue-bottles, and stable flies may travel over water. Science, n. s. xxxviii, p. 513.
**Honeij, J. A.** and **Parker, R. R.** 1914. Leprosy: flies in relation to the transmission of the disease. Journ. Med. Research, Boston, xxx, p. 127-130.
**Hooker, W. A.** 1908 a. Life history, habits, and methods of study of the Ixodoidea. Jour, Econ. Ent. i, p. 34-51.
——— 1908 b. A review of the present knowledge of the rôle of ticks in the transmission of disease. ibid., i, p. 65-76.
**Hope. F, W.** 1837. On insects and their larvæ occasionally found in the human body. Trans. Ent. Soc., London, ii, p. 256-271.
**Hough, G. de N.** 1899 a. Synopsis of the Calliphorinæ of the United States. Zoological Bulletin, ii, p. 283-290.
——— 1899 b. Some Muscinæ of North America. Biological Bulletin i, p. 19-33.
——— 1899 c. Some North American Genera of Calliphorinæ. Entom. News, x, p. 62-66.
**Hovarth, G.** 1912. Revision of the American Cimicidæ. Ann. Mus. Nat. Hungarici, x, p. 257-262.
**Howard, C. W.** 1908. A list of the ticks of South Africa, with descriptions and keys to all the forms known. Ann. Transvaal Mus. I, p. 73-170.
**Howard, C. W.** and **Clark, P. F.** 1912. Experiments on insect transmission of the virus of poliomyelitis. Journ. Exper. Med. xvi, p. 805-859.
**Howard, L. O.** 1899. Spider bites and kissing bugs. Pop. Sci. Mo. lv, p. 31-42.
——— 1900. A contribution to the study of the insect fauna of human excrement. Proc. Wash. Acad. Sci. ii, p. 541-604.
——— 1901. Mosquitoes, how they live, how they carry disease, how they are classified, how they may be destroyed. 8vo. New York, Doubleday, Page & Co. (xv + 241 p.)
——— 1909. Economic loss to the people of the United States, through insects that carry disease. U. S. Dept. Agric. Bur. of Ent. Bul. 78, p. 1-40.
**Howard, L. O., Dyar, H. G.** and **Knab, F.** 1913-. The mosquitoes of North and Central America and the West Indies. Vol. I. A general consideration of mosquitoes, their habits, and their relations to the human species. 4°. Carnegie Institution of Washington (vii + 520 p.).
**Howard, L. O.** and **Marlatt, C. L.** 1902. The principal household insects of the United States. U. S. Dept. Agric., Bur. Ent. Bul. 4.
**Huebner, W.** 1907. Ueber das Pfeilgift der Kalahari. Arch. exper. Path. und Pharm., lvii, p. 358-366.
**Hunter, S. J.** 1913. Pellagra and the sand-fly. Jour. econ. Ent. vi, p. 96-99.
**Hunter, W. D.** 1913. American interest in medical entomology. Jour. econ. Ent. vi, p. 27-39.
**Hunter, W. D.** and **Bishopp, F. C.** 1910. Some of the more important ticks of the United States. U. S. Dept. Agric. Yearbook 1910, p. 219-230, pls. xv-xvi.
——— 1911. The Rocky Mountain spotted fever tick. With special reference to the problem of its control in the Bitter Root Valley in Montana. U. S. Dept. Agric., Bur. Ent. Bul. 105, p. 1-47.
**Hutchison, R. H.** 1914. The migratory habit of housefly larvæ as indicating a favorable remedial measure. An account of progress. U. S. Dept. Agric., Bul. 14, p. 1-11.
**Jennings, A. H.** 1914. Summary of two years' study of insects in relation to pellagra. Journ. of Parasitology, i, p. 10-21.

Jennings, A. H. and King, W. V. 1913. One of the possible factors in the causation of pellagra. Journ. Amer. Med. Assoc., lx, p. 271–274.
Jepson, F. P. 1909. Notes on colouring flies for purposes of identification. Rep't to the Local Gov't Board on Publ. Health, n. s. 16, p. 4–9.
Johannsen, O. A. 1903. Aquatic Nematocerous Diptera. N. Y. State Mus. Bul., 68, p. 328–448, pls. 32–50.
―――― 1905. Aquatic Nematocerous Diptera II. (Chironomidæ). ibid. 86, p. 76–330, pls. 16–37.
―――― 1908. North America Chironomidæ. ibid., 124, p. 264–285.
―――― 1911. The typhoid fly and its allies. Maine Agric. Exp. Sta. Bul., 401, p. 1–7.
―――― 1911. Simulium and pellagra. Insect Notes for 1910. Maine Agr Exper. Station. Bul, 187, p 4.
Kellogg, V. L. 1915. Spider poison. Jour. of Parasitology, i p. 107+
Kelly, H. A. 1907. Walter Reed and yellow fever. 8vo. New York, McClure, Phillips & Co. (xix + 310 p.).
Kephart, Cornelia F. 1914. The poison glands of the larva of the browntail moth (Euproctis chrysorrhoea Linn.). Journ. Parasit., i, p.
Kieffer, J. J. 1906. Chironomidæ. Genera Insectorum. Fasc. 42, p. 1–78.
―――― 1913. Nouv. étude sur les Chironomides de l'Indien Museum de Calcutta. Records of the Indian Mus., ix, p. 119–197.
King, A. F. A. 1883. Insects and disease—mosquitoes and malaria. Pop. Sci. Mo. xxiii, p. 644–658.
Kirkland, A. H. 1907. Second annual report of the Superintendent for supressing the gypsy and browntail moths. 8vo. Boston. 170 p.
Kleine, E. 1909. Postive Infektionsversuche mit *Trypanosoma brucei* durch *Glossina palpalis*. Deutsche med. Wochenschr., xxxv, p. 469–470.
Weitere wissenschaftliche Beobachtungen über die Entwicklung von Trypanosomen in Glossinen. ibid. p. 924–925.
Weitere Untersuchungen über die Ætiologie der Schlafkrankheit. ibid., p. 1257–1260.
Weitere Beobachtungen über Tsetsefliegen und Trypanosomen. ibid., p. 1956–1958.
Kling, C. and Levaditi, C. 1913. Études sur la poliomyélite aiguë épidémique. Ann. Inst. Pasteur, xxvii, p. 718–749, 739–855.
Knab, F. 1912. Unconsidered factors in disease-transmission by blood-sucking insects. Journ. Econ. Ent., v, p. 196–200.
―――― 1913 a. The species of Anopheles that transmit human malaria. Amer. Journ. Trop. Dis. and Preventive Med., i, p. 24–43.
―――― 1913 b. Anopheles and malaria. ibid., i, p. 217.
―――― 1913 c. The life history of *Dermatobia hominis*. ibid., i, p. 464-468
Knab, F. See Howard, Dyar, and Knab.
Kobert, R. 1893. Lehrbuch der Intoxikationen. 4°. Stuttgart, Enke. (xxii + 816 p.). 2d ed. in 2 vols., 1906.
―――― 1901. Beiträge zur Kenntniss der Giftspinnen. 8°. Stuttgart, Enke. (viii + 191 p.).
Kolbe, H. J. 1894. Der Pfeilgiftkäfer der Kalahari-Wüste, *Diamphidia simplex*. Stett. Ent. Zeitg., iv, p. 79–86.
Krause, M. 1907. Untersuchungen über Pfeilgifte aus unseren africanischen Kolonien. Verhand. deutsche Kolonien kong. 1905. p. 264–288.
Lallier, P. 1897. Étude sur la myase du tube digestif chez l'homme. Thesis, Paris, 8°. 120 p.
Langer, J. 1897. Ueber das Gift unserer Honigbiene. Archiv. exper. Path. und Pharm., xxxviii, p. 381–396.
Lavinder, C. H. 1911. Pellagra; a précis. U. S. Publ. Health Service Bul. 48, 37 p.
Leidy, J. 1847. History and anatomy of the hemipterous genus *Belostoma*. Journ. Acad. Philad. (2), i, p. 57–67.
Leiper, R. T. 1907. The etiology and prophylaxis of dracontiasis. British Med. Journ. 1907, p. 129–132.

**Leishman, W. B.** 1910 a. Observations on the mechanism of infection in tick fever and on the hereditary transmission of *Spirochæta duttoni* in the tick. Trans. Soc. Trop. Med. Hyg., iii, p. 77–95. Abstr. in Bul. Inst. Pasteur, viii, p. 312–313.
———— 1910 b. On the hereditary transmission and mechanism of infection in tick fever and on the hereditary transmission of *Spirochæta duttoni* in the tick. Lancet., clxxvii, p. 11.
**Linnell, R. McC.** 1914. Notes on a case of death following the sting of a scorpion. Lancet, 1914, o. 1608–1609.
**Livingstone, D.** 1857. Missionary travels and researches in South Africa.
**Lucas, H.** 1843. (note) *Latrodectus malmignatus* Bul. Soc. Ent., France, 1843, p. viii.
**Ludlow, C. S.** 1914. Diesase bearing mosquitoes of North and Central America, the West Indies and the Philippine Islands. War Dept., Offlce of Surgeon General. Bul. No. 4, 1–96.
**Lugger,** 1896. Insects injurious in 1896. Agr. Exp. Sta. Bul. 48.p. 33 to 270.
**MacCallum, W. C.** 1898. On the hæmatozoan infection of birds. Journ. Exp. Med. iii, p. 117.
**MacGregor, M. E.** 1914. The posterior stigmata of dipterous larvæ as a diagnostic character. Parasitology, vii, p. 176–188.
**Macloskie, G.** 1888. The poison apparatus of the mosquito. Amer. Naturalist, xxii, p. 884–888.
**Malloch, J. P.** 1913. American black-flies or Buffalo gnats. U. S. Dept. Agric. Bur. Ent. Tech. Bul. 26, p. 1–72.
———— 1914. Notes on North American Diptera. Bul. Illinois State Lab. Nat. Hist., x, p. 213–243.
**Manson, P.** 1911. Tropical diseases: a manual of the diseases of warm climates. 8°. London, Cassell & Co. (xx + 876 p.). 4 ed. (1907). Reprinted.
**Marchoux, E. and Couvy, L.** 1913. Argas et spirochætes (1 mémoire). Les granules de Leishman. Ann. Inst. Pasteur, xxvii, p. 450–480. 2 mémoire. Le virus chez l'acarien. ibid. p. 620–643.
**Marchoux, E. and Selimbeni, A.** 1903. La spirillose des poules. Ann. Inst. Pasteur, xvii, p. 569–580.
**Marchoux, E. and Simond, P. L.** 1905. Études sur la fièvre jaune. Ann. Inst. Pasteur, xx, pp. 16–40, 104–148, 161–205.
**Marlatt, C. L.** 1902. (See Howard, L. O. and Marlatt, C. L.)
———— 1907. The bed-bug ( *Cimex lectularius* L.) U. S. Dept. Agric., Bur. Ent., Circ. No. 47, revised ed., 8 pp.
**Martin, G. Leboeuf, and Roubaud.** 1909. Rapport de la mission d'études de la maladie du sommeil au Congo francais. 4°. Paris, Masson & Cie. (vi + 722 p., 8 pls. and map.).
**Maver, Maria B.** 1911. Transmission of spotted fever by other than Montana and Idaho ticks. Journ. Infec. Dis., viii, p. 322–326.
**McClintic, T. B.** 1912. Investigations of and tick eradications in Rocky Mountain spotted fever. Publ. Health Repts., Washington, xxvii, p. 732–760.
**Meckel, H.** 1847. Uber schwarzes Pigment in der Milz und im Blute einer Geisteskranken. Allgem. Zeitschr. f. Psychiatrie, iv, p. 198–226.
**Megni, P.** 1906. Les insectes buveurs de sang. 12mo. Paris, Rudeval. (150 p.).
**Melnikoff, N.** 1869. Ueber die Jugendzustände der *Tænia cucumerina*. Arch. f. Naturg., xxxv, p. 62–70.
**Mense, C.** 1913. Handbuch der Tropenkrankheiten. 1 Band. 4°. Leipzig, Barth (xv + 295 p.) Entomological parts by A. Eysell, and by Doerr and Russ.
**Minchin, E. A.** 1912. An introduction to the study of the Protozoa, with special reference to the parasitic forms. 8°. London. Arnold (xi + 517 p.).
**Mitchell, Evelyn G.** 1907. Mosquito life. 8vo. New York, Putmans. (xxii + 281 p.).
**Mitzmain, M. B.** 1910. General observations on the bionomics of the rodent and human flies. U. S. Publ. Health Service. Bul., 38, p. 1-34.

———— 1912. The rôle of *Stomoxys calcitrans* in the transmission of *Trypanosoma evansi*. Philippine Journ. Sci., vii, p. 475-519, 5 pls.

———— 1913 a. The biology of *Tabanus striatus* Fabricius, the horsefly of the Philippines, ibid., vii, B. p. 197-221.

———— 1913 b. The mechanical transmission of surra. ibid., viii, sec. B., p. 223-229.

———— 1914 a. Experimental insect transmission of anthrax. U. S. Public Health Repts. xxix, p. 75-77.

———— 1914 b. I. Collected studies on the insect transmission of *Trypanosoma evansi*. II. Summary of experiments in the transmission of anthrax by biting flies. U. S. Pub. Health Service, Hyg. Lab. Bul., 94, p. 1-48.

**Miyake, H.** and **Scriba, J.** 1893. Vorläufige Mitteilung über einen neuen Parasit des Menschen. Berl. klin. Wochenschr., xxx, p. 374.

**Mollers, B.** 1907. Experimentelle Studien über die Uebertragung des Rückfallfiebers durch Zecken. Zeitschr. für Hyg. u. Infektionskrankheiten, lviii, p. 277-286.

**Mote, D. C.** 1914. The cheese-skipper (*Piophila casei*). Ohio Naturalist xiv, p. 309-310.

**Neiva, A.** 1910. Beiträge zur Biologie der *Conorhinus megistus* Burm. Memorias de Institute Oswaldo Cruz., ii, p. 206-212.

**Neveu-Lemaire, M.** 1907. Un nouveau cas de parasitisme accidental d'un myriapode dans le tube digestif de l'homme. C. R. Soc. der Biol., lxiii p. 305-308.

———— 1908. Précis de parasitologie humaine. 8vo. Paris, Rudeval. (v + 712 p.).

**Newstead, R.** 1911. The papataci flies (Phlebotomus) of the Maltese Islands. Bul. of Ent. Research, ii, p. 47-78, pls. 1-3.

**Nicoll, W.** 1911. On the part played by flies in the disposal of the eggs of parasitic worms. Repts. to the Local Gov't. Board on Publ. Health and Med. Subjects, n. s. No. 53, p. 13-30.

**Nicolle, C.** 1910. Recherches expérimentales sur la typhus exanthématique entreprises a l'Institut Pasteur de Tunis pendant l'année 1909. Ann. Inst. Pasteur, xxiv, p. 243-275.

———— 1911. Recherches expérimentales sur la typhus exanthématique entreprises a l' Institut Pasteur de Tunis pendant l'année 1910. ibid., xxv, p. 1-55, 97-154.

**Nicolle, C., Blaizot, A.,** and **Conseil, E.** 1912 a. Étiologie de la fièvre récurrente. Son mode de transmission par le pou. C. R. Acad. Sci., cliv, p. 1636-1638.

———— 1912 b. Conditions de transmission de la fièvere récurrente par le pou. ibid., clv., p. 481-484.

**Nicolle, C.** and **Catouillard, G.** 1905. Sur le venin d'un scorpion commun de Tunisie (*Heterometrus maurus*). C. R. Soc. Biol. lviii: p. 100-102.

**Noe, G.** 1901. Sul ciclo evolutivo della *Filaria bancrofti* e della *Filaria immitis*. Ricerche labr. anat. comp. norm. Univ. di Roma., viii, p. 275-353.

**Norman, W. W.** 1896. The effect of the poison of centipedes. Trans. Texas Acad. Sci.,i , p. 118-119.

**Nuttall, G. H. F.** 1899. On the rôle of insects, arachnids, and myriapods as carriers in the spread of bacterial and parasitic diseases of man and animals. Johns Hopkins Hosp. Repts., viii, 154 p., 3 pls.

———— 1908 a. On the behavior of Spirochætæ in *Acanthia lectularia*. Parasitology, i, p. 143-151.

———— 1908 b. The transmission of *Trypanosoma lewisi* by fleas and lice. ibid., i, p. 296-301.

———— 1908 c. The Ixodoidea or ticks, spirochætosis in man and animals, piroplasmosis. Journ. Roy. Inst. Publ. Health, xvi, p. 385-403, 449-464, 513-526.

———— 1914. Tick paralysis in man and animals. Parasitology, vii, p. 95-104.

**Nuttall, G. H. F.** and **Jepson, F. P.** 1909. The part played by *Musca domestica* and allied (non-biting) flies in the spread of infective diseases. A summary of our present knowledge. Rept. to the Local Gov't Board on Publ. Health and Med. Subjects, n. s. 16, p. 13-41.
**Nuttall, G. H. F.** and **Shipley, E. A.** 1901-03. Studies in relation to malaria. The structure and biology of Anopheles. Journ. Hyg., vols. i, ii, and iii.
**Orth. J.** 1910. Ueber die Beziehungungen der Haarsackmilbe zu Krebsbildungen in der Mamma. Berliner klin. Wochenschr., xlvii, p. 452-453.
**Osborn, Herbert.** 1896. Insects affecting domestic animals. U. S. Dept. Agric., Bur. of Ent. Bul., 5, n. s., 302 p.
——— 1902. Poisonous insects. Article in Reference Handbook. Med. Sci., v, p. 158-169.
**Osler, W.** 1887. An address on the Hæmatozoa of malaria. British Med. Jour. i. p. 556.
**Osten Sacken, C. R.** 1875-78. Prodrome of a Monograph of North American Tabanidæ. Mem. Boston Soc. Nat. Hist., ii, p. 365-397, 421-479, and 555-566.
**Oudemans, A. C.** 1910. Neue Ansichten über die Morphologie des Flohkopfes, sowie über die Ontogenie, Phylogenie und Systematik der Flöhe. Novit. Zool., xvi, p. 133-158.
**Patton, W. S.** 1907. Preliminary report on the development of the Leishman-Donovan body in the bed-bug. Sci. Mem., Med. and Sanitary Dept., Gov't of India, 28, p. 1-19.
**Patton, W. S.** and **Cragg, F. W.** 1913. A textbook of medical entomology. 4°. London, Christian Literature Society for India. (xxxiv + 764 p.)
**Pawlowsky, E.** 1906. Ueber den Steck- und Saug-apparat der Pediculiden. Zeitschr. wiss. Insektenbiol., ii, p. 156-162, 198-204.
**Pawlowsky, E.** 1913. Scorpiotomische Mitteilungen. I. Ein Beitrag zur Morphologie des Giftdrüsen der Skorpione. Zeitschr. wiss. Zool., cv., p. 157-177. Taf. x-xi.
**Pepper, W., Schnauss, F. W.,** and **Smith, A. J.** 1908. Transient parasitism in men by a species of *Rhizoglyphus*. Univ. of Pa. Med. Bul. xxi, p. 274-277.
**Petrovskaia, Maria.** 1910. Sur les myases produites chez l'homme par les Oestrides (Gastrophilus et Rhinœstrus). Thèse, Fac. de médecine, Paris, 79 p.
**Pettit, A.** and **Krohn, A.** 1905. Sur la structure der glandes salivaire du Notonecte (*Notonecta glauca*). Arch. anat. micr. Paris, vii, p. 351-368, pl. 13.
**Phisalix, Mme.** 1900. Un venin volatil. Sécrétion cutanée du *Iulus terrestris*. C. R. Soc. Biol. Paris, 1900, p. 1033-1036.
——— 1912. Effets physiologiques du venin de la Mygale de Haïti, le *Phormictopus cancerides* Pocock. Effets physiologiques du venin de la Mygale de Corse (*Cteniza sauvaga* Rossi); Bul. Mus. Paris, 1912: 134-138.
**Portschinsky, I. A.** 1908. *Rhinœstrus purpureus*, a parasite of horses which deposits its larvæ in the eyes of man. Mss. transl. by Miss S. L. Weissman, in library of Ent. Dept., Cornell University.
——— 1910. Biology of *Stomoxys calcitrans* and other coprophagous flies. Monograph in Russian. Mss. summarized transl. by Miss S. L. Weissman, in Library of Ent. Dept., C. U.
——— 1911. *Gastrophilus intestinalis*. Mss. transl. by Miss S. L. Weiseman, in library of Ent. Dept., C. U.
——— 1913 a. The sheep gad-fly, *Oestrus ovis*, its life, habits, methods of combating it, and its relation to man. Russian. Mss. summarized trans. by Miss S. L. Weissman, in library of Ent. Dept., C. U.
——— 1913 b. *Muscina stabulans*. A monograph in Russian. Mss., trans. by J. Millman, in library of Ent. Dept., Cornell Univ.
**Prowazek, S.** 1905. Studien über Säugetiertrypanosomen. Arb. aus dem kais. Gesundheitsamte xxii, p. 351-395.
**Pusey, W. A.** 1911. The principles and practice of dermatology. 2 ed, 8vo. Appleton & Co. (1079 p.)

**Rabinowitsch, L.** and **Kempmer, W.** 1899. Beitrag zur Kentniss der Blutparasiten, speciell der Ratten trypanosomen. Zeitschr. f. Hyg. xxx, p. 251-291.

**Ransom, B. H.** 1904. An account of the tape worms of the genus *Hymenolepis* parasitic in man. Bul. No. 18, Hyg. Lab., U. S. Pub. Health and Mar.-Hosp. Serv., Wash., p. 1–138.

———— 1911. The life history of a parasitic nematode, *Hebronema muscæ*. Science n. s. xxxiv, p. 690–692.

———— 1913. The life history of *Habronema muscæ*, (Carter), a parasite of the horse transmitted by the house-fly. U. S. Dept. Agric. Bur. Animal, Ind. Bul. 163, p. 1–36.

**Reaumur, R. A. F. de.** 1738. Mémoires pour servir a l'histoirie des insectes. Histoire des cousins, iv, p. 573–636.

**Reed, Walter.** 1900. The etiology of yellow fever. Philadelphia Med. Jour. Oct. 27, 1900, vi, p. 790–796.

**Reed, W.** and **Carroll, J.** 1901. The prevention of yellow fever. Med. Record, Oct. 26, 1901, p. 441–449.

**Reuter, Enzio.** 1910. Acari und Geschwulstätiologie. Centralbl. Bakt. Jena. Abt. I, lvi,: Originale 339–344.

**Reuter, O. M.** 1912. Bemerkungen über mein neues Heteropterensystem. Ofv. Finska Vetensk. Soc. Förh., liv. Afd. A. vi, p. 1–62.

**Ribaga, C.** 1897. Sopra un organo particolare della Cimici dei letti (*Cimex lectularius* L.). Rivista di Patologia Vegetale, v, p. 343–352.

**Ricardo, Gertrude.** 1900. Notes on the Pangoninæ. Ann. and Mag. Nat. Hist. v, p. 97–121.

———— 1901. Further Notes on the Pangoninæ. ibid. viii, p. 286–315.

———— 1904. Notes on the smaller genera of the Tabanidæ. ibid. xiv, p. 349–373.

**Ricketts, H. T.** 1906–1910. Contributions to medical sciences by Howard Taylor Ricketts. 1870–1910. Univ. of Chicago Press. 1911.

———— 1909. A microorganism which apparently has a specific relationship to Rocky Mountain spotted fever. A preliminary report. Jour. Amer. Med. Assoc. iii, p. 373–380.

———— Spotted fever reports 1 and 2. In the 4th Bien. Rept. State Board of Health, Montana, 1909, p. 87–191.

**Ricketts, H. T.** and **Wilder, R. M.** 1910. The transmission of the typhus fever of Mexico (tabardillo) by means of the louse, *Pediculus vestimenti*. Journ. Am. Med. Assoc. liv. p. 1304.

**Riley, C. V.** and **Howard, L. O.** 1889. A contribution to the literature of fatal spider-bites. Insect life, Washington, i. p. 204–211.

**Riley, W. A.** 1906. A case of pseudoparasitism by dipterous larvæ. Canadian Ent. xxxviii, p. 413.

———— 1910 a. Earlier references to the relation of flies to disease. Science n. s. xxxi, p. 263–4.

———— 1910 b. *Dipylidium caninum* in an American child. Science n. s. xxxi, p. 349–350.

———— 1911. The relation of insects to disease. Cornell Countryman ix, p. 51–55.

———— 1912 a. Notes on the relation of insects to disease. 8vo. Ithaca, N. Y. 51 p.

———— 1912 b. Notes on animal parasites and parasitism. 8vo. Ithaca, N. Y. 55 p.

———— 1913. Some sources of laboratory material for work on the relations of insects to disease. Ent. News. xxiv, p. 172–175.

———— 1914. Mr. Nott's thory of insect causation of disease- Jour. of Parasitology. i, p. 37–39.

**Rosenau, M. J.** and **Brues, C. T.** 1912. Some experimental observations on monkeys, concerning the transmission of poliomyelitis through the agency of *Stomoxys calcitrans*. Monthly Bul. Mass. State Board of Health. Vol. vii, p. 314–317.

**Ross, R.** 1904. Researches on Malaria. The Nobel Medical Prize Lecture for 1902, Stockholm, Norstedt & Söner. 89 p. 9 pls. In "Les Prix Nobel en 1902."
——— 1910. The prevention of malaria. 4°. New York. Dutton & Co. (xx + 669 p.).
**Rothschild, N. C.** 1905 a. North American Ceratophyllus. Novitates Zoologicæ xii, p. 153–174.
——— 1905 b. Some further notes on *Pulex canis* and *P. felis.* ibid. xii, p. 192–193.
**Roubaud, E.** 1911. Les Choeromyies. C. R. Acad. Sci. Paris, cliii, p. 553.
——— 1913. Recherches sur les Auchméromyies. Bul. Sci. France et Belg. Paris, p. 105–202.
**Sachs, Hans.** 1902. Zur Kentniss der Kreuzspinnengiftes. Beitr. Chem. hysiol.ii, p. 125–133. Abstr. Centralbl. Bakter. 1. Abth. xxxi., Referate, p. 788.
**Sambon, L. W.** 1908. Report presented at the International Conference on Sleeping Sickness.
——— 1910. Progress report on the investigation of pellagra. Reprinted from the Journ. Trop. Med. and Hyg.; London; Bale, Sons and Danielsson, 12°. 125 p.
**Sanderson, E. D.** 1910. Controlling the black-fly in the White Mountains. Jour. Econ. Ent. iii, p. 27–29.
**Saul, E.** 1910. Untersuchungen über Beziehungen der Acari zur Geschwulstätiologie. Centralbl. Bakt. Jena, Abt. 1, lv Originale, p. 15–18.
**Saul, E.** 1913. Beziehungen des Helminthen und Acari. zur Geschwulstätiologie. ibid., Abt. 1, lxxi, Originalie, p. 59–65.
**Sawyer, W. A.** and **Herms, W. B.** 1913. Attempts to transmit poliomyelites by means of the stable-fly (*Stomoxys calcitrans*). Journ. Amer. Med. Assoc. lxi, p. 461–466.
**Schaudinn, F.** 1904. Generations- und Wirtwechsel bei *Trypanosoma* und Spirochæte. Arb. aus dem kais. Gesundheitsamte xx, p. 387–493.
**Schiner, J. R.** 1862–64. Fauna Austriaca. Diptera, Vienna, I, lxxx + 674; II, xxxii + 658.
**Schnabl, J.** and **Dziedzicki, H.** 1911. Die Anthomyiden 4to. Halle. p. 1-306.
**Schweinitz, G. E. de** and **Shumway, E. A.** 1904. Conjunctivitis nodosa, with histological examination. Univ. of Pa. Med. Bul., Nov. 1904.
**Sergent, E.** and **Foly, H.** 1910. Recherches sur la fièvre récurrente et son mode de transmission, dans une épidémie algérienne. Ann. Inst. Pasteur xxiv, p. 337–373.
——— 1911. Typhus récurrent Algérien. Sa transmission par les poux. Sa guérison par l'arsénobenzol. C. R. Soc. Biol. Paris. lxiii, p. 1039–1040.
**Shipley, E. A.** 1914. Pseudo-parasitism. Parasitology, vi, p. 351–352
**Siler, J. F., Garrison, P. E.,** and **MacNeal, W. J.** 1914. Further studies of the Thompson-McFadden Pellagra Commission. A summary of the second progress report. Journ. Amer. Med. Assoc. lxiii, pp. 1090–1093.
**Skelton, D. S.** and **Parkham, J. G.** 1913. Leprosy and the bed-bug. R. A. M. C. Journ., xx, p. 291.
**Skinner, H.** 1909. A remedy for the house-fleas. Journ. Econ. Ent. ii, p. 192.
**Smith, G. U.** 1909. On some cases of relapsing fever in Egypt and the question of carriage by domestic vermin. Résumé in Ann. Inst. Pasteur xxiv, p. 374–375.
**Smith, J. B.** 1904. Report upon the mosquitoes occurring within the State, their habits, life history, etc. N. J. Agric. Exp. Sta. 1904, p. 1–482.
——— 1908. The house mosquito, a city, town, and village problem. N. J. Agric. Exp. Sta. Bul. No. 216, p. 1–21.
**Smith, T.** and **Kilbourne, F. L.** 1893. Investigations into the nature, causation, and prevention of Texas or southern cattle fever. U. S. Dept. Agric., Bur. Animal Ind. Bul. 1, p. 1–301. 10 pls.
**Speiser, P.** 1903. Studien über Diptera pupipara. Zeitschr. Syst. Hymenopterologie und Dipt., iii, p. 145–180.

**Spuler, A.** 1906. Ueber einen parasitisch lebenden Schmetterling, *Bradypodicola hahneli*. Biol. Centralbl., xxvi, p. 690–697.
**Stiles, C. W.** 1905. A zoological investigation into the cause, transmission, and source of Rocky Mountain fever. U. S. Public Health and Marine Hosp. Serv. Hyg. Labr. Bul. 14, 121 p.
─── 1907. Diseases caused by animal parasites. Osler's Modern Medicine, i, p. 525-637.
─── 1910 a. The sanitary privy: its purpose and construction. Public Health Bul. No. 37. U. S. Pub. Health and Marine Hosp. Service, p. 1–24.
─── 1910 b. The taxonomic value of the microscopic structure of the stigmal plates in the tick genus *Dermacentor*. Bul. No. 62; Hyg. Lab., U. S. Pub. Health and Mar. Hosp. Serc., Washington, p. 1–72. 43 pls.
**Stiles, C. W.** and **Gardner.** 1910. Further observations on the disposal of excreta. Public Health Repts. Washington. xxv, p. 1825–1830.
**Stiles, C. W.** and **Keister, W. S.** 1913. Flies as carriers of Lamblia Spores. The contamination of food with human excreta. Public Health Repts. Washington, xxviii, p. 2530–2534.
**Stiles, C. W.** and **Lumsden, L. L.** 1911. The sanitary privy. U. S. Dept. Agric., Farmers Bul. 463, 32 p.
**Strickland, C.** 1914. The biology of *Ceratophyllus fasciatus* Bosc., the common rat-flea of Great Britain. Jour. Hygiene, xiv, p. 139–142.
**Strong, R P.** and **Teague, O.** 1912. Infectivity of the breath. Rept. of Intern. Plague Conf. held at Mukden, Apr. 1911, p. 83–87.
**Strong, R. P., Tyzzer, E. E.,** and **Brues, C. T.** 1913. Verruga peruviana, Oroya fever and uta. Journ. Amer Med.. Assoc. lxi, p. 1713–1716.
**Stryke, Anna C.** 1912. The life-cycle of the malarial parasite. Entom. News. xxiii, p. 221–223.
**Surcouf, J.** 1913. La transmission du ver macaque par un moustique. C. R. Acad. Sci., Paris, clvi, p. 1406–1408.
**Taschenberg, O.** 1909. Die giftigen Tiere. 8vo. Stuttgart, Enke. (xv + 325 p.).
**Taute, M.** 1911. Experimentelle Studien über die Beziehungen der *Glossina morsitans* zur Schlafkrankheit. Zeitschr. f. Hyg. lxix, p. 553–558.
**Temple, I. U.** 1912. Acute ascending paralysis, or tick paralysis. Medical Sentinel, Portland, Oregon. Sept. 1912. (Reprint unpaged.)
**Theobald, F. V.** 1901+ A monograph of the Culicidæ of the World. Five volumes. London.
**Thebault, V.** 1901. Hémorrhagie intestinale et affection typhiode causée par des larves de Diptère. Arch. Parasit. iv, p. 353–361
**Thompson, D.** 1913. Preliminary note on bed-bugs and leprosy. British Med. Journ. 1913, p. 847.
**Tiraboschi, C.** 1904. Les rats, les souris et leurs parasites cutanés dans leurs rapports avec la propagation de la peste bubonique. Arch. Parasit. viii, p. 161–349.
**Topsent, E.** 1901. Sur un cas de myase hypodermique chez l'homme. Arch. Parasit., iv. p. 607–614.
**Torrey, J. C.** 1912. Numbers and types of bacteria carried by city flies. Journ. of Inf. Dis., x, p. 166–177.
**Townsend, C. H. T.** 1908. The taxonomy of the Muscoidean flies. Smithsonian Misc. Col., p. 1–138.
─── 1911. Review of work by Pantel and Portchinski on reproductive and early stage characters of Muscoid flies. Proc. Ent. Soc., Washington, xiii, p. 151–170.
─── 1912. Muscoid names. ibid., xiv, p. 45.
─── 1913 a. Preliminary characterization of the vector of verruga, *Phlebotomus verrucarum* sp. nov. Insecutor Inscitiæ Menstruus, Washington, i, p. 107–109.
─── 1913 b. The transmission of verruga by *Phlebotomus*. Journ. Amer. Med. Assoc., lxi, p. 1717.

――― 1914 a. The relations between lizards and *Phlebotomus verrucarum* as indicating the reservoir of verruga. Science n. s., xl, p. 212–214.
――― 1914 b. Progress of verruga work with *Phlebotomus verrucarum* T. Journ. Econ. Ent., vii. p. 357–367.
**Trouessart, E.** 1902. Endoparasitisme accidental chez l'homme d'une espèce de Sarcoptidæ détriticole, (*Histiogaster spermaticus*). Arch. Parasit., v, p. 449–459.
**Tsunoda, T.** 1910. Eine Milbenart von *Glyciphagus* als Endoparasit. D. med. Wochenscher., xxxvi, p. 1327–1328.
**Tyzzer, E. E.** 1907. The pathology of the brown-tail moth dermatitis. In 2d Rept. of the Supt. for Suppressing the Gypsy and Brown-tail Moths, Boston, 1907, p. 154–168.
**Vaughan,**
**Verdun, P.** and **Bruyant, L.** 1912. Un nouveau cas de pseudo-parasitsme d'un myriapode, (*Chætachlyne vesuviana*) chez l'homme. C. R. Soc. Biol., Paris, lxiv, p. 236–237.
**Verjbitski, D. T.** The part played by insects in the epidemiology of plague. Transl. from Russian in Jour. Hyg., viii, p. 162–208.
**Villeneuve, J.** 1914. Quelques réflexions au sujet de la tribu des Calliphorinæ Bul. Soc. Ent., France, No. 8, p. 256–258.
**Ward, H. B.** 1905. The relation of animals to disease. Science n. s. xxii, p. 193–203.
**Watson, J. J.** 1910. Symptomology of pellagra and report of cases. Trans. Nat. Conference on Pellagra, Columbia, S. C., Nov. 3 and 4, 1909, p. 207–218.
**Weed, C. M.** 1904. An experiment with black-flies. U. S. Dept. Agric., Bur. Ent. Bul. n. s., 46, p. 108–109.
**Wellman, F. C.** 1906. Human trypanosomiasis and spirochætosis in Portuguese Southwest Africa, with suggestions for preventing their spread in the Colony. Journ. Hyg., vi, p. 237–345.
**Werner, F.** 1911. Scorpions and allied annulated spiders. Wellcome Trop. Research Laboratories, 4th Rept., vol. B, p. 178–194. Pls. xiv–xv.
**Whitfield, A.** 1912. A method of rapidly exterminating pediculi capitis. Lancet 1912 (2), p. 1648. See notes.
**Williston, S. W.** 1908. Manual of the North American Diptera, New Haven, p. 1–405.
**Wilson, G. B.** and **Chowning, W. M.** 1903. Studies in *Piroplasmosis hominis*. Journ. Inf. Dis., iv, p. 31–57.
**Wilson, W. H.** 1904. On the venom of scorpions. Rec. Egyptian Gov't School of Medicine, Cairo, ii, p. 7–44.

# INDEX

| | PAGE |
|---|---|
| Abscess | 178 |
| Acanthia | 87 |
| Acariasis | 58 |
| Acarina | 23, 58, 131, 259 |
| Acarus dysenteriæ | 132 |
| Accidental parasites | 131, 132, 134 |
| Aedes | 194, 293 |
| Aedes calopus | 182, 201, 205, 206, 208 |
| Aedes cantator | 101 |
| Aedes sollicitans | 101 |
| Aedes tœniorhynchus | 101 |
| Aerobic bacteria | 152 |
| Aestivo-autumnal | 186 |
| African Relapsing Fever | 230 |
| Akis spinosa | 177 |
| Alternation of Generations | 175 |
| Amblyomma | 264 |
| Amblyomma americanum | 67 |
| Amblyomma cajennense | 67 |
| American dog tick | 228 |
| Amœboid organism | 189 |
| Anisolabis annulipes | 177 |
| Anterior poliomyelitis | 241 |
| Anopheles | 194, 291 |
| Anopheles crucians | 199 |
| Anopheles maculipennis | 182 |
| Anopheles punctipennis | 198 |
| Anopheles quadrimaculatus | 197 |
| Anopheline | 192 |
| Anthocoris | 279 |
| Anthomyiidæ | 300 |
| Anthomyia | 138 |
| Anthrax | 165 |
| Antipruritic treatment | 72 |
| Ants | 42 |
| Aphiochæta | 295 |
| Apis mellifica | 36 |
| Arachnida | 258 |
| Araneida | 6 |
| Argas | 64 |
| Argas persicus | 63, 235, 237 |
| Argasidæ | 62 |
| Argopsylla | 317 |
| Argus | 259 |

| | PAGE |
|---|---|
| Arilus | 284 |
| Arthopods, poisonous | 6 |
| Asopia farinalis | 177 |
| Assassin-bugs | 31, 219 |
| Auchmeromyia | 117 |
| Automeris io | 47 |
| Avicularoidea | 12 |
| | |
| Babesia | 226 |
| Babesia bovis | 223 |
| Babesia ovis | 225 |
| Babesiosis | 221–222 |
| Bacilli | 170 |
| Bacillus icteroides | 202, 205 |
| Bacillus pestis | 166 |
| Bacillus typhosus | 153 |
| Back swimmers | 30 |
| Bdellolarynx | 304 |
| Beauperthuy, Louis Daniel | 2 |
| Bed-bug | 86, 88, 90, 173, 219–220 |
| Bed-bug, cone-nosed | 92 |
| Blister beetles | 54 |
| Belostoma | 28, 277 |
| Belostoma americana | 31 |
| Belostomatidæ | 30 |
| Bengalia | 314 |
| Bird-spiders | 10 |
| Black death | 1, 166 |
| Black flies | 33, 104, 247 |
| Black heads | 80 |
| Blaps mortisaga | 134 |
| Blepharoceridæ | 286 |
| Boophilus | 264 |
| Boophilus annulatus | 67, 223–225 |
| Bot-flies | 112 |
| Blue bottle flies | 140 |
| Brill's disease | 238 |
| Brown-tailed moth | 48 |
| Bruck | 34 |
| Buthus quinquestriatus | 21 |
| | |
| Cabbage butterfly | 56 |
| Calliphora | 136, 140, 312 |
| Calliphora erythrocephala | 141 |

## Index

Calobata ..................... 296
Camponotinæ ................. 43
Cancer ....................... 254
Cantharidin .................. 54
Cantharidin poison............. 55
Canthariasis ................. 134
Capsidæ ...................... 280
Carriers, simple...............4, 144
Carriers of disease............ 144
Carrion's fever............... 253
Caterpillar rash.............. 45
Cat flea...................... 172
Cattle ticks.................. 222
Causative organism............ 170
Cellia........................ 291
Centipedes..................25, 257
Ceratophyllus............120, 316
Ceratophyllus acutus.......... 123
Ceratophyllus fasciatus..122, 172, 213
Ceratopogon................... 108
Cheese-fly ................... 137
Cheyletus eruditus............ 271
Chigger .....................60, 70
Chigoes ...................... 126
Chilopoda..................25, 257
Chiracanthium nutrix.......... 18
Chironomidæ .................. 107
Chorioptes ................... 270
Chrysomelid................... 55
Chrysomyia................136, 308
Chrysomyia macellaria......117, 140
Chrysops ..................... 294
Chylous dropsy................ 179
Chyluria ..................... 178
Cicadidæ...................... 55
Cimex L....................... 278
Cimex boueti.................. 92
Cimex columbarius............. 92
Cimex hemipterus............91, 220
Cimex hirundinis.............. 92
Cimex inodorus................ 92
Cimex lectularius...........87, 219
Citheronia regalis............ 44
Clinocoris ................... 87
Coleoptera................134, 274
Comedons...................... 80
Complete metamorphosis........ 80
Compressor muscle............. 20

Compsomyia ................... 117
Cone-nosed bed-bug............ 92
Conjunctivitis, nodular....... 52
Conorhinus.................... 282
Conorhinus megistus......93, 219–220
Conorhinus rubrofasciatus..... 220
Conorhinus sanguisugus......32, 92
Copra itch.................... 72
Cordylobia ................... 118
Coriscus ..................... 280
Coriscus subcoleoptratus...... 32
Creeping myasis............... 112
Crustacea .................... 257
Cryptocystis ................. 176
Cryptotoxic................. 54–55
Cteniza sauvagei.............. 13
Ctenocephalus......120, 172, 213, 317
Culex..................194, 201, 293
Culex pipiens...............35, 98
Culex quinquefasciatus........ 180
Culex sollicitans............. 200
Culex territans............... 101
Culicidæ...................33, 97
Culicin ...................... 34
Culicoides................109, 288
Cyclops...................183, 257
Cynomyia..................136, 311

Dance, St. Vitus ............. 8
Dancing mania................. 8
Deer-flies ................... 110
Definitive host............... 192
Demodecidæ ................... 78
Demodex ...................... 259
Demodex folliculorum.......... 78
Dermacentor .................. 262
Dermacentor andersoni......67, 228
Dermacentor occidentalis...... 227
Dermacentor variabilis........ 67
Dermacentor venustus........24, 228
Dermanyssidæ ................. 68
Dermanyssus .................. 266
Dermanyssus gallinæ........... 68
Dermatitis..............72, 77, 85
Dermatobia................115, 298
Dermatobia cyaniventris....... 163
Dermatophilus................. 317
Dermatophilus penetrans.....60, 126

## Index

Diamphidia simplex............ 55
Dimorphism.................. 65
Direct inoculators............. 4
Diplopoda..................25, 257
Diptera...................33, 94, 274
Dipterous Larvæ.............. 135
Dipylidium................175, 221
Dipylidium canium........4, 175–176
Dog flea..................... 172
Dracunculus.................. 257
Dracunculus medinensis........ 182
Drosophila................... 296
Dum-dum fever............... 220
Dysentery ................... 154

Ear-flies .................... 110
Earwig ...................... 177
Echidnophaga ................ 317
Echinorynchus................ 185
Elephantiasis ............178–179
Empoasca mali............... 33
Empretia .................... 46
English Plague Commission...... 171
Epeira diadema............... 18
Epizootic .................... 170
Eristalis ..................137, 295
Essential hosts...............4, 165
Eumusca..................... 307
European Relapsing Fever....... 233
Euproctis chrysorrhœa.......... 48
Eusimulium .................. 286

Facultative parasites........... 131
Fannia............136, 138, 145, 300
Federal Health Service.......... 169
Fever, lenticular .............. 237
  African Relapsing........230, 234
  Carrion's................... 253
  dum-dum .................. 154
  European Relapsing.......... 233
  pappatici .................. 96
  red water.................. 220
  Rocky Mt. Spotted........... 226
  three day .................. 96
  Typhus .................... 237
Filaria...................178, 221
  immitis.................... 182
Filariasis ................... 178

Flannel-moth larvæ............ 44
Fleas...................119, 166, 213
  cat ....................... 172
  dog ....................... 172
  human ..................172, 176
  rodent.....................123, 172
  rat ....................... 171
Flesope ..................... 125
Formaldehyde ................ 91
Fomites................. 199, 204
Fulgoridæ ................... 28
Fumigation .................. 320

Gamasid .................... 68
Gangrene ................... 129
Gastrophilus ............113, 297
Giant crab spiders............. 13
Giant water bugs.............. 30
Gigantorhynchus.............. 185
Glossina..............117, 297, 303
Glossina morsitans.........214, 217
  palpalis............215, 217, 218
Glyciphagus ................. 267
Grain moth................... 69
Grocer's itch................. 72
Guinea-worm ................ 182

Habronema muscæ..........156, 183
Hæmatobia .............166, 304
  irritans ................... 146
Hæmatobosca ............... 304
Hæmatomyidium ............. 288
Hæmatopinus spinulosus....... 213
Hæmatopota ................. 294
Hæmatosiphon ............... 279
Hæmoglobinuria .............. 220
Hæmozoin ................... 189
Harpactor.................... 284
Harvest mites................ 60
  effect of................... 59
Head-louse .................. 173
Helminthiasis................. 138
Helophilus .................. 295
Hemiptera..........27, 86, 273–275
Heteropodidæ ............... 13
Heuchis sanguinea............ 55
Hexapod larvæ............... 58
Hexapoda............27, 80, 258

Hippelates .................... 297
Hippobosca.. ................. 285
Histiogaster ................... 269
   spermaticus ................. 132
Homalomyia........... 136, 138, 300
Honey bee.................... 36
   poison of................... 37
Hornets....................... 43
Horn-fly .............. 137, 304, 308
Horse-fly..........'.......... 110, 165
House-fly.......... 137–139, 144, 183
   control of................ 156, 160
Human flea.................... 124
Host, definitive................ 175
   intermediate................. 175
   primary..................... 175
Hyalomma ................... 264
   ægypticum ............. 224–225
Hydrocyanic Acid Gas.......... 318
Hydrotæa .................... 300
Hymenolepis diminuta.......... 176
Hymenoptera................ 36, 275
Hypoderma ............... 113, 298
   diana ...................... 113
   lineata ..................... 113
Hypopharynx ................. 80

Immunity from stings........... 39
Incomplete metamorphosis...... 80
Infantile paralysis........... 162,241
   splenic ..................... 220
   Direct inoculation............ 164
Insects ...................... 258
   blood-sucking................ 170
Intermediate host.......... 192, 203
Intestinal infestation........ 112, 133
   myasis ..................... 137
Isosoma ..................... 69
Itch ...................... 73–74
   mite ...................... 73
   Norwegian .................. 77
Ixodes ...................... 260
   ricinus................... 66, 225
   scapularis ................... 66
Ixodidæ.................... 64–65
Ixodoidea .................... 62

Janthinosoma lutzi............. 116

Jigger ....................... 60
Johannseniella ............ 110, 288
Journal of Tropical Medicine and
   Hygiene ................... 36
Julus terrestris ................ 25
June bug..................... 185

Kala-azar..................... 220
Kara, kurte................... 14
Katipo ...................... 14
King, A. F. A................. 3
Kircher, Athanasius ......... 1, 8
Kissing-bug .................. 31

Labium .................... 29, 80
Labrum.................... 28, 80
Lachnosterna ................ 185
Lælaps ...................... 266
Lœmopsylla .................. 172
Lagoa crispata................ 45
Lamblia intestinalis............ 154
Langer, Josef.................. 37
Larder beetles................. 135
Latrodectus.............. 12, 14, 17
   mactans .................... 15
Leishmanioses ................ 220
Lenticular fever................ 237
Lepidoptera .................. 274
Lepidopterous larvæ............ 134
Leprosy...................... 252
Leptidæ ..................... 112
Leptis ...................... 295
Leptus................... 60, 273
Lice ....................... 80
Linguatulina ................. 258
Liponyssus .................. 265
Lone star tick................. 228
Louse, body.................. 84
   crab ...................... 85
   dog ....................... 176
   head ...................... 82
   pubic ..................... 85
Lœmopsylla............... 172, 317
Lucilia................... 136, 312
Lycosa tarantula............... 10
Lycosidæ .................... 10
Lyctocoris.................... 279
Lygus pratensis................ 33

## Index

Lymphangitis............. ...... 67
Lymph scrotum................ 178
Lyperosia .................... 304
Lyperosiops .................. 305

Macloskie .................... 34
Maggots, rat-tail.............. 137
Magnes sive de Arte Magnetica... 8
Malaria ...................... 186
Malmigniatte ................. 14
Mandibles ..................28, 80
Mange......................73–75
Margaropus ..............237, 264
   annulatus .................. 223
Masked bed-bug hunter......... 32
Mastigoproctus giganteus......19, 80
Maxillae ..................... 28
Meal infesting species........... 135
Melanin granules............... 189
Melanolestes .................. 280
   picipes .................... 32
Mena-vodi .................... 14
Mercurialis .................. 1
Merozoites ................... 190
Metamorphosis ................ 80
Miana bug.................... 63
Microgametoblast ............. 192
Midges ...................... 107
Migratory ookinete............. 192
Millipedes..................25, 257
Mites......................23, 58
Monieziella................... 269
Mosquitoes.......33, 97, 178, 196, 250
   treatment for bites of....34, 36, 102
Musca ....................137, 307
   domestica....139, 145, 146, 157, 162
Muscidæ ..................... 117
Muscina..............137, 146, 307
   stabulans .................. 140
Mutualism ................... 57
Myasis ..................112, 135
   intestinal ...............135–140
   nasal ..................... 141
Mycterotypus ................. 287
Myiospila ................146, 307
Myriapoda ...........25, 132, 257

Nagana ..................165, 214

Nasal infestation............114, 133
Necrobia .................... 135
Nematode parasite............ 182
Nepa ....................... 28
Nephrophages sanguinarius...... 132
Nettling insects............... 43
   larvæ, poison of............. 53
Neurasthenia ................ 89
Nits ........................ 86
North African Relapsing Fever.. 234
Norwegian itch............... 77
No-see-ums .................. 109
Notœdres .................... 269
   cati ....................... 78
Notonecta.. .................28, 277
Notonectidæ ................. 30
Nott, Dr. Josiah............... 2
Nuttall ...................... 34

Occipital headaches............ 138
Oecacta ..................... 288
Oeciacus .................... 279
Œsophageal diverticula......... 35
Oestridæ ................112, 136
Oestris ovis.................. 113
Oestrus ..................... 298
   oocyst ..................... 192
   ookinete ................... 192
Opsicoetes personatus.......... 32
Opthalmia ................... 155
   nodosa..................... 52
Oriental sore................. 221
Ornithodoros ...............65, 260
   moubata ...............220, 230
Orthotylus flavosparsus........ 33
Ornithomyia ................. 286
Oroya ...................... 253
Oscinus ..................... 297
Otiobius .................... 259
   megnini.................... 65
Otodectes ...................271

Pangonia .................... 294
Pappatici fever............... 96
Parasimulium ................ 286
Parasite .........3, 57, 131, 134, 182
   accidental..............3, 131, 134
   facultative.............3, 57, 131

## Index

Parasite, nematode.............. 182
   stationary ................... 57
   temporary ................... 57
   true......................... 3
Parasitism, accidental............ 134
Pathogenic bacteria.............. 152
   organisms ................144, 164
Pawlowsky .................... 81
Pediculoides ................... 267
   ventricosus ................69, 72
Pediculosis..................... 81
Pediculus...................... 275
   corporis ..............84, 233, 238
   humanus ..................82, 173
Pellagra ..................162, 246
Pernicious fever................. 186
Pest ......................... 166
Phidippus audax................ 19
Philæmatomyia ................ 306
Phisalix ....................13, 43
Phlebotomus ................... 289
   papatasii ................... 94
   verrucarum ................. 254
   vexator ..................... 95
Phora ........................ 295
Phormia ...................... 136
Phormictopus carcerides......... 13
Phthirus pubis................85, 275
Phortica ...................... 296
Pieris brassicæ.................. 56
Piophila ...................... 297
Piophila casei.............. 136, 137
Piroplasmosis .................. 222
Plague ....................... 166
   bubonic............. 166, 169, 170
   pneumonic .................. 167
Plasmodium ................... 186
Platymetopius acutus............ 33
Plica palonica................... 83
Pneumonic ................... 166
   plague ..................167, 173
Poisoning by nettling larvæ...... 53
Poison of spiders................ 7
Pollenia....................... 308
   rudis ...................146, 147
primary gland.................. 28
Prionurus citrinus............... 20
Prosimulium ................... 286

Protocalliphora ............136, 312
Protozoan blood parasite........ 165
Pseudo-tubercular ............. 52
Psorophora .................... 293
Psoroptes ..................... 270
Psychodidæ ................... 94
Pulex.........120, 124, 126, 172, 317
   cheopis ..................... 172
   irritans ..................... 124
   penetrans ................... 126
   serraticeps .................. 120
Pulvillus ...................... 150
Punkies ...................... 109
Pycnosoma ................... 308

Rasahus ...................... 280
   thoracicus .................. 32
Rat fleas..............120, 124, 171
Rat louse...................... 213
Red bugs....................70–72
Reduviidæ .................... 31
Reduviolus .................... 280
Reduvius ..................... 282
   personatus .................. 32
Redwater fever................. 220
Relapsing fever............230, 233
Rhinœstrus nasalis.............. 115
Rhipicentor ................... 264
Rhipicephalus ................. 264
Rhizoglyphus .................. 269
Rhodnius ..................... 280
Rocky Mountain Spotted Fever.. 226
   spotted fever tick............ 67
Russian gad-fly................. 115

St. Vitus's or St. John's dance.... 8
Salivary syringe................. 28
Sand-flies ................109, 250
Sanguinetti.................... 11
Sarcophaga............ 136, 142, 143
Sarcophila .................... 302
Sarcopsylla ................... 317
   penetrans ................... 126
Sarcoptes ..................... 270
   minor ...................... 78
   scabiei ..................... 73
Sarcoptidæ ................... 72
Scabies...............72, 73, 74, 75

| | |
|---|---|
| Scaurus striatus | 177 |
| Schaudinn | 34 |
| Schizont | 189, 190 |
| Scholeciasis | 134 |
| Scolopendra morsitans | 26 |
| Scorpions | 20 |
|   poison of | 21 |
| Screw worm fly | 140 |
| Sepsidæ | 296 |
| Sepsis | 136, 297 |
| Shipley | 34 |
| Sibine | 46 |
| Silvius | 294 |
| Simple carriers | 4, 144 |
| Simuliidæ | 33, 104 |
| Simulium | 247, 249, 286, 321 |
|   pictipes | 104 |
| Siphonaptera | 119, 274, 316 |
| Siphunculata | 80, 275 |
| Sitotroga cerealella | 69 |
| Skippers | 137 |
| Sleeping sickness | 166, 215 |
| Snipe-flies | 112 |
| Solpugida | 22 |
| Spanish fly | 54 |
| Spermatozoa | 192 |
| Spinose ear-tick | 65 |
| Spirochœta | 35 |
|   berberi | 234 |
|   duttoni | 234 |
| Spirochætosis | 235 |
| Sporozoite | 189 |
| Spotted fever | 67, 226 |
| Squirrel flea | 123 |
| Stable-fly | 137, 160, 163, 165 |
| Stegomyia | 182, 293 |
|   calopus | 206 |
|   fasciata | 206 |
| Stomoxys | 137, 305 |
|   calcitrans | 117, 146, 160, 161, 165, 242 |
| Straw-worm | 69 |
| Stygeromyia | 305 |
| Sucking stomach | 35 |
| Sulphur ointment | 77 |
| Surra | 165 |
| Symbiosis | 57 |
| Symphoromyia | 112, 295 |

| | |
|---|---|
| Tabanidæ | 110 |
| Tabanus | 110, 166, 294 |
|   striatus | 165 |
| Taenia | 175 |
| Tapeworm | 4, 176 |
| Tarantella | 8 |
| Tarantism | 8 |
| Tarantula | 10 |
| Tarsonemidæ | 69 |
| Tarsonemus | 267 |
| Tenebrionid beetles | 127 |
| Tersesthes | 110, 288 |
| Tetanus | 129 |
| Tetranychus | 273 |
| Texas fever | 220-223 |
| Three-day fever | 96 |
| Tick | 23, 226 |
|   bites, Treatment of | 68 |
|   fever | 230 |
|   paralysis | 67 |
| Treatment, | |
|   Bee stings | 36, 41 |
|   Bites of, | |
|     Bed-bugs | 90, 93 |
|     Blackflies | 107 |
|     Buffalo flies | 107 |
|     Bugs | 31, 33 |
|     Centipedes | 26, 27 |
|     Chiggers | 127 |
|     Chigoes | 127 |
|     Fleas | 127 |
|     Harvest mites | 61 |
|     Jiggers | 129 |
|     Lice | 83, 85 |
|     Mosquitoes | 34, 36, 102 |
|     Phlebotomus flies | 97 |
|     Sand flies | 96, 107, 109 |
|     Scorpions | 22, 23 |
|     Spiders | 19 |
|     Ticks | 61, 68, 72 |
|     Ticks, ear | 65 |
|   Blister beetle poison | 55 |
|   Brown-tail moth rash | 45 |
|   Cantharidin poison | 55 |
|   Caterpillar rash | 45 |
|   Ear ticks | 65 |
|   House fly control | 156, 160 |
|   Itch | 77 |

Itch, grocer's.................. 72
Lice ....................... 85
Nasal myasis................. 143
Rocky Mt. spotted fever... 228, 229
Rash, caterpillar.............. 45
Scabies ..................... 77
Sleeping sickness control...... 218
Spotted fever..............228, 229
Stings, bee..................36, 41
Typhus fever, prophylaxis..... 239
Trichodectes canis............... 176
Trichoma .................... 82
Trineura .................... 295
Trochosa singoriensis.............. 11
Trombidium................. 60, 273
True insects.................. 80
Trypanosoma.................. 35
Trypanosoma, brucei........... 165
Trypanosoma cruzi.............. 219
Trypanosoma lewisi............. 213
Trypanosomiases................ 212
Trypanosomiasis ...........165, 219
Tsetse flies.........117, 166, 214, 219
Tsetse flies disease.............. 165
Tuberculosis.................. 155
Tumbu-fly ................... 118
Tydeus ..................... 271
Typhoid .................... 155

Typhoid fever................. 154
Typhus ..................... 237
Typhus fever.................. 237
Tyroglyphus............72, 131, 268
Dr. Tyzzer................... 49

Uranotænia .................. 292

Vancoho ..................... 14
Varicose groin glands........... 178
Verruga peruviana............. 253
Vescicating insects............. 54

Wanzenspritze ................ 29
Warble-flies .................. 112
Wasps ...................... 43
Whip-scorpions ............... 19
Wohlfahrtia.............143, 302
Wolf-spiders ................. 10
Wyeomyia smithii ......... 101, 293

Xenopsylla ..............172, 317
Xenopsylla cheopis .........171, 124
Xestopsylla .................. 317

Yaws ....................... 2
Yellow fever ......... 196, 203, 205